ULTIMATE GUIDE TO
STRENGTH TRAINING

Thunder Bay Press
An imprint of Printers Row Publishing Group
10350 Barnes Canyon Road, Suite 100, San Diego, CA 92121
www.thunderbaybooks.com • mail@thunderbaybooks.com

Printers Row Publishing Group is a division of Readerlink Distribution Services, LLC.
Thunder Bay Press is a registered trademark of Readerlink Distribution Services, LLC.

Correspondence regarding the content of this book should be sent to Thunder Bay Press,
Editorial Department, at the above address. Author and illustration inquiries should
be addressed to Moseley Road Inc., info@moseleyroad.com.

Thunder Bay Press
Publisher: Peter Norton
Associate Publisher: Ana Parker
Senior Developmental Editor: April Graham Farr
Senior Product Manager: Kathryn C. Dalby
Production Team: Jonathan Lopes, Rusty von Dyl

Produced by Moseley Road Inc., www.moseleyroad.com
President: Sean Moore
Art and Editorial Director: Lisa Purcell
Production Director: Adam Moore
Editor: Ann Kay
Designer: Tina Vaughan
Photography: Naila Ruechel, www.nailaruechel.com

Library of Congress Cataloging-in-Publication data available on request.

ISBN: 978-1-64517-043-3

Printed in China

24 23 22 21 20   2 3 4 5 6

ULTIMATE GUIDE TO
STRENGTH TRAINING

WITH DETAILED INSTRUCTIONS AND ANATOMICAL ILLUSTRATIONS FOR 245 STRENGTH EXERCISES

Hollis Liebman

THUNDER BAY
P·R·E·S·S

San Diego, California

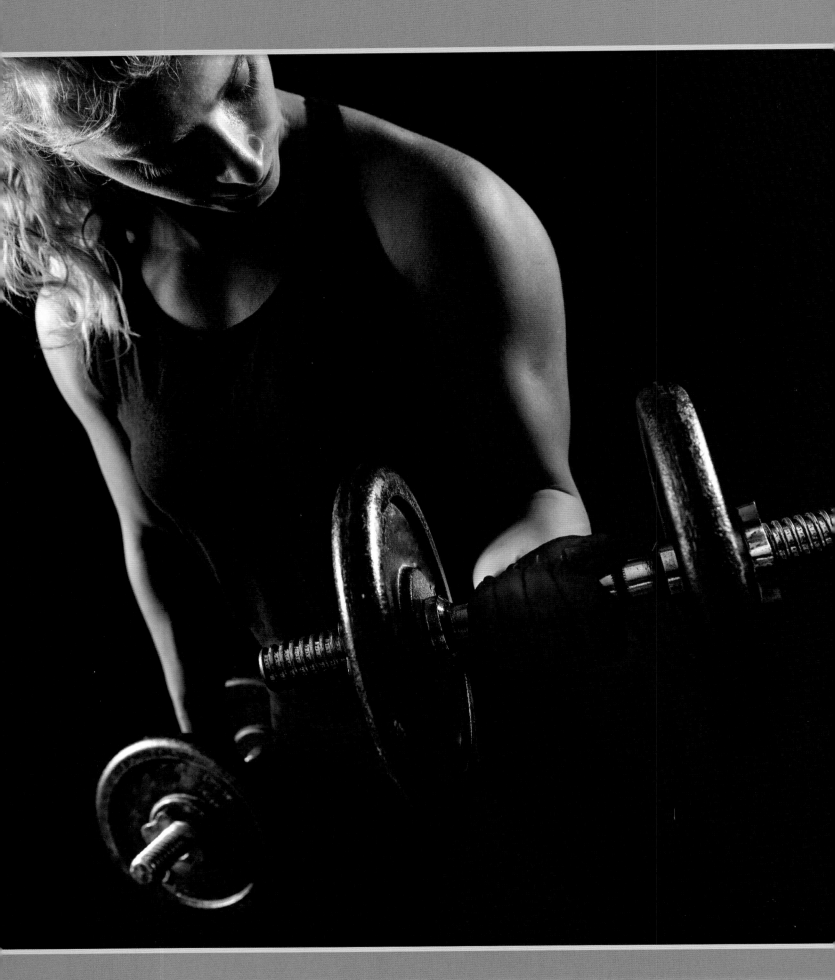

CONTENTS

06 Introduction
22 Full-Body Anatomy

24 CHAPTER ONE
FLEXIBILITY EXERCISES

26 Arm, Shoulder, and Chest Stretches
28 Hip, Leg, and Glutes Stretches
34 Torso and Upper-Arm Stretches
38 Core Stretches

46 CHAPTER TWO
BODY-WEIGHT EXERCISES

48 Back Exercises
60 Arm and Shoulder Exercises
68 Chest Exercises
74 Core Exercises
94 Leg and Glutes Exercises
112 Total-Body Exercises

132 CHAPTER THREE
WEIGHTED EXERCISES

134 Back Exercises
152 Arm and Shoulder Exercises
174 Chest Exercises
184 Core Exercises
192 Leg and Glutes Exercises
210 Total-Body Exercises

218 CHAPTER FOUR
EQUIPMENT EXERCISES

220 Back Exercises
234 Arm and Shoulder Exercises
250 Chest Exercises
262 Core Exercises
286 Leg and Glutes Exercises
304 Total-Body Exercises

316 CHAPTER FIVE
WORKOUT ROUTINES

318 Body Routines
338 Sports Routines
354 Something-for-Everyone Routines

378 Glossary
382 Icon Index
394 Index
400 Credits & Acknowledgments

What Is Strength Training?

The answer to this question is simple—essentially this kind of training increases your muscle strength. In recent years the image of strength training has been moving away from the muscle-bound superhero physique and toward a recognition that strength work is an invaluable component of any kind of fitness regimen, for anyone.

Strength training has been around for a very long time. Impressive tales of lifting great weights date far back in many different cultures. The Nordic Icelandic Sagas tell us of men carrying huge ship masts; some scholars have suggested that the stone *halteres* used in ancient Greek sports may have been an early forerunner of the dumbbell. Modern dumbbells appeared in the late 1800s, along with other strength equipment such as barbells. The 1960s brought exercise machines onto the scene.

WORKING AGAINST RESISTANCE

Strength training is often also called "resistance training." The two aren't exactly the same, but basically strength training uses resistance techniques to strengthen your muscles. What you are doing here is moving your body against an external force of some kind that resists this movement.

These external forces can be all kinds of things—your own body weight, dumbbells, a Swiss ball, rubberized bands, or a cable machine, for example.

It is working against this resistance that causes your muscles to contract and builds strength and endurance.

TARGETING MUSCLES

Exercises such as those in this book can be devised to target specific muscles or muscle groups, large areas of the body, or even much of the whole body. Strength training can be focused to improve tone and shape, or to enhance posture or balance.

Because of the complex interconnectedness of the human body, great things can be achieved. So, actively working and strengthening one set of muscles may help to stabilize another set. Many of us appreciate how stronger abdominal muscles can make our whole upper body work and feel better.

POWER AND PRECISION

Athletes of all types can vouch for the performance-boosting properties of strength training. This approach improves muscles' range of motion. It makes them "fire" faster, more powerfully, and with greater precision. Who wouldn't want a share of some of this?

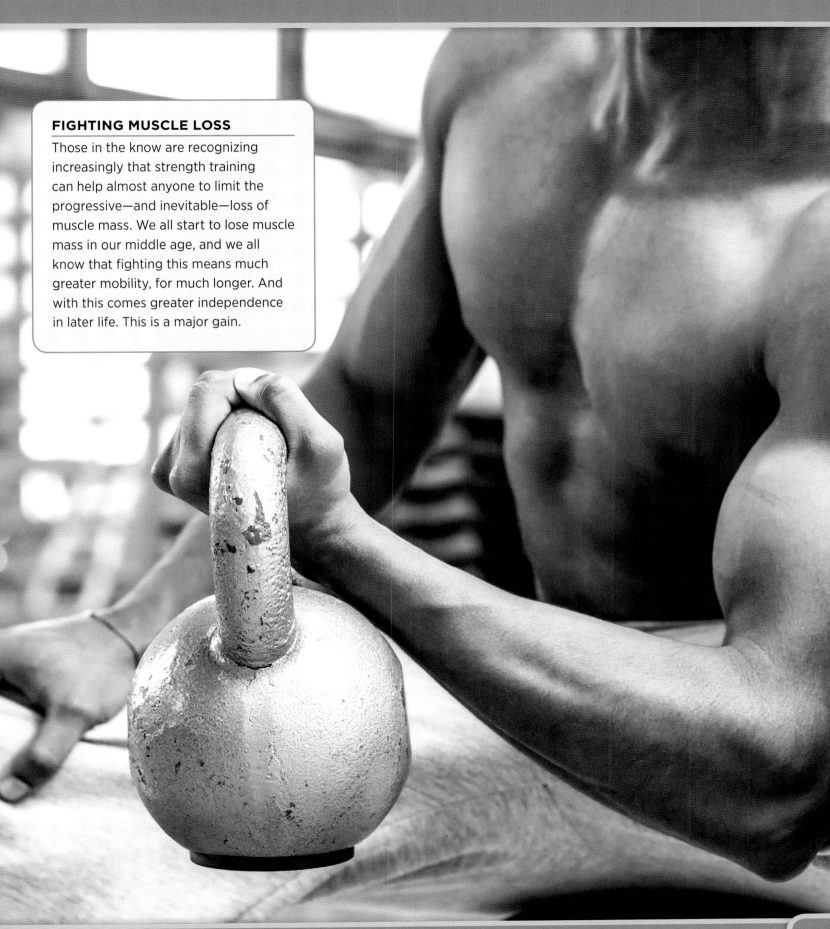

FIGHTING MUSCLE LOSS

Those in the know are recognizing increasingly that strength training can help almost anyone to limit the progressive—and inevitable—loss of muscle mass. We all start to lose muscle mass in our middle age, and we all know that fighting this means much greater mobility, for much longer. And with this comes greater independence in later life. This is a major gain.

First Principles

This section introduces some basic issues you should consider. This is helpful if you're new to strength training, and worth being reminded about if you're not. The foundational messages are: listen to your body; keep breathing; warm up and cool down. You'll also find some notes on specialist terms.

Getting into the habit of understanding your body will reap rich rewards for your strength training. Before you start a session, take some time out to think about how you're feeling that day. Are you full of energy and raring to go, after a great night's sleep? Or perhaps your energy levels are low and you have certain physical discomforts. Always pay attention to this.

LISTEN TO YOUR BODY

Never push yourself if you are tired, and never try movements that might strain a part of you that is inherently weak or is feeling sore that day. One of the main things to say about strength training is: *Never lift a weight heavier than you feel you can manage comfortably.*

Avoiding going outside this comfort zone is especially relevant when you are new to this kind of exercise, or haven't done much exercise before or recently. Always build up gradually as you gain strength. If you have any doubts, or specific health issues, ask your physician and a fitness professional for tailored advice.

KEEP BREATHING

So much is said about the best ways to breathe while exercising—much of it contradictory. In fact, it's best not to get overly obsessed with whether you're inhaling (or breathing in) and exhaling (breathing out) in the right places, especially when you're starting out. However, breathing is an important issue. The principal takeaway from breathing advice is that you must keep breathing well and evenly while you exercise, even if you're not doing it in some accepted way.

So, don't hold your breath or forget to breathe, as this can cause injury. It could even make you pass out if you are putting your body under some strain—such as following a taxing workout routine at speed—by causing spikes in blood pressure. This is because your body isn't getting enough oxygen, needed to produce energy. It's actually quite common to hold your breath while you focus on a task like lifting a weight, and you may have even seen weightlifters do it—but just don't!

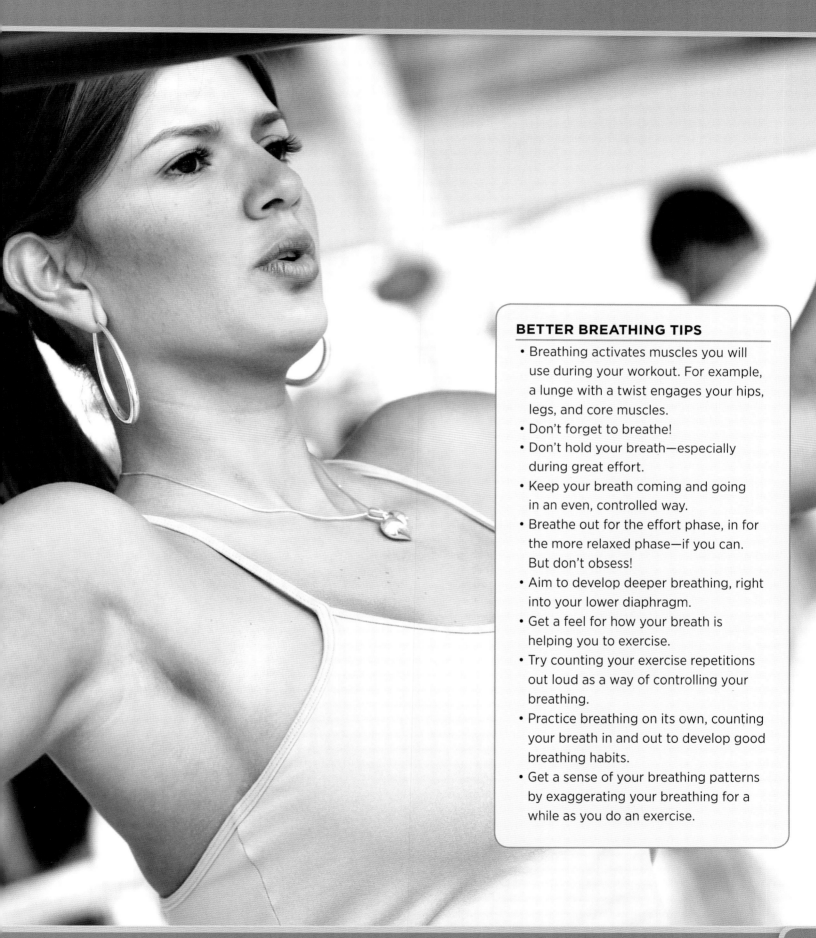

BETTER BREATHING TIPS

- Breathing activates muscles you will use during your workout. For example, a lunge with a twist engages your hips, legs, and core muscles.
- Don't forget to breathe!
- Don't hold your breath—especially during great effort.
- Keep your breath coming and going in an even, controlled way.
- Breathe out for the effort phase, in for the more relaxed phase—if you can. But don't obsess!
- Aim to develop deeper breathing, right into your lower diaphragm.
- Get a feel for how your breath is helping you to exercise.
- Try counting your exercise repetitions out loud as a way of controlling your breathing.
- Practice breathing on its own, counting your breath in and out to develop good breathing habits.
- Get a sense of your breathing patterns by exaggerating your breathing for a while as you do an exercise.

INS AND OUTS

There is a good general rule that says you should exhale during the hardest effort (the *concentric* phase of activity) and inhale when you're doing something more relaxed like returning to your starting position (the *eccentric* phase). So, for strength training, you might exhale as you lift a barbell, and inhale as you bring it back down to the floor.

You'll find that breathing well makes it progressively easier to do exercises, or to take exercises that little bit further. Try just practicing breathing on its own, taking deep breaths and really feeling the activity in your torso. Stand with your hands on the front of your torso, below your chest. Breathe in and out deeply to feel your rib cage move up and out on the inhale, and down and in as you exhale.

Note that specific breathing advice isn't given in this book for each exercise—although the occasional breathing tip might be given. So just find your own comfortable, helpful pattern and stick to it if you can.

WARM UP, COOL DOWN

You've no doubt heard it many times before, but you should always follow a warm-up and cooldown routine at the start and end of any exercise session. Warm-up exercises do just that—prepare your muscles for further work so that they respond better to load and effort.

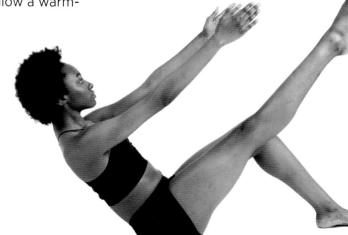

You will perform better and, by reducing stiffness, will also lessen your chances of injury.

Simple exercises to get your body moving well are key to a warm-up—squats or lunges are great for warming up the lower body, for example. Warm-ups will get your heart working, circulating plenty of oxygen-rich blood efficiently around your body; they make muscle-nerve linkages "fire" more quickly, so your muscles respond faster and more precisely.

Cooldowns are essential for bringing a body that has been under stress gradually back to non-exercise mode. This helps the body deal with waste products such as lactic acid, which may well have built up. You need to relax your muscles and reduce your temperature. A gentle jog can be a good way to do this, plus perhaps a little light stretching.

SEE IT THROUGH

Another point worth making is that you should always complete an entire exercise. Each exercise in this book has been devised to take certain muscles through a complete range of motion—or ROM, as it's often called. This involves one or more muscles moving from being fully stretched to fully contracted. So don't be tempted to do just half of an exercise—or cheat by taking shortcuts. You will gain far less than if you complete the whole thing, and could even injure yourself.

SOME TERMS USED

Here are some brief notes about terminology used in the book or linked with strength training.

Abdominals Commonly abbreviated to "abs," or "six-pack" (or more than six if more are clearly visible). People often use this term to refer just to the rectus abdominis, the distinctive pair of vertical parallel muscles on the front of the torso. However, in this book "abdominals" is frequently used as a general term to refer to all of the major abdominal muscles, including the obliques. Where the rectus abdominis or the obliques need to be mentioned in particular, those specific terms have been used.

Cardio Another word for "aerobic."

Clean (as in "kettlebell clean") Moving something from a lower to a higher position. For example, lifting kettlebells from the ground toward your upper body.

Clean and jerk A two-stage process, as in lifting a barbell. Typically, the *clean* movement moves the barbell from the floor to the lifter's upper body. The *jerk* then moves it from there upward to be held over the lifter's head.

Deadlift A lift in which a weight is lifted off the floor up to around your hips, and then lowered down to the ground again.

Dumbbells/Hand weights Lighter dumbbell-type weights are often referred to as "hand weights." The exercises in this book, however, use dumbbells as a catchall term, regardless of size or weight.

Fly (also flye) A weight exercise—holding weights or using a machine—where the arms move through an arc, while the elbow keeps the same angle.

Free weight Weighted objects such as dumbbells, barbells, kettlebells, and medicine balls that are not fixed, as opposed to weight machines.

Hammer-grip Holding something as you would if you picked up a hammer.

Row Movements where the arm action pulls back as if rowing a boat.

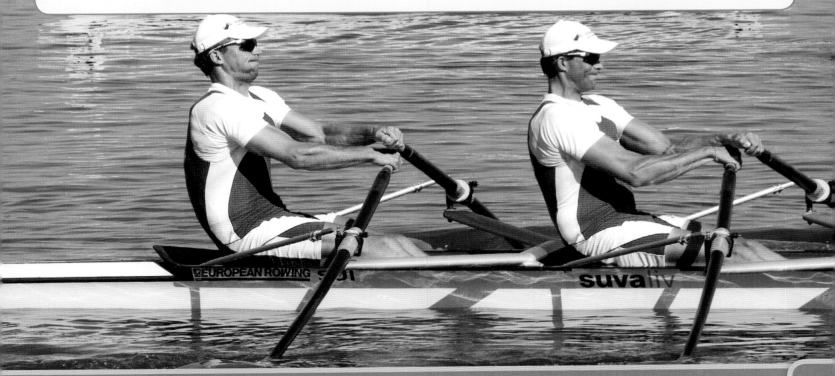

How Your Muscles Work

How muscle tissue works is a fascinating and complex affair. Understanding a little about what happens during exercise and loading of your muscles should certainly enhance your strength-training workouts. This brief introduction to the topic provides some of the essentials.

There are certain key actions and protagonists involved in moving skeletal muscles—the muscles that we are concerned with when it comes to movement and exercise. *Concentric* actions involve a muscle's shortening as it contracts to make effort, as in lifting a weight up in a biceps curl. *Eccentric* actions see the muscle lengthen and relax as it goes back to its pre-contraction state—lowering the weight again.

The main protagonist in a movement is the agonist (or "prime mover")—for example, the biceps muscle in the biceps curl. But agonists also need *antagonist* muscles to act against them. Antagonists often stay relaxed and stop or slow actions down, helping to stabilize joints. Your triceps does this in the biceps curl. *Synergist* muscles are those that help out less directly with an action.

MUSCLE FIBERS

Skeletal muscles consist of bundles of fine fibers. These are rich in proteins called actin and myosin, which cause muscle contraction by sliding over one another. Strength training doesn't magically

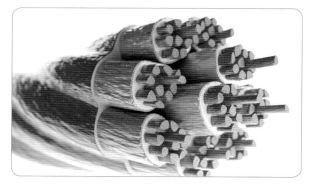

create more fibers but it brings more fibers into play for a specific move. It also makes fibers larger, helping to increase muscle mass and size.

Fibers are divided into slow-twitch (ST) and fast-twitch (FT). ST types typically contract more slowly, use oxygen for energy, and are engaged in less intense aerobic endurance activities such as running. Fast-contracting FT types come to the fore with shorter-term intense anaerobic activities that stress strength, as in lifting weights. They tend to get larger more easily but tire faster. In reality, any good strength-training program—such as the varied exercises in this book—combines both aspects to build both muscle strength and endurance.

MUSCLE-NERVE UNITS

Your muscles are fired into action by *motor nerves*. Each muscle fiber is a single cell, and together a nerve cell and 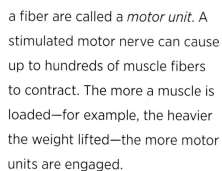 a fiber are called a *motor unit*. A stimulated motor nerve can cause up to hundreds of muscle fibers to contract. The more a muscle is loaded—for example, the heavier the weight lifted—the more motor units are engaged.

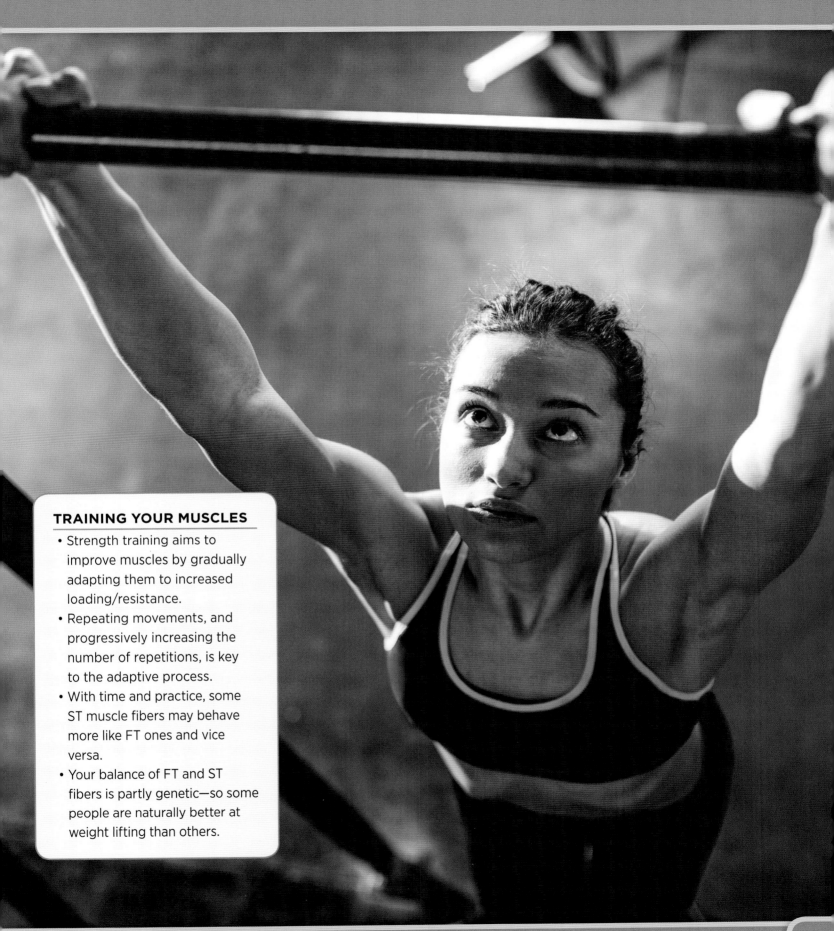

TRAINING YOUR MUSCLES

- Strength training aims to improve muscles by gradually adapting them to increased loading/resistance.
- Repeating movements, and progressively increasing the number of repetitions, is key to the adaptive process.
- With time and practice, some ST muscle fibers may behave more like FT ones and vice versa.
- Your balance of FT and ST fibers is partly genetic—so some people are naturally better at weight lifting than others.

Nutrition

There is endless debate about which are the best nutrition plans for health and fitness. Plus your goals will differ depending on how you approach strength training—as part of an all-around plan for better health, or to build a more muscular body with greatly superior strength. However, some basics do emerge.

It has been said on numerous occasions, but the main thing to keep in mind is that a basic health requirement is to eat a good variety of foods. These should offer the wide range of nutrients needed by the body for optimal health and be as fresh and unprocessed as possible.

THE FAT/MUSCLE EQUATION

In order to get the most from strength training—and in fact, from life—you need to aim for lean muscles and minimize your excess body fat. There is a key fact here: if you take in more calories than you burn, your body creates fat and you will gain weight. Fat is essential for functions such as those in your nervous and immune systems, and having fat at around 20% of your body weight (just below for a man, just above for a woman) is seen as healthy for an average fit person. If it drops to around 5%, though, this might make you ill.

To keep your muscles lean and healthy, protein is very important—and you need to replenish stocks regularly as it's not straightforwardly stored by the body. Lean meat, poultry, fish, eggs, and pulses are effective sources. Foods such as nuts and grains are other sources but might not always supply enough.

BUILDING AND KEEPING MUSCLE

If you want to just maintain lean muscle mass and incorporate strength training into an average fitness regimen, then you probably need less protein than those looking to significantly enlarge or develop their muscles. That said, muscle building does not benefit from massive protein intake, as only so much can be taken in at a time.

Experts argue about levels of required protein, but you might look at protein making up around 15–20% of your calorie intake. Take into consideration also that one common recommendation suggests that adults with sedentary lifestyles need about 50–60 grams of protein per day. You may also need to have extra calories overall in your diet if you really want to build lean muscle. As long as you are actively strength training, perhaps look at around 300 calories on top of recommended healthy amounts.

CARBS—BEATING THE "RUSH"

Carbohydrates—sugary or starchy foods—are where we gain most of our energy. Classic examples include pasta, potatoes, and bread, while fruit contains simple sugars that are carbs too. The main issue here is where foods fall on the glycemic index, or GI. High-GI foods cause blood-sugar levels to soar (the famed "sugar rush"), then plummet. This is bad for your energy levels—especially if you are engaged in demanding exercise such as strength training—and harmful to overall health. Low-GI foods release energy in a slower, more sustained way, which is good news for everyone.

Giving catchall carb intake guidelines is always difficult, but you might look at having around 45–65% of your daily calories as carbs. Don't forget, too, that high-fiber foods are great at helping to control blood-sugar levels, as well as all the other health benefits they bring.

COMMON SENSE

Ultimately, the strength trainer's nutritional approach needn't be dramatically different from good eating for the average, healthy, exercising person. That said, if you want to undergo a really rigorous strength-training, bodybuilding, or weight-lifting program, seek expert nutritional advice.

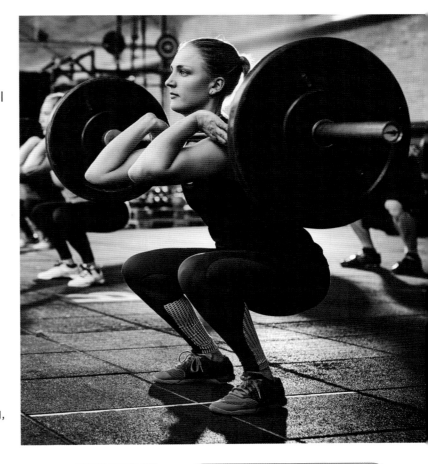

DOES MUSCLE TURN TO FAT?

People often talk about muscle turning into fat if you stop exercising—or even about turning fat into muscle. No! One kind of tissue cannot turn into a totally different one. What may happen, however, is that you might be eating more calories because you are exercising a great deal and then you decrease your exercise level but keep eating at the same level, and so gain weight/fat. And of course less exercise will mean your muscles will change by losing strength and mass.

KEEPING IT LOW

The following is a small selection of low-GI foods—with a score of 55 or under out of 100 on the GI scale.

- Oatmeal, oat bran, muesli
- Stone-ground whole wheat bread, spelt breads
- Whole wheat pasta, "converted" rice, bulgur wheat
- Peas, legumes, lentils
- Most fresh fruits and non-starchy vegetables

EATING ESSENTIALS

- Don't take in more calories than you use.
- Eat regular, balanced, not overly large meals.
- Don't skip breakfast.
- Stick to minimum snacking between meals.
- Keep hydrated.
- Favor low-GI foods over "energy spike" ones.
- Choose fresh, not processed.

Equipment

Using your own body weight alone works well to provide resistance for certain strength-training exercises. Add some equipment, though, and you can dramatically increase your exercising range to enjoy what's in this book fully, and embrace strength training completely. A selection of equipment options are offered here.

If all you did was purchase one inexpensive pair of dumbbells—or used a couple of filled water bottles instead—and borrowed a small inflatable ball from your kids, you'd still increase the range of what you could get from your training by a mile. Handheld equipment options are now more affordable and accessible than ever before. Plus there are plenty of good-value gym day-passes and deals that give you access to sophisticated weight machines.

TOOLS OF THE TRADE

The box "Equipment Featured in This Book" lists the equipment found in this book's exercises. Certain pieces have been picked out for further discussion on these pages.

All equipment, however, and especially heavy-duty items, should be bought with care so that it is safe and doesn't do more harm than good. In many cases, especially if you are new to strength training or lifting weights, it is a good idea to seek expert advice or use equipment within the monitored environment of a gym. Beware also certain homemade equivalents. Pulling yourself up on something too flimsy to take your weight could cause serious injury.

DUMBBELLS AND KETTLEBELLS

Many strength-training exercises use either of these. They're an easy way to add extra valuable resistance to a movement, and can be used in many cases where a weight is called for—either singly or as a pair.

• **Dumbbells** You'll often see the term "hand weights" used for the smallest ones, although *dumbbells* is the general term. You might start out with very light dumbbells weighing around 2 pounds (0.9 kilograms) and work your way up to heavier ones. Light homemade substitutes could be filled water bottles or unopened cans or packets of food.

If you decide to buy dumbbells that are all-in-one pieces with no extra added-on weights, then think about buying a set so you can work with different weight levels. For those where weight can be added on, make sure you choose ones with a solid locking mechanism. This makes it quick and simple to add or remove weight discs.

• **Kettlebells** Like dumbbells, if you are buying these, you might like to invest in a few different weights so you can progress. For beginners, women could look at starting with 18 pounds (8 kilograms), and beginner men at around 26 pounds (12 kilograms).

Some things to avoid with kettlebells include: sharp uncomfortable handles, attached bases that might dig in to you, or certain plastic coatings that make the handle too slippery. Also bear in mind that "competition" kettlebells have room for only one hand. These are less versatile than ones with room for two hands if you want to do two-handed kettlebell exercises.

SWISS BALL

This invaluable aid goes by other names, too, such as "fitness ball," "exercise ball," "stability ball," or "balance ball." This is a large, sturdy inflatable ball known for really working your core and improving your balance by introducing an element of instability. Available in diameters ranging between about 18 and 30 inches (46–76 centimeters), it's important that you pick one that suits your height (and weight).

RESISTANCE BANDS

Again, other names abound, including "exercise bands," "fitness bands," "Thera-Bands," "Dyna-Bands," and "stretching bands." Whatever the name, these are essentially simple, stretchy bands that are fantastic at adding resistance to all kinds of movements. They are also lightweight and easily portable. There are now many types, but the two basic divisions are those with handles and those without. Both appear in this book. Bands work by creating tension for your muscles to work against (as opposed to gravity, which supplies resistance when working with weights).

EQUIPMENT FEATURED IN THIS BOOK	
Barbell	Incline bench/similar
Body bar	Kettlebells
Cable machine	Mat for floor work
Dumbbells	Medicine ball (weighted ball)
Flat bench/similar	Plyo box(es)/block(s)
Foam roller	Pull-up bar
Half-dome balance ball (aka a Bosu ball or balance trainer)	Resistance bands
	Small inflatable ball/ Pilates ball
	Step/bench/platform
	Swiss ball

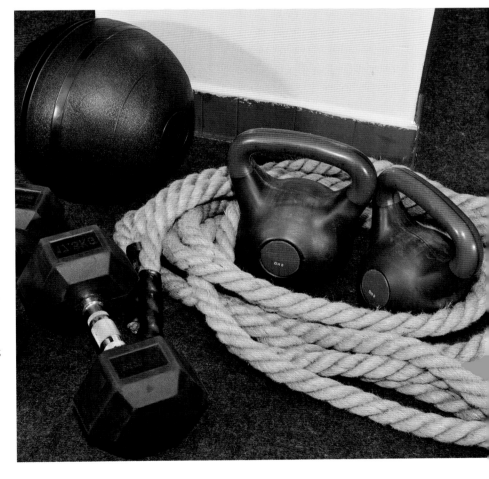

Creating a Workout Schedule

It's always best with fitness regimens to follow a plan, but where to start with strength training? This section addresses some of the vital questions you need to ask yourself as you sit down to create the most effective personalized workout schedule for you.

The first question you need to ask yourself is what you want to get from your strength training. Much bigger muscles and much greater strength (emphasizing anaerobic activity)? Or leaner, toned muscles and a strengthened, generally fitter body (more aerobic activity)? Do you also want to improve your self-confidence and positivity in life? This is step one.

REPS AND YOUR "REP"

People often get embarrassed about their level of ability and may feel that they have a reputation of some kind to uphold. Try to forget about that, especially if you're a beginner. Never be tempted to go too far or too fast—you could hurt yourself and then no training will be possible.

At each stage, feel that you can comfortably manage what you are doing before you step things up.

The main thing that any program should do is allow you to start at a very comfortable level for you and then progress in gradual increments that provide you with sufficient achievements to keep you motivated. Build up the number of repetitions that you do, and then the number of sets of "reps." Add in easier or harder modifications along the way—plenty are suggested in this book.

ACTIVITY AND RECOVERY

Just as you should always build warm-up and cooldown time into workouts (pages 8–11), build in suitable recovery time, too. Your body needs recovery time to repair itself—especially as you get older—so again don't push yourself too much. You should be spending more time not training than training. One estimate is that a muscle needs a couple of days to recover after a strength-training workout, so two or three sessions a week is perfect. And, typically, the higher the intensity, such as using very heavy weights, the shorter your activity session should be, time-wise.

The *work-to-rest ratio* is often talked about, which is your time spent active in relation to your time spent resting. So, if an activity took you 30 seconds and you then rest for 2 minutes, the ratio is 1:4. The more intense the workout, such as strenuous pull-ups or lifting a heavy barbell, the longer the recovery time required.

This ratio should be considered in tandem with your 1RM, or "one-repetition maximum"—the maximum weight you can lift comfortably during an exercise without losing form at all. The best way to arrive at your 1RM for a specific activity is by: 1) warming up; 2) then gradually building up the weight lifted from a modest starting point, resting for a generous time between lifts, until you reach your comfortable max.

FROM A MUSCULAR VIEWPOINT

When devising your schedules, think about how muscles work. A muscle's *strength* relates to how much weight it can lift. Its *power* equals strength plus speed, so while you must work within your ability zone and never rush, certain strength-training exercises recommend that you pick up pace as you perform them. If not actual speed, then certainly a smoothness and ease of execution and of transitioning from one part of the move to the next. Muscular *endurance* is how long muscles can keep working—in other words,

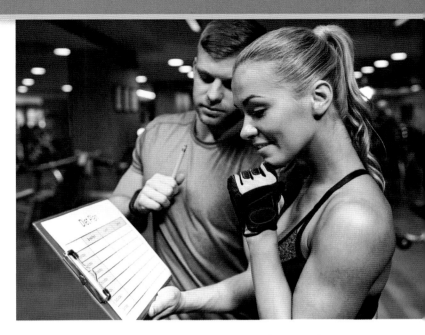

contracting when faced with a load or resistance. For example, can your biceps manage 10 repetitions of a curl, or 15? A good strength-training program should develop all three aspects: strength, power, and endurance.

ISOLATING OR COMPOUND?

An effective strength-training schedule should involve some activity that isolates specific muscles and works them. However, make sure you do plenty of "compound" work that engages multiple muscles or muscle groups. Don't overdo your repetitions, and have some sessions where you take it easy and others where you push yourself a little harder. This variety will help you understand your limitation zones more easily—and make training more enjoyable!

SOME BIG QUESTIONS

- What are my goals—physical and psychological?
- What is my ability/strength/confidence level now?
- What time do I have available?
- Which kind of equipment do I have access to?
- What kind of exercises do I enjoy doing most?
- Would I benefit from a training "buddy"?

AEROBIC VERSUS ANAEROBIC

- *Aerobic exercise*—a metabolic process that stresses oxygen use and includes low-intensity, high-endurance activity, such as distance running
- *Anaerobic exercise*—high-intensity, short-burst activity, such as lifting heavy weights

How to Use This Book

This book features step-by-step instructions for around 150 exercises specially selected to fit into a well-rounded strength-training regimen.

For all the exercises, you'll find a short overview, photos with step-by-step instructions, tips on form, and anatomical illustrations that highlight key muscles. Some exercises have variations, shown in a modification box. There is also a quick-read panel that features key points.

CHAPTER BREAKDOWNS

Chapter One: Flexibility Exercises Here you will find a selection of exercises to promote the general flexibility that will help with your strength-training workouts.

Chapter Two: Body-Weight Exercises Featuring exercises that rely on your own body weight only, you can take this chapter anywhere.

Chapter Three: Weighted Exercises Get out your dumbbells and kettlebells for this chapter. This challenging group uses weights for resistance.

Chapter Four: Equipment Exercises This chapter offers you a selection of exercises that use a variety of fitness equipment. From gym classics such as the chest press and cable fly, to at-home favorites such as Swiss ball bridges and aerobic step-work, you will find effective tools to help you build a better body.

Chapter Five: Workout Routines Once you've familiarized yourself with the featured exercises, turn to this chapter to learn how to combine them into strength workouts.

KEY

EXERCISE SPREADS

1 Category
Gives the body areas targeted: for example your chest, your legs and glutes, or your whole body.

2 Exercise Info
Gives the name of the exercise and a general overview of some key helpful details.

3 How to Do It
Step-by-step instructions explaining how to perform the exercise.

4 Step-by-Step Photos
Images of the key steps to the exercise.

5 Do It Right
Tips to help you perfect your form.

6 Fact File
A quick list of key facts: the exercise's main targets, equipment needed to perform it, its principal benefits, and any cautions that may apply.

7 Anatomical Illustration
Highlights the key working muscles. May also include an inset showing muscles not illustrated in the main image.

8 Modification
Shows you modifications that may be easier, harder, or of a similar difficulty.

WORKOUT SPREADS

1 Routine info
Gives the name of the routine and some key details you need to know about it.

2 Exercise Info
Shows the exercise name, pages where you can find it, and information on repetitions and timings.

3 Photo Icon
A quick view of the exercise.

4 Fact File
A quick list of key facts about the routine: body areas targeted, equipment needed, and general benefits.

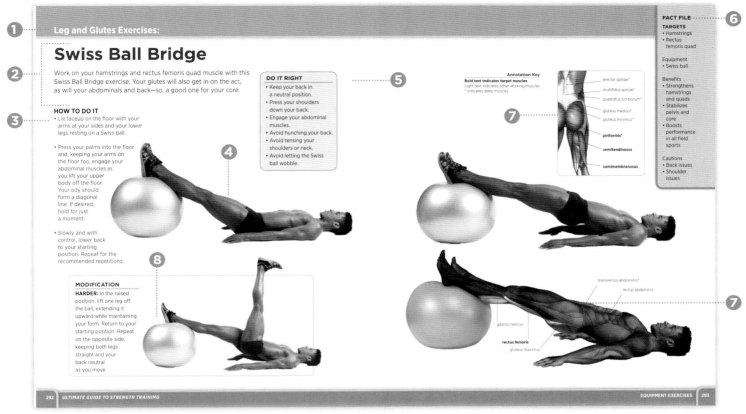

Swiss Ball Bridge

Work on your hamstrings and rectus femoris quad muscle with this Swiss Ball Bridge exercise. Your glutes will also get in on the act, as will your abdominals and back—so, a good one for your core.

HOW TO DO IT
- Lie faceup on the floor with your arms at your sides and your lower legs resting on a Swiss ball.

- Press your palms into the floor and, keeping your arms on the floor too, engage your abdominal muscles as you lift your upper body off the floor. Your ody should form a diagonal line. If desired, hold for just a moment.

- Slowly and with control, lower back to your starting position. Repeat for the recommended repetitions.

MODIFICATION
HARDER: In the raised position, lift one leg off the ball, extending it upward while maintaining your form. Return to your starting position. Repeat on the opposite side, keeping both legs straight and your back neutral as you move.

DO IT RIGHT
- Keep your back in a neutral position.
- Press your shoulders down your back.
- Engage your abdominal muscles.
- Avoid hunching your back.
- Avoid tensing your shoulders or neck.
- Avoid letting the Swiss ball wobble.

Annotation Key
Bold text indicates target muscles
Light text indicates other working muscles
* indicates deep muscles

erector spinae*
multifidus spinae*
quadratus lumborum*
gluteus medius*
gluteus minimus*
piriformis*
semitendinosus
semimembranosus

transversus abdiomnis*
rectus abdominis
gastrocnemius
rectus femoris
gluteus maximus

FACT FILE
TARGETS
- Hamstrings
- Rectus femoris quad

Equipment
- Swiss ball

Benefits
- Strengthens hamstrings and quads
- Stabilizes pelvis and core
- Boosts performance in all field sports

Cautions
- Back issues
- Shoulder issues

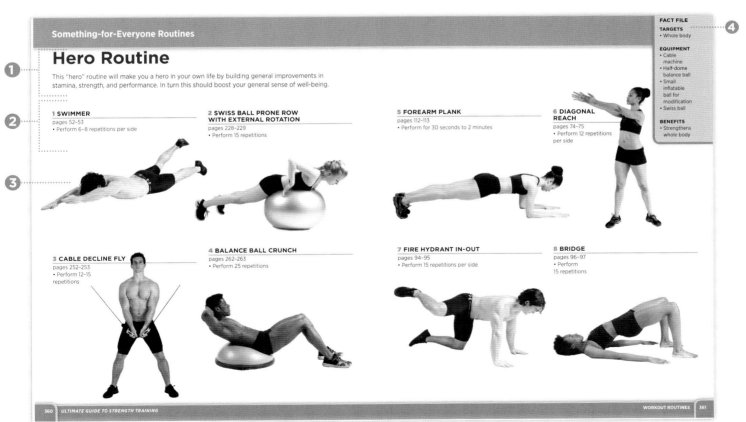

Hero Routine

This "hero" routine will make you a hero in your own life by building general improvements in stamina, strength, and performance. In turn this should boost your general sense of well-being.

1 SWIMMER
pages 52–53
- Perform 6–8 repetitions per side

2 SWISS BALL PRONE ROW WITH EXTERNAL ROTATION
pages 228–229
- Perform 15 repetitions

3 CABLE DECLINE FLY
pages 252–253
- Perform 12–15 repetitions

4 BALANCE BALL CRUNCH
pages 262–263
- Perform 25 repetitions

5 FOREARM PLANK
pages 112–113
- Perform for 30 seconds to 2 minutes

6 DIAGONAL REACH
pages 74–75
- Perform 12 repetitions per side

7 FIRE HYDRANT IN-OUT
pages 94–95
- Perform 15 repetitions per side

8 BRIDGE
pages 96–97
- Perform 15 repetitions

FACT FILE
TARGETS
- Whole body

EQUIPMENT
- Cable machine
- Half-dome balance ball
- Small inflatable ball for modification
- Swiss ball

BENEFITS
- Strengthens whole body

Full-Body Anatomy

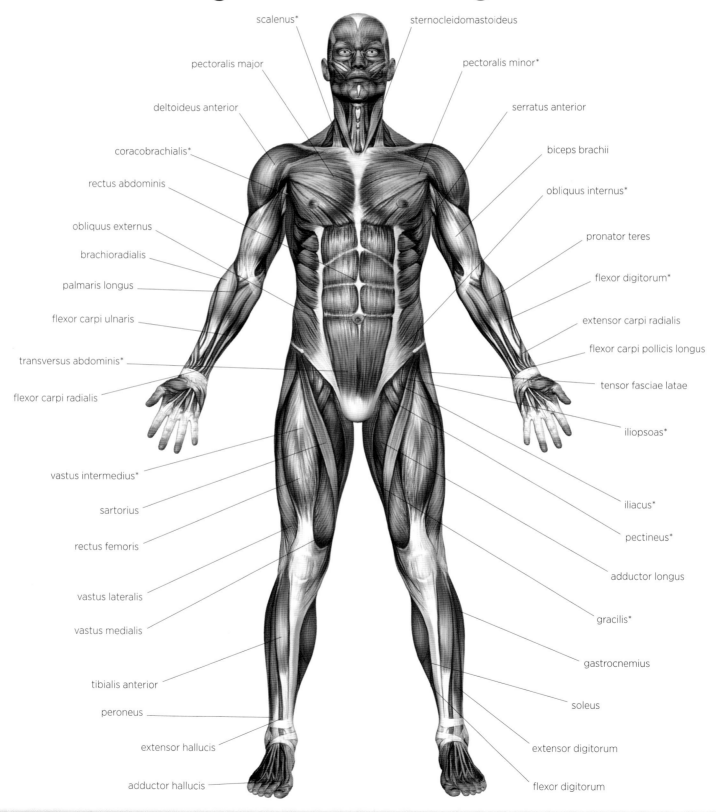

scalenus*

sternocleidomastoideus

pectoralis major

pectoralis minor*

deltoideus anterior

serratus anterior

coracobrachialis*

biceps brachii

rectus abdominis

obliquus internus*

obliquus externus

pronator teres

brachioradialis

flexor digitorum*

palmaris longus

extensor carpi radialis

flexor carpi ulnaris

flexor carpi pollicis longus

transversus abdominis*

tensor fasciae latae

flexor carpi radialis

iliopsoas*

vastus intermedius*

iliacus*

sartorius

pectineus*

rectus femoris

adductor longus

vastus lateralis

gracilis*

vastus medialis

gastrocnemius

tibialis anterior

soleus

peroneus

extensor hallucis

extensor digitorum

adductor hallucis

flexor digitorum

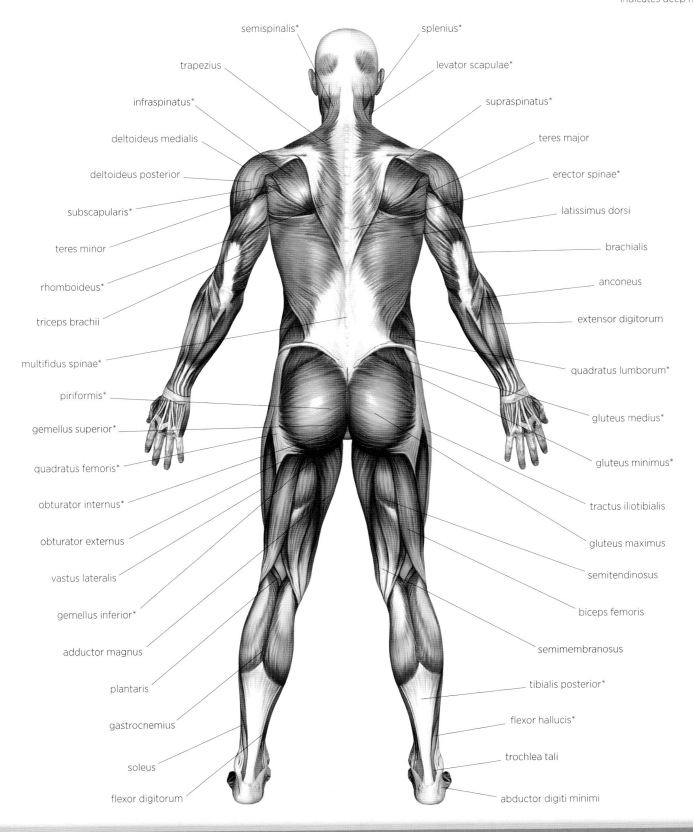

semispinalis*

splenius*

trapezius

levator scapulae*

infraspinatus*

supraspinatus*

deltoideus medialis

teres major

deltoideus posterior

erector spinae*

subscapularis*

latissimus dorsi

teres minor

brachialis

rhomboideus*

anconeus

triceps brachii

extensor digitorum

multifidus spinae*

quadratus lumborum*

piriformis*

gluteus medius*

gemellus superior*

quadratus femoris*

gluteus minimus*

obturator internus*

tractus iliotibialis

obturator externus

gluteus maximus

vastus lateralis

semitendinosus

gemellus inferior*

biceps femoris

adductor magnus

semimembranosus

plantaris

tibialis posterior*

gastrocnemius

flexor hallucis*

soleus

trochlea tali

flexor digitorum

abductor digiti minimi

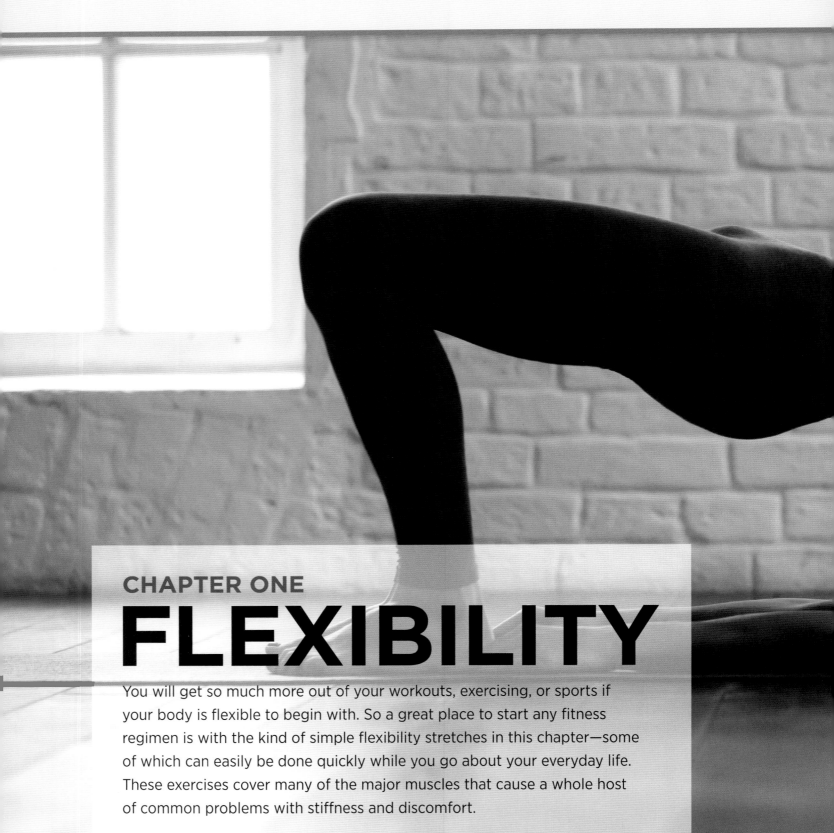

CHAPTER ONE
FLEXIBILITY

You will get so much more out of your workouts, exercising, or sports if your body is flexible to begin with. So a great place to start any fitness regimen is with the kind of simple flexibility stretches in this chapter—some of which can easily be done quickly while you go about your everyday life. These exercises cover many of the major muscles that cause a whole host of common problems with stiffness and discomfort.

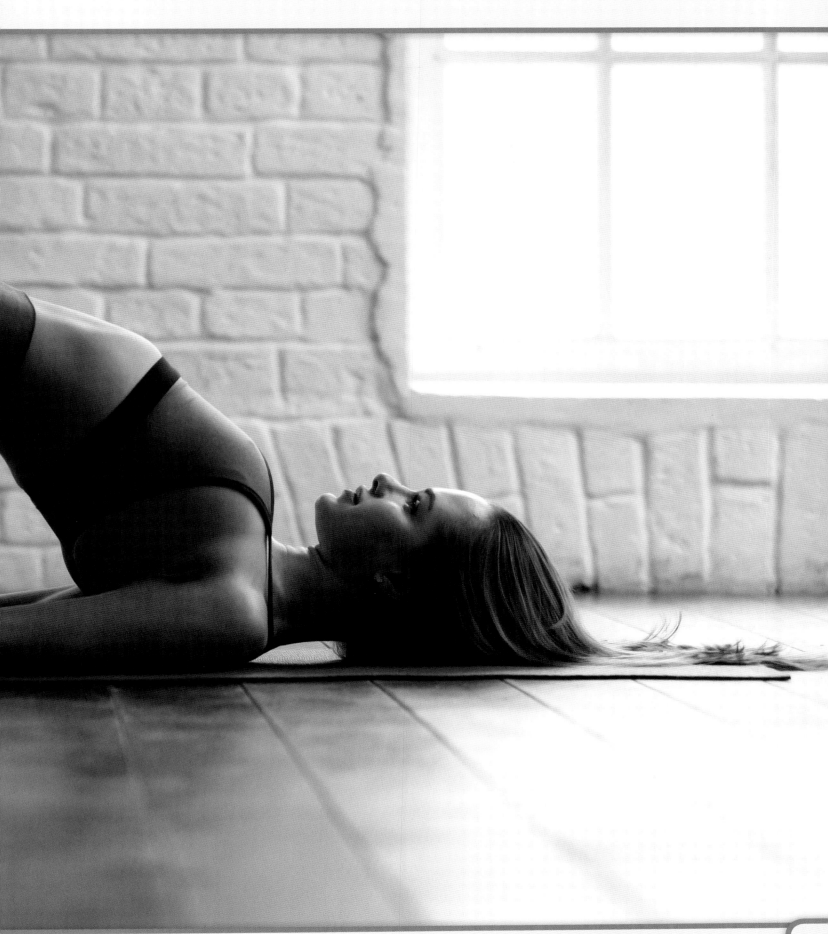

Triceps Stretch

The Triceps Stretch is easy to do anytime, anywhere. It improves shoulder and upper-body flexibility, fends off muscle soreness, and extends your range of motion while building durability.

HOW TO DO IT

- Stand with your legs and feet parallel and shoulder-width apart. Bend your knees very slightly, and shift your pelvis slightly forward.

- Reach your right arm up behind your head. Bend from the elbow, aiming to bring your elbow toward the middle of the back of your head. Your right hand should fall between your shoulder blades.

- Grab your right elbow with your left hand, and gently pull down to intensify the stretch.

- Hold for the recommended time, release the stretch, and then repeat on the opposite side.

DO IT RIGHT

- Keep your shoulders pressed down and back, away from your ears.
- Maintain a firm, stable midsection, keeping your pelvis slightly tucked.
- Avoid tilting your head or neck forward.

FACT FILE

TARGETS
- Triceps brachii

EQUIPMENT
- None

BENEFITS
- Increases upper-arm mobility
- Relaxes tight shoulder joints

CAUTIONS
- Shoulder issues

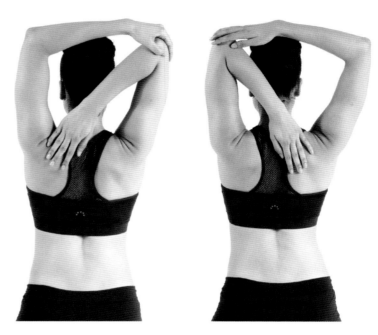

triceps brachii

deltoideus posterior

infraspinatus

teres major

teres minor

Annotation Key
Bold text indicates target muscles
Light text indicates other working muscles
* indicates deep muscles

Biceps-Pecs Stretch

This stretch opens up the upper-front part of your body. Working the chest and upper arms together, it counteracts tightening caused by bad habits such as slouching.

HOW TO DO IT

- Stand with your legs and feet parallel and shoulder-width apart. Shift your pelvis slightly forward.

- Clasp your hands together behind your back with your fingers interwoven. If you want an extra stretch, twist your hands and wrists so that your palms are pulled in toward your buttocks and your thumbs point downward.

- Hold for the recommended time, release the stretch, and then repeat for the recommended repetitions.

FACT FILE

TARGETS
- Biceps brachii
- Shoulders
- Chest

EQUIPMENT
- None

BENEFITS
- Stretches and strengthens arms
- Opens chest

CAUTIONS
- Shoulder issues
- Wrist issues

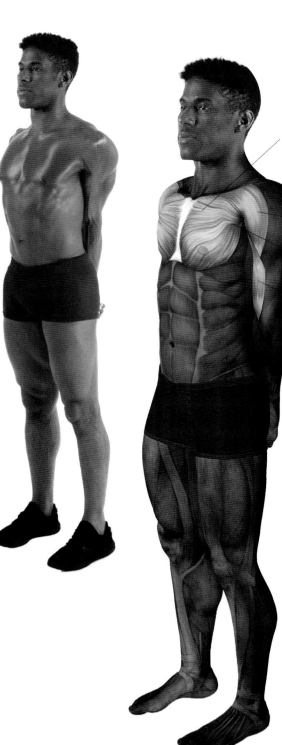
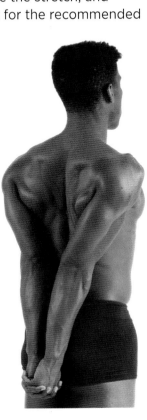

pectoralis major

deltoideus anterior

pectoralis minor*

biceps brachii

DO IT RIGHT

- Keep your shoulders pressed down and back, away from your ears.
- Avoid collapsing your chest forward.

Annotation Key

Bold text indicates target muscles
Light text indicates other working muscles
* indicates deep muscles

Lateral Lunge Stretch

Sideway lunges tone key muscles in your thighs and buttocks, helping to free up movement in your legs and hips as well as stabilizing your knees.

HOW TO DO IT

- Begin bent over, with your feet planted far apart. Allow your arms to dangle toward the floor in front of you.

- Bend your right knee while keeping your left leg straight. Place most of your weight on your bent leg, feeling the stretch in your lengthened leg.

- Hold for the recommended time, release the stretch, and then repeat on the opposite side.

DO IT RIGHT

- Extend your leg fully while in the stretch position.
- Gaze toward the floor throughout the stretch.
- Keep your feet flat on the floor.
- Avoid twisting your torso.
- Avoid curving your back forward.
- Avoid arching your back or neck.

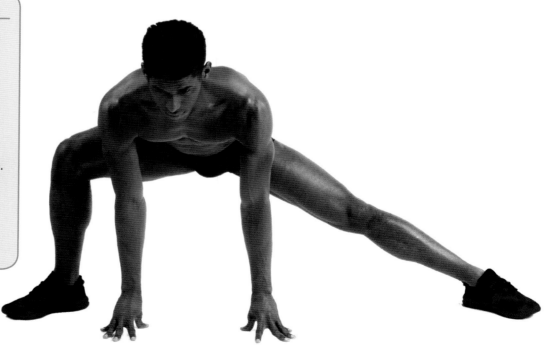

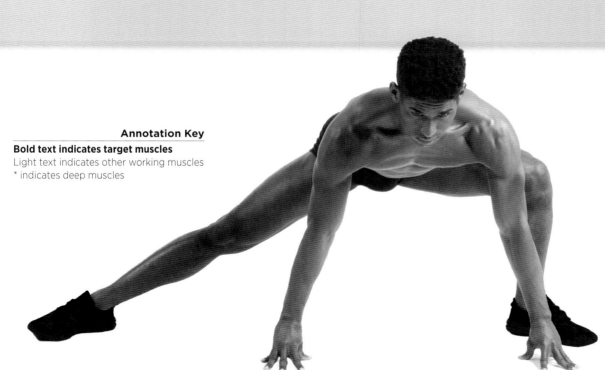

FACT FILE

TARGETS
- Glutes
- Inner thighs
- Quadriceps

EQUIPMENT
- None

BENEFITS
- Stretches leg muscles

CAUTIONS
- Knee issues

Annotation Key

Bold text indicates target muscles
Light text indicates other working muscles
* indicates deep muscles

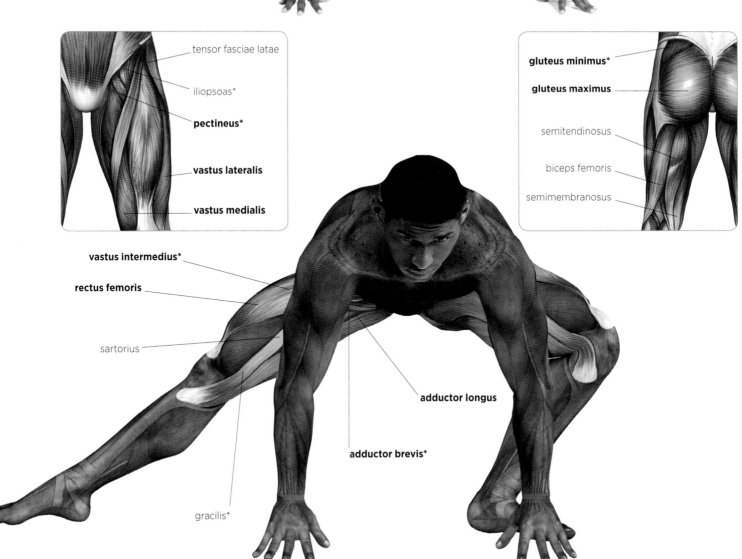

tensor fasciae latae

iliopsoas*

pectineus*

vastus lateralis

vastus medialis

gluteus minimus*

gluteus maximus

semitendinosus

biceps femoris

semimembranosus

vastus intermedius*

rectus femoris

sartorius

gracilis*

adductor longus

adductor brevis*

Standing Quadriceps Stretch

FACT FILE

TARGETS
• Quadriceps

EQUIPMENT
• None

BENEFITS
• Helps to keep thigh muscles flexible

CAUTIONS
• Knee issues

The Standing Quadriceps Stretch relieves stiffness by giving the front and sides of your thighs a strong stretch while also releasing hip flexor muscles and improving balance and posture.

HOW TO DO IT

• Stand with your legs and feet parallel and shoulder-width apart. Tuck your pelvis slightly forward, lift your chest, and press your shoulders downward and back.

• Bend your right knee behind you so that your ankle is raised toward your buttocks.

• Reach down with your right hand to grab your foot just below your ankle, and gently pull as you stretch.

• Hold for the recommended time, release the stretch, and then repeat on the opposite side

DO IT RIGHT

• Keep your torso upright.
• Pull your foot toward your buttocks gently, stretching only as far as you feel comfortable.
• Gaze forward.
• Avoid leaning forward.
• Avoid arching your back.
• Avoid hunching your shoulders.

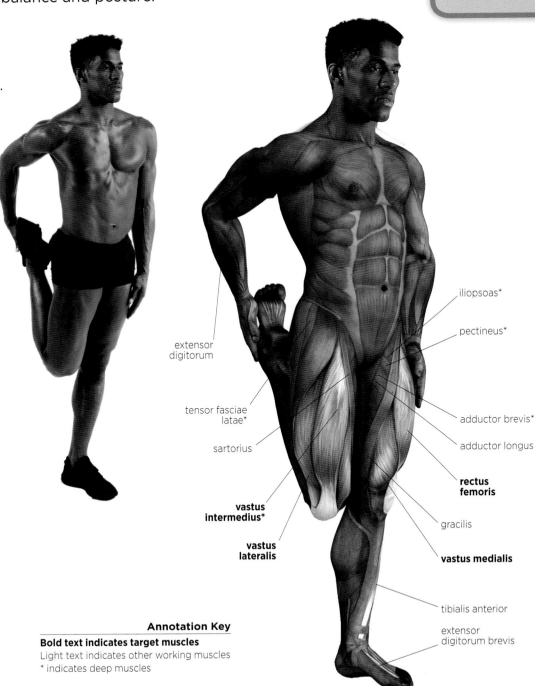

iliopsoas*

pectineus*

extensor digitorum

tensor fasciae latae*

sartorius

adductor brevis*

adductor longus

rectus femoris

vastus intermedius*

gracilis

vastus lateralis

vastus medialis

tibialis anterior

extensor digitorum brevis

Annotation Key
Bold text indicates target muscles
Light text indicates other working muscles
* indicates deep muscles

Standing Hamstrings Stretch

A simple, effective way to counteract the common problem of tight muscles at the back of the thigh, this stretch should benefit both your calves and your lower back.

HOW TO DO IT

- Stand with your right leg bent and your left leg extended in front of you with the heel on the floor.

- Lean over your left leg, resting both hands above your knee. Place the majority of your body weight on your front heel while feeling the stretch in the back of your thigh.

- Hold for the recommended time, release the stretch, and then repeat on the opposite side.

FACT FILE

TARGETS
• Hamstrings

EQUIPMENT
• None

BENEFITS
• Helps to keep hamstring muscles flexible

CAUTIONS
• Lower-back issues
• Knee issues

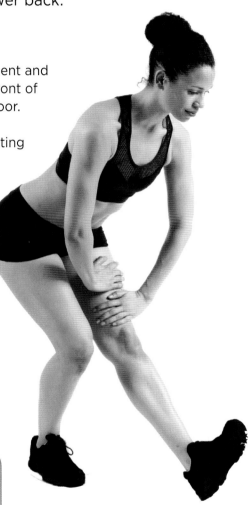

DO IT RIGHT
- Keep your front leg straight.
- Flex the foot of your front leg as you stretch.
- Avoid arching your back or rounding it forward.
- Avoid hunching your shoulders.

Annotation Key
Bold text indicates target muscles
Light text indicates other working muscles
* indicates deep muscles

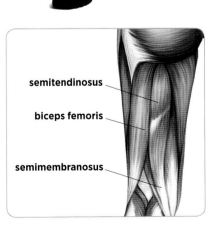

semitendinosus

biceps femoris

semimembranosus

Iliotibial Band Stretch

The tractus iliotibialis, commonly called the iliotibial band or ITB, is a band of tissue linking your hips and shins and interconnecting with major muscles. This stretch counters common problems in the knees, hips, or thighs.

HOW TO DO IT

- Stand upright, with your arms along your sides. Cross your right foot in front of your left.

- Bending at your waist, gradually reach toward the floor with your hands.

- Hold for the recommended time, release the stretch, and then slowly roll up to the starting position. Repeat on the opposite side.

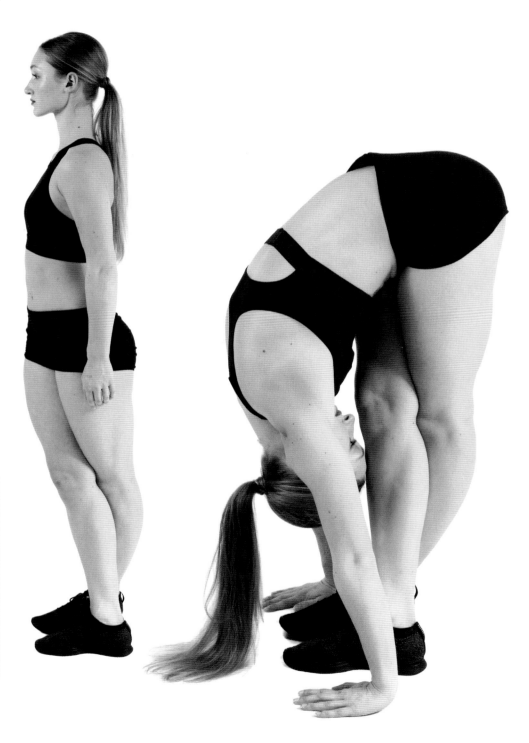

DO IT RIGHT

- Keep your knees straight, yet soft, throughout the exercise.
- Let your head drop.
- Avoid bending or locking your knees.
- Avoid twisting your neck, shoulders, or torso to either side.

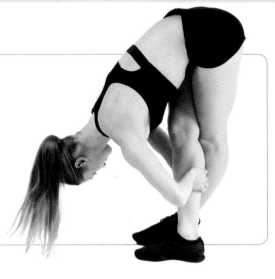

MODIFICATION

EASIER: If you find it difficult to reach the floor with your hands while maintaining your form, hold the stretch when your hands are only partway to the floor, or hold onto your straight leg. Try to reach slightly lower each time you stretch.

FACT FILE

TARGETS
- Iliotibial band
- Glutes
- Hamstrings

EQUIPMENT
- None

BENEFITS
- Stretches IT band
- Counteracts effects of wearing high heels
- Boosts performance in running, skiing, and cycling

CAUTIONS
- Neck issues
- Lower-back pain

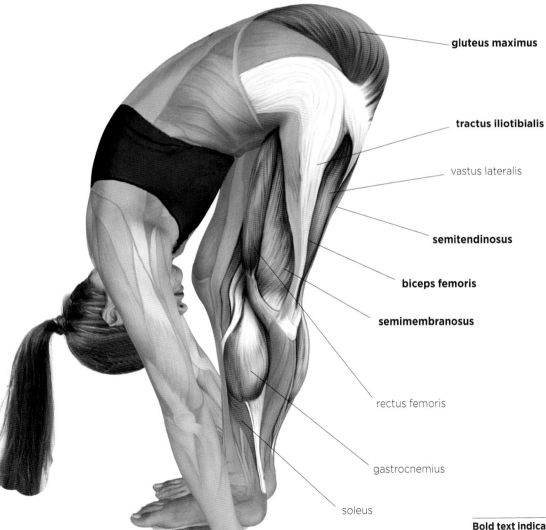

gluteus maximus

tractus iliotibialis

vastus lateralis

semitendinosus

biceps femoris

semimembranosus

rectus femoris

gastrocnemius

soleus

Annotation Key
Bold text indicates target muscles
Light text indicates other working muscles
* indicates deep muscles

Cat-to-Cow Stretch

The Cat-to-Cow is a simple, deep stretch that eases out your spine.
It also works your neck and shoulders and opens up your chest and hips.

HOW TO DO IT

- To perform the Cat Stretch, kneel on all fours, with your hands planted directly below your shoulders and your knees aligned beneath your hips. Your hips should be in a neutral position and the tops of your feet on the floor.

- Spread your fingers, grounding down through your thumb and index finger. Externally rotate your arms, thinking of opening your right upper arm clockwise and your left upper arm counterclockwise.

- Drop your head as you round your upper back, and then draw your belly into your spine. Gazing down at the floor or toward your navel, hold for the recommended time, and then release the stretch.

- To move into the Cow Stretch, lift your sternum, and arch your upper back, raising your sit bones toward the ceiling. Hold for the recommended time, and then release the stretch.

- Alternate Cat and Cow for the recommended repetitions.

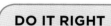

DO IT RIGHT

- Allow your shoulder blades to separate and breathe more space into your upper spine.
- Keep your shoulders over your wrists as you round your back.
- Avoid bringing your weight back toward your knees as you round your spine.

TARGETS
• Spine
• Chest
• Neck

EQUIPMENT
• None

BENEFITS
• Stretches
  upper body
  and back
• Strengthens
  hand and
  wrist muscles
• Massages
  spine
• Increases
  mobility

CAUTIONS
• Neck issues
• Wrist issues

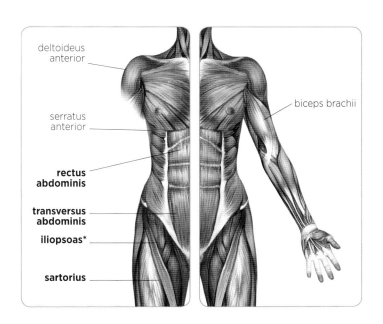

deltoideus
anterior

serratus
anterior

**rectus
abdominis**

**transversus
abdominis**

iliopsoas*

sartorius

biceps brachii

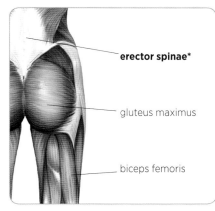

erector spinae*

gluteus maximus

biceps femoris

Annotation Key

Bold text indicates target muscles
Light text indicates other working muscles
* indicates deep muscles

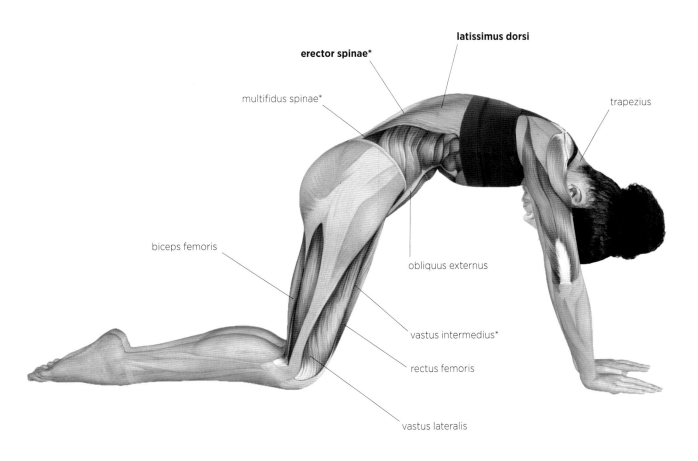

latissimus dorsi

erector spinae*

multifidus spinae*

trapezius

biceps femoris

obliquus externus

vastus intermedius*

rectus femoris

vastus lateralis

Cobra Stretch

As well as promoting spinal flexibility, this yoga-inspired stretch builds strength in your back and shoulders and also in your abdominals, buttocks, and chest.

HOW TO DO IT

- Lie facedown. Bend your elbows, placing your hands flat on the floor beside your chest. Extend your legs, and press down into the floor with your thighs and the tops of your feet.

- Inhaling, lift your chest off the floor, pressing your palms downward.

- Continue lifting your chest as you straighten your arms.

- Hold for the recommended time, and then, on an exhalation, lower yourself to the floor.

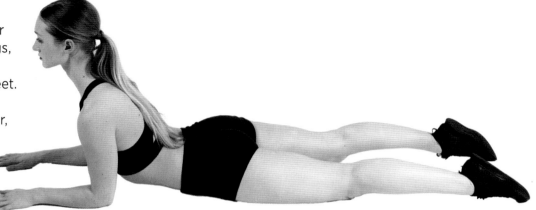

DO IT RIGHT

- Gaze forward.
- Keep your elbows pulled in toward your body.
- Lift from your chest and back, rather than depending too much on your arms to create the arch in your back.
- Keep your shoulders and elbows pressed back.
- Press your pubic bone into the floor as you lift.
- Avoid tensing your buttocks.
- Avoid splaying your elbows out to the sides.
- Avoid lifting your hips off the floor.
- Avoid twisting your neck.

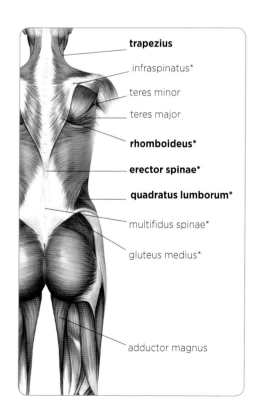

trapezius
infraspinatus*
teres minor
teres major
rhomboideus*
erector spinae*
quadratus lumborum*
multifidus spinae*
gluteus medius*
adductor magnus

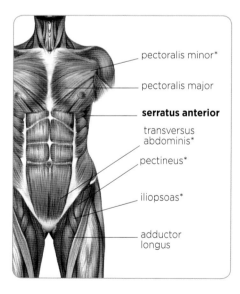

pectoralis minor*
pectoralis major
serratus anterior
transversus abdominis*
pectineus*
iliopsoas*
adductor longus

Annotation Key
Bold text indicates target muscles
Light text indicates other working muscles
* indicates deep muscles

FACT FILE

TARGETS
• Abdominals
• Back
• Chest
• Glutes
• Shoulders
• Triceps

EQUIPMENT
• None

BENEFITS
• Strengthens spine and glutes
• Stretches chest, abdominals, and shoulders
• Boosts performance in all sports

CAUTIONS
• Lower-back issues/pain

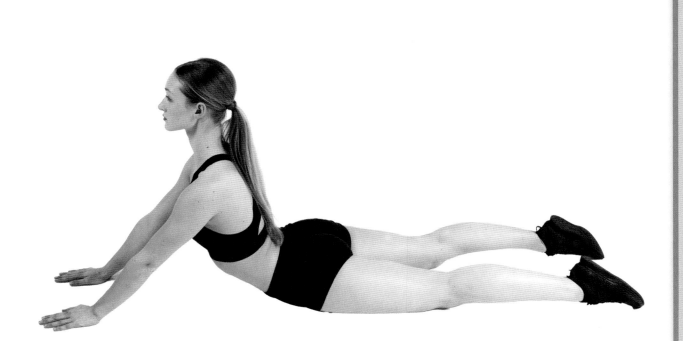

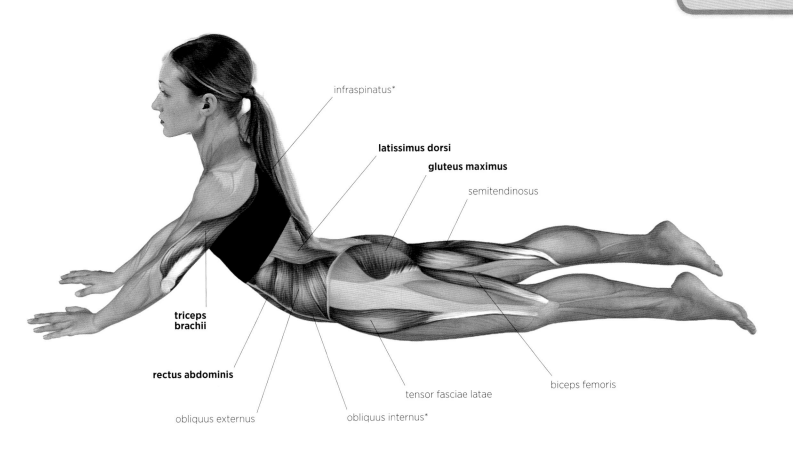

infraspinatus*

latissimus dorsi

gluteus maximus

semitendinosus

triceps brachii

rectus abdominis

biceps femoris

tensor fasciae latae

obliquus externus

obliquus internus*

Bird-Dog

A great stretch for developing core body strength, this works your back, abdominals, and glutes, with the added bonus of improving balance and smooth coordination.

HOW TO DO IT

- Begin on your hands and knees, with your back straight and your abdominals pulled in.

- Keeping your torso stable and your abdominals engaged, contract your right arm and your left leg into your body.

- Extend your right arm and left leg outward. Hold the extended position for the recommended time.

- Return to the starting position, and repeat on the opposite side.

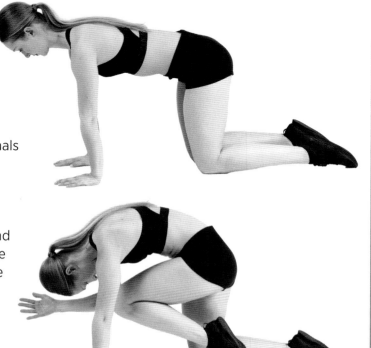

DO IT RIGHT

- Move slowly and with control.
- Keep your neck relaxed and your gaze toward the floor.
- Tuck your chin slightly while contracting your arm and leg inward.
- Keep your abs pulled in throughout the stretch.
- Avoid arching your back while your arm and leg are extended.
- Avoid twisting your torso.
- Avoid arching your neck.

MODIFICATION

HARDER: From the starting position, extend one arm and the opposite leg straight out to the side. Hold, release, and repeat on the opposite side.

HARDER: Begin facedown on top of a Swiss ball, with your core and upper thighs supported. Your hands should be on the floor and your legs extended with toes on the floor.

Slowly and with control, lift one arm and the opposite leg upward, keeping the rest of your body stable. Hold, release, and repeat on the opposite side.

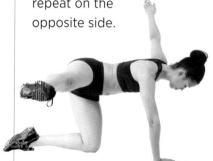
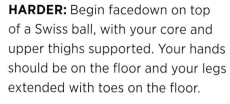
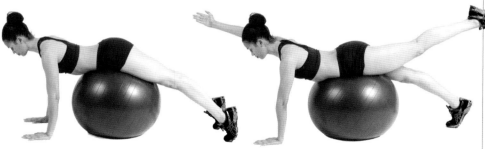

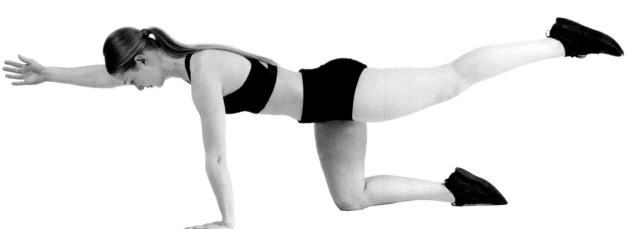

FACT FILE

TARGETS
- Abdominals
- Back
- Glutes

EQUIPMENT
- None/Swiss ball for modification

BENEFITS
- Stretches and tones abdominals, arms, and legs
- Aids balance and coordination

CAUTIONS
- Wrist pain
- Lower-back pain
- Knee injury

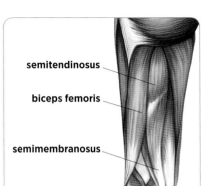

semitendinosus

biceps femoris

semimembranosus

Annotation Key
Bold text indicates target muscles
Light text indicates other working muscles
* indicates deep muscles

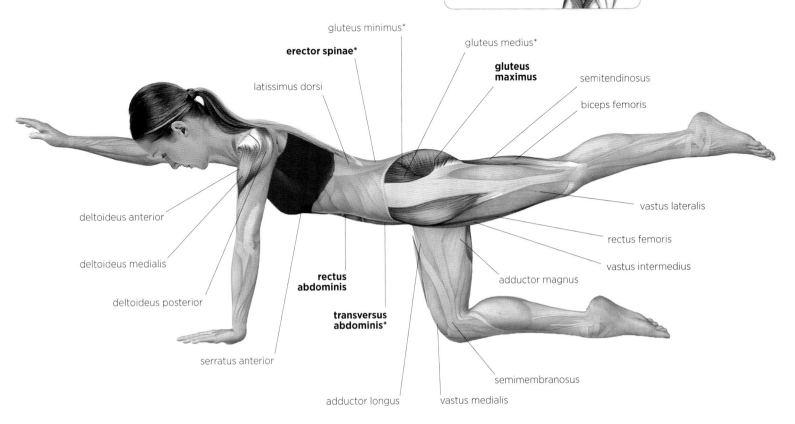

gluteus minimus*

erector spinae*

latissimus dorsi

gluteus medius*

gluteus maximus

semitendinosus

biceps femoris

deltoideus anterior

deltoideus medialis

deltoideus posterior

rectus abdominis

transversus abdominis*

serratus anterior

adductor longus

vastus medialis

semimembranosus

adductor magnus

vastus intermedius

rectus femoris

vastus lateralis

Half-Kneeling Rotation

This warm-up stretch brings important benefits to your general spinal mobility, improves both your posture and balance, and boosts your core rotation.

HOW TO DO IT

- Kneel on your left leg with your right leg bent at 90 degrees in front of you, foot on the floor. Place your hands beside your head so that your elbows flare outward.

- Keeping your back straight, rotate your left shoulder so that your upper body turns to the right.

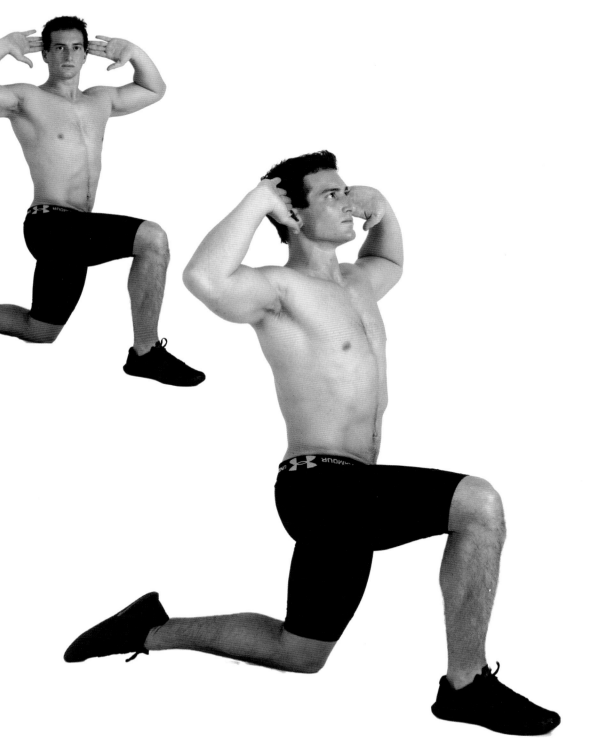

- Hold for the recommended time, release the stretch, and then repeat on the opposite side.

DO IT RIGHT

- Keep your back straight.
- Avoid rotating too far.
- Avoid letting your stomach bulge outward as your upper body rotates from one side to the other.

TARGETS
- Obliques
- Spine

EQUIPMENT
- None

BENEFITS
- Increases spinal rotation
- Improves posture

CAUTIONS
- Knee issues

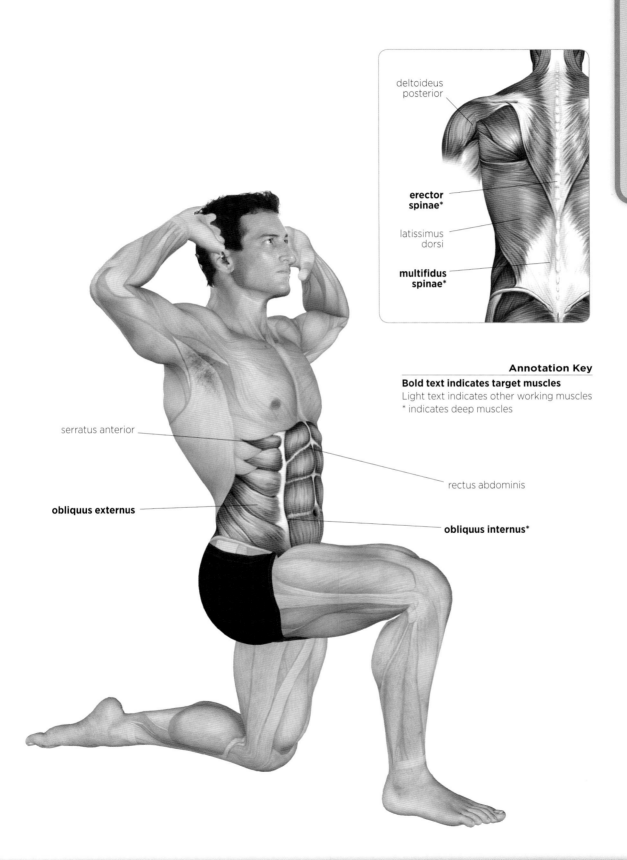

deltoideus posterior

erector spinae*

latissimus dorsi

multifidus spinae*

Annotation Key

Bold text indicates target muscles
Light text indicates other working muscles
* indicates deep muscles

serratus anterior

rectus abdominis

obliquus externus

obliquus internus*

Side Bending

This straightforward standing exercise stretches out the top half of your body and helps to counteract the poor, hunched posture that comes with sedentary lifestyles.

HOW TO DO IT

- Stand, keeping your neck, shoulders, and torso straight.

- Raise both arms above your head, and clasp your hands together, with your fingers interlocked and palms facing upward.

- Leaning from the hips, slowly drop your torso to the right.

- Keeping a smooth flow, lean your torso to the left.

- Continue alternating sides for the recommended repetitions.

DO IT RIGHT

- Elongate your arms and shoulders as much as possible.
- Avoid dropping to the side too quickly.

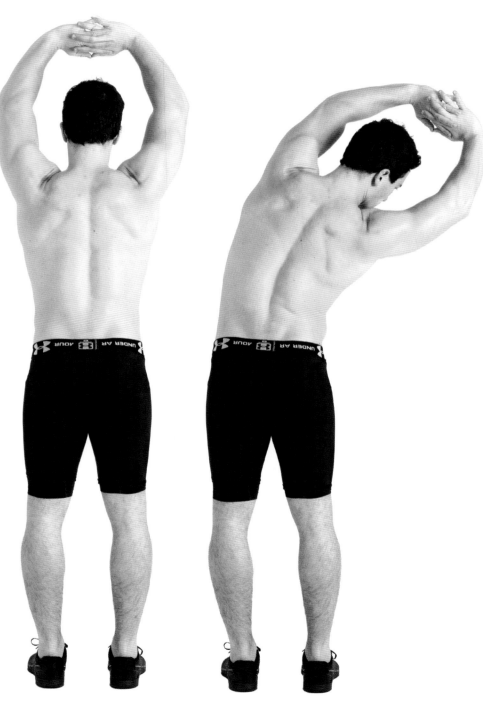

FACT FILE

TARGETS
• Upper back
• Obliques

EQUIPMENT
• None

BENEFITS
• Increases upper-body mobility
• Improves posture

CAUTIONS
• Lower-back pain

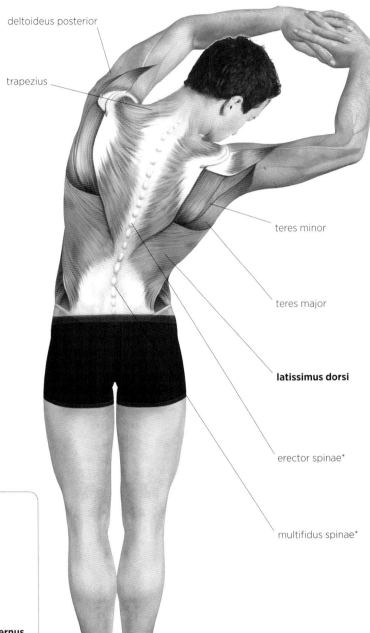

deltoideus posterior

trapezius

teres minor

teres major

latissimus dorsi

erector spinae*

multifidus spinae*

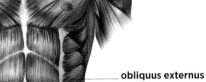

obliquus externus

obliquus internus*

Annotation Key

Bold text indicates target muscles
Light text indicates other working muscles
* indicates deep muscles

Swiss Ball Abdominal Stretch

A thorough toning and stretching workout for the muscles around your abdomen, this strong stretch is also an excellent routine for building core strength.

HOW TO DO IT

• Lie with a Swiss ball beneath your back. Your arms should be extended diagonally behind your head, your feet planted shoulder-width apart, and your knees bent.

• Slowly reach downward with your arms until your fingers rest on the floor.

• While keeping your lower back on the ball, lower your hips and stretch your abdominals toward the ceiling.

• Hold for the recommended time, release the stretch, and then repeat for the recommended repetitions.

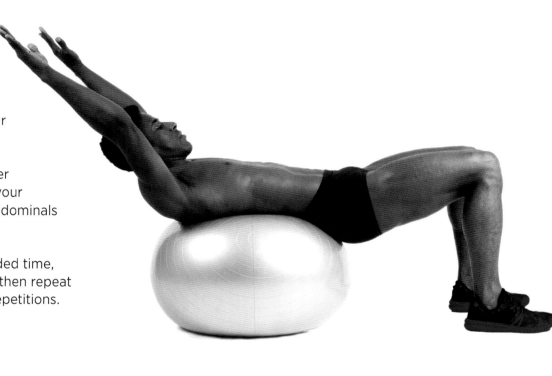

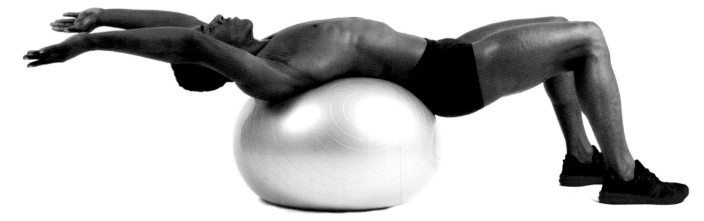

TARGETS
• Upper abdominals

EQUIPMENT
• Swiss ball

BENEFITS
• Stretches upper abdominals
• Improves balance

CAUTIONS
• Lower-back pain
• Shoulder issues
• Balancing difficulties

DO IT RIGHT
• Keep your torso planted on the ball.
• Avoid overextending your pelvis as you raise it.

Annotation Key
Bold text indicates target muscles
Light text indicates other working muscles
* indicates deep muscles

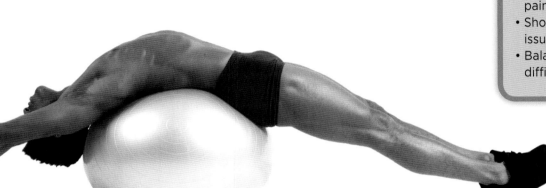

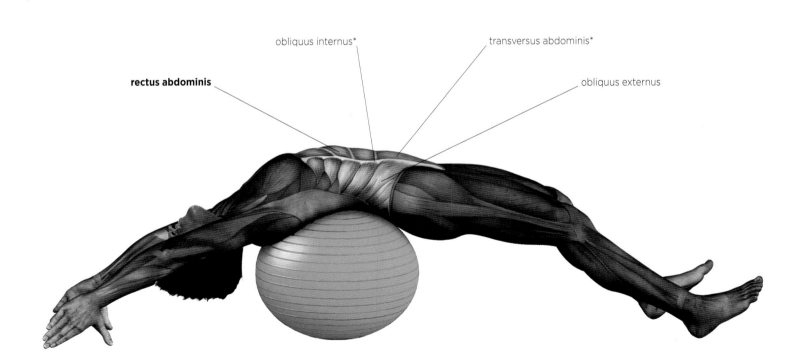

obliquus internus*

transversus abdominis*

rectus abdominis

obliquus externus

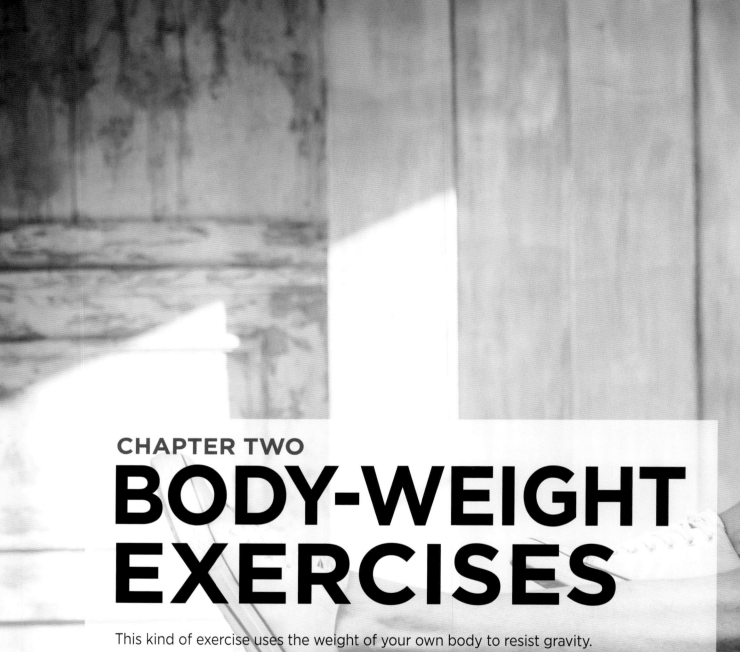

CHAPTER TWO
BODY-WEIGHT EXERCISES

This kind of exercise uses the weight of your own body to resist gravity. Body-weight exercises are an excellent way to build strength. They also increase staying power while improving your balance and flexibility. Many body-weight exercises work several muscle sets at the same time. This means you'll really feel a difference in your everyday movement, as well as in sports and workouts, and be more likely to resist injuries.

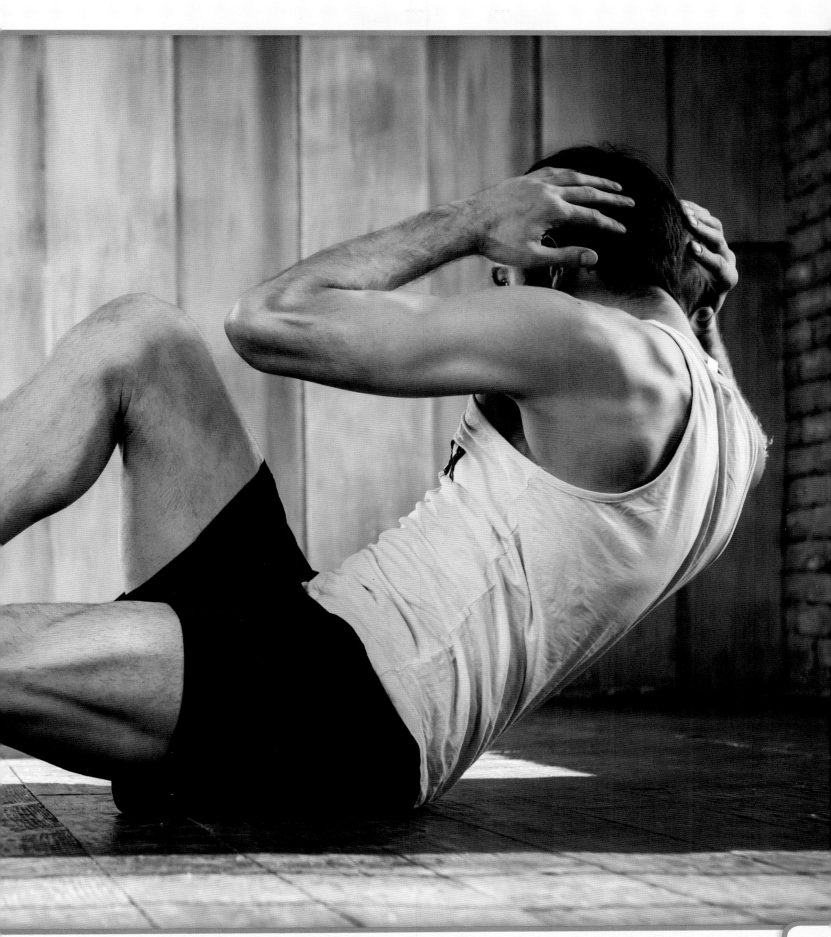

Thread the Needle

This spine-strengthener is popular in all kinds of training regimens. Thread the Needle gives your body a thorough rotation, with the arm movement building your core stability.

HOW TO DO IT

- Begin on all fours with your back flat and palms downward, directly below your shoulders.

- Turn your left hand over, so the back of your hand is now on the floor. Slide this hand behind your right arm and out to your right side, keeping the back of your hand on the floor. Bend your supporting arm as you slide your left hand out farther.

- Continue sliding until your left shoulder rests on the floor and your supporting arm is bent perpendicular. The side of your head should be resting on the floor with your gaze to the right.

- Hold for the recommended time, return to your starting position, and repeat on the opposite side.

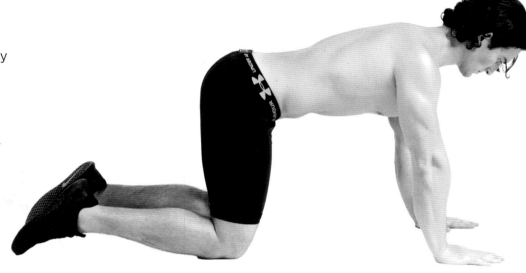

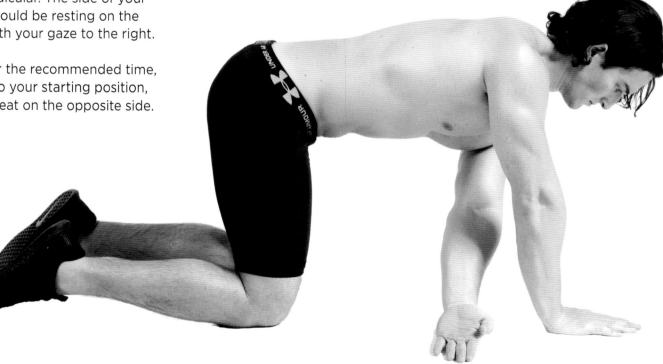

TARGETS
• Back

EQUIPMENT
• None

BENEFITS
• Improves back
  and shoulder
  mobility
• Increases
  spinal
  flexibility

CAUTIONS
• Lower-back
  pain
• Wrist or
  elbow pain
• Shoulder
  issues

DO IT RIGHT

• Rotate evenly throughout.
• Move slowly through the
  exercise to complete the
  full range of motion.
• Keep your supporting
  arm engaged to maintain
  balance.

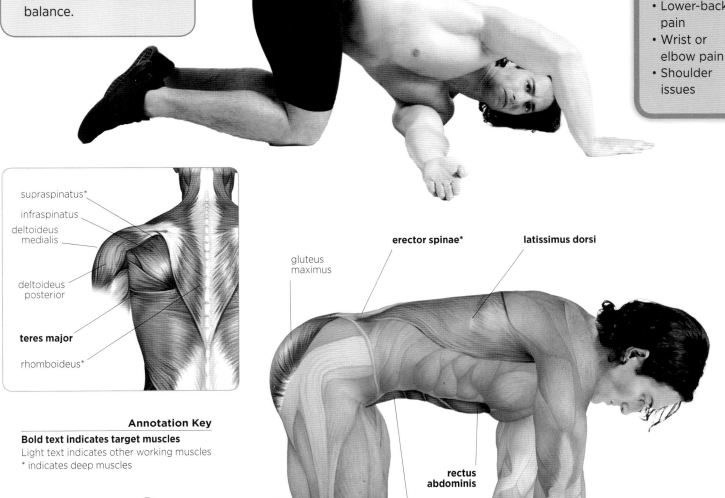

supraspinatus*
infraspinatus
deltoideus
medialis

deltoideus
posterior

teres major

rhomboideus*

gluteus
maximus

erector spinae*

latissimus dorsi

**rectus
abdominis**

**transversus
abdominis***

Annotation Key

Bold text indicates target muscles
Light text indicates other working muscles
* indicates deep muscles

Hip Crossover

The Hip Crossover effectively consolidates your core. As with many core exercises, aim for controlled movements. You want your muscles—not momentum—to move you.

HOW TO DO IT

- Lie on your back with your arms lengthened away from your body and your legs bent at a 90-degree angle and lifted off the floor.

- Brace your abs, and lower your knees to your right side, dropping them as close to the floor as possible without lifting your shoulders off the floor.

- Return to the starting position, hold for the recommended time, and repeat on the opposite side.

DO IT RIGHT
- Keep your core centered.
- Move carefully and with control.
- Avoid swinging your legs excessively.

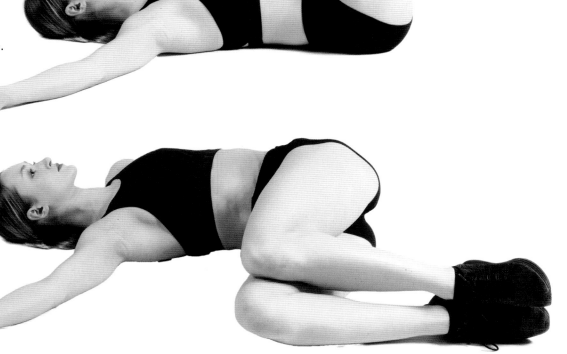

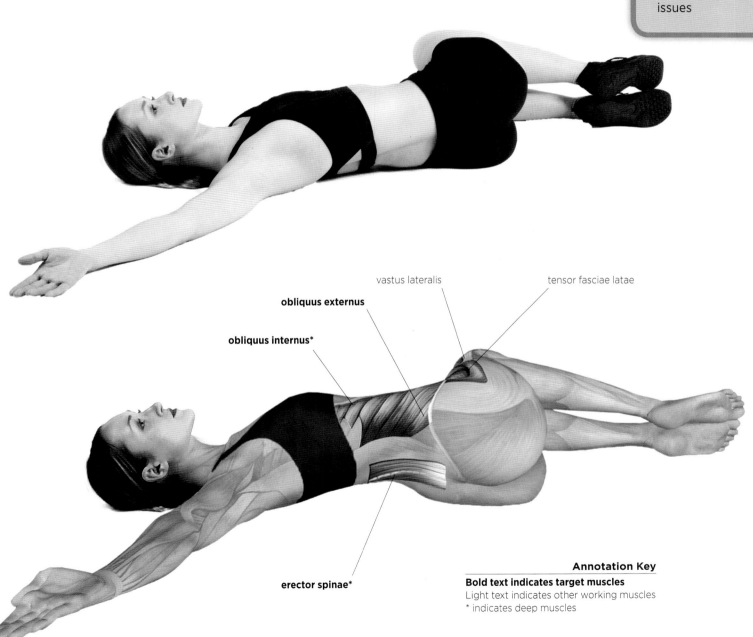

FACT FILE

TARGETS
• Lower back
• Obliques

EQUIPMENT
• None

BENEFITS
• Tones
  abdominals
• Stabilizes core

CAUTIONS
• Lower-back
  issues

vastus lateralis   tensor fasciae latae

obliquus externus

obliquus internus*

erector spinae*

Annotation Key

Bold text indicates target muscles
Light text indicates other working muscles
* indicates deep muscles

Swimmer

The Swimmer engages pretty much every muscle in your body, but it is especially effective at strengthening both your hip extensors and the muscles that support your spine.

HOW TO DO IT

- Lie facedown with your legs hip-width apart. Stretch your arms beside your ears on the floor. Engage your pelvic floor, and draw your navel into your spine.

- Extend through your upper back as you lift your left arm and right leg simultaneously. Lift your head and shoulders off the floor.

- Lower your arm and leg to the starting position, maintaining a stretch in your limbs throughout.

- Extend your opposite arm and leg off the floor, lengthening and lifting your head and shoulders.

- Elongate your limbs as you return to the starting position. Repeat, alternating sides for the recommended repetitions.

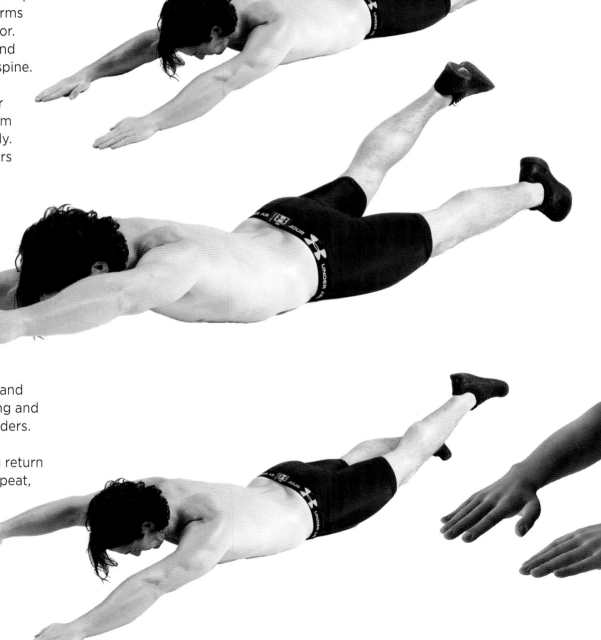

TARGETS
- Hips
- Spine

EQUIPMENT
- None

BENEFITS
- Strengthens hip and spine extensors
- Challenges stabilization of the spine against rotation

CAUTIONS
- Lower-back pain
- Extreme curvature of upper spine
- Curvature of lower spine

MODIFICATION

HARDER: Instead of lifting the opposite leg and arm, lift both arms and legs simultaneously, continuing to draw your navel into your spine. This version of the exercise is known as the Superman.

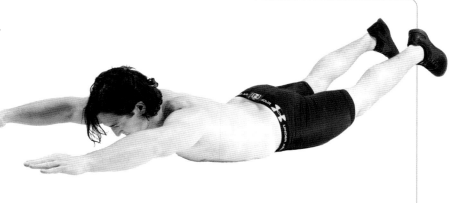

Annotation Key

Bold text indicates target muscles
Light text indicates other working muscles
* indicates deep muscles

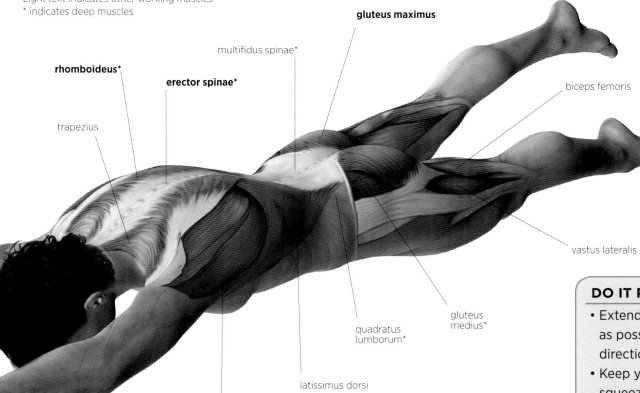

gluteus maximus

multifidus spinae*

rhomboideus*

erector spinae*

trapezius

biceps femoris

vastus lateralis

gluteus medius*

quadratus lumborum*

latissimus dorsi

deltoideus

DO IT RIGHT

- Extend your limbs as long as possible in opposite directions.
- Keep your glutes tightly squeezed and your navel drawn in.
- Keep your neck long and relaxed.
- Avoid allowing your shoulders to lift toward your ears.

Breaststroke

If you tend to slouch, Breaststroke is a great exercise. The arm rotation and lifting action strengthens the scapular muscles around your shoulder blades and your spine.

HOW TO DO IT

- Lie facedown with your legs extended and feet pointed. Bend your arms, holding your hands palms down and raised a few inches off the floor.

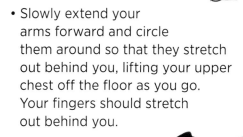

- Slowly extend your arms forward and circle them around so that they stretch out behind you, lifting your upper chest off the floor as you go. Your fingers should stretch out behind you.

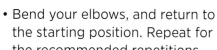

- Bend your elbows, and return to the starting position. Repeat for the recommended repetitions.

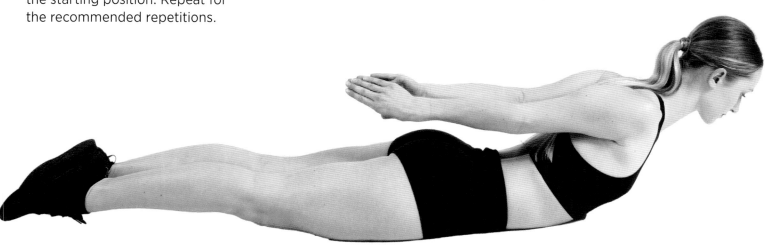

TARGETS
- Shoulders
- Rotator cuffs
- Spine
- Upper back
- Middle back

EQUIPMENT
- None

BENEFITS
- Increases upper-back and spine mobility
- Strengthens back, spine, and core
- Engages shoulders, upper arms, hips, and glutes

CAUTIONS
- Shoulder issues
- Neck issues

DO IT RIGHT

- Keep your arms raised from the floor.
- Keep your wrists engaged.
- Keep your hip and pubic bones on the floor.
- Squeeze your legs together to engage your core.
- Align the back of your head and neck with your spine.
- Avoid lifting your torso higher than the bottom of your ribcage.

Annotation Key

Bold text indicates target muscles
Light text indicates other working muscles
* indicates deep muscles

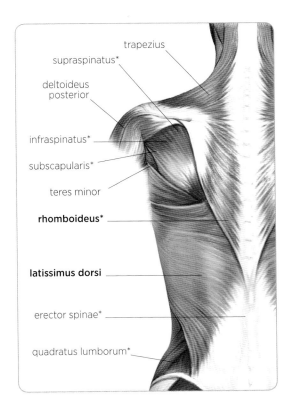

trapezius
supraspinatus*
deltoideus posterior
infraspinatus*
subscapularis*
teres minor
rhomboideus*
latissimus dorsi
erector spinae*
quadratus lumborum*

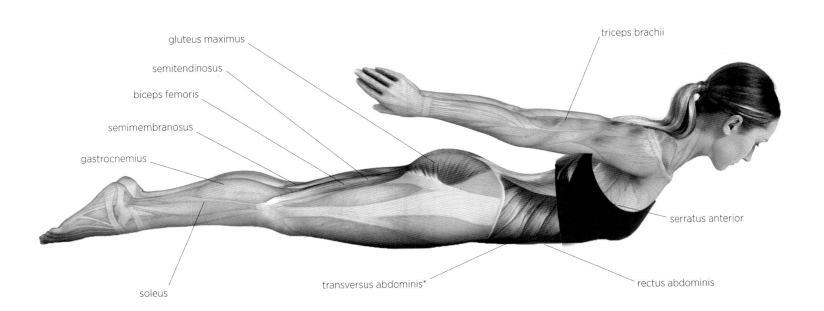

gluteus maximus
semitendinosus
biceps femoris
semimembranosus
gastrocnemius
soleus
transversus abdominis*
triceps brachii
serratus anterior
rectus abdominis

Back Burner

The Back Burner strengthens your lower back as well as all of your abdominal muscles. With regular practice, you'll build a strong core while enhancing your posture.

HOW TO DO IT

- Lie on your stomach with your arms extended in front of you. Your legs should be weighted into the floor with feet pointed. Press your navel to your spine and your shoulders down your back.

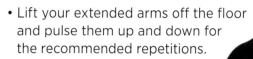

- Lift your extended arms off the floor and pulse them up and down for the recommended repetitions.

- Reposition your arms so that they are at 10:00 and 2:00 on an imaginary clock. Perform a further recommended number of pulses from this position.

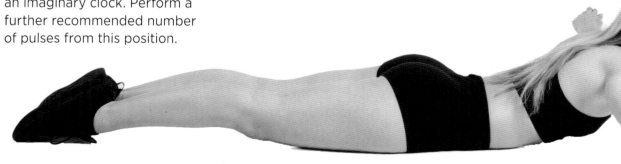

- Keeping your shoulders down, move your arms to the 3:00 and 9:00 position. Perform a further recommended number of pulses from this position.

- Bring both arms behind you, angled slightly with palms inward. With the action originating from your shoulders, perform a further recommended number of pulses from this position.

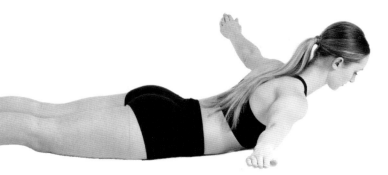

TARGETS
- Lower back
- Abdominals
- Glutes

EQUIPMENT
- None

BENEFITS
- Strengthens lower-back muscles
- Strengthens abdominals
- Improves posture

CAUTIONS
- Lower-back issues
- Other back issues
- Shoulder issues

DO IT RIGHT

- Keep your abdominals strong and your hips stable.
- Look toward the floor to elongate your neck.
- Keep your torso and legs still throughout.
- Move your arms from under your shoulder blades.
- Avoid hunching your shoulders.
- Avoid lifting your feet off the floor.

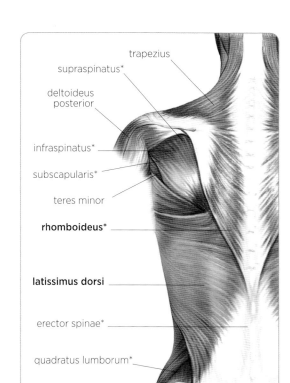

trapezius
supraspinatus*
deltoideus posterior
infraspinatus*
subscapularis*
teres minor
rhomboideus*
latissimus dorsi
erector spinae*
quadratus lumborum*

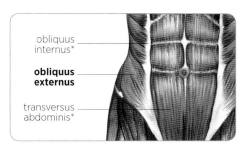

obliquus internus*
obliquus externus
transversus abdominis*

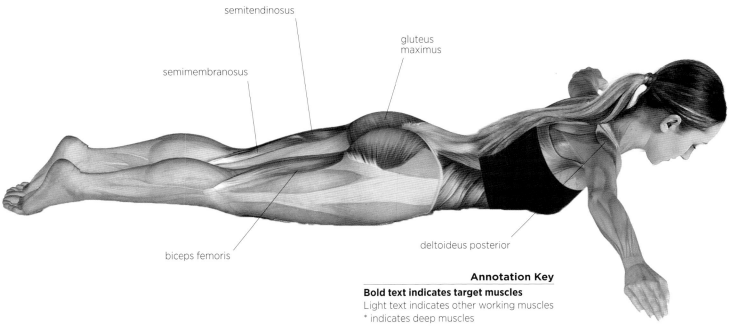

semitendinosus
gluteus maximus
semimembranosus
biceps femoris
deltoideus posterior

Annotation Key
Bold text indicates target muscles
Light text indicates other working muscles
* indicates deep muscles

Alligator Crawl

In the fun but challenging Alligator Crawl, you imitate an alligator stalking its prey. The movements work your chest, shoulders, back, and arms.

HOW TO DO IT

- Begin in a high plank position with your palms on the floor and your back straight.

- Lower into a half push-up position, keeping your back straight.

- Keeping your body low to the floor, bring your right knee to your right elbow while walking your left hand forward.

- Repeat on the opposite side by walking your right hand forward and bringing your left knee to your left elbow.

- Continue moving forward, alternating your hand and knee positions. Perform for the recommended time.

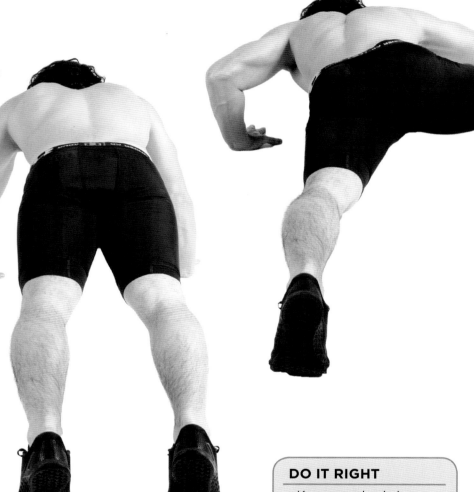

DO IT RIGHT

- Keep your body in a hover position close to the floor, with your elbows at 90 degrees during the entire exercise.
- Avoid allowing your hips to rise.
- Avoid straightening your arms.

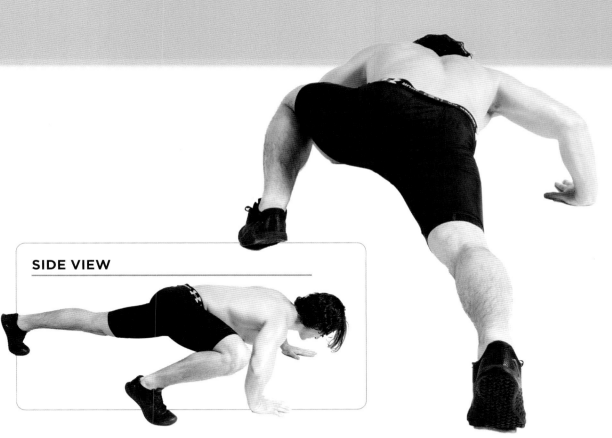

FACT FILE

TARGETS
• Pectorals
• Deltoids
• Back
• Biceps
• Triceps

EQUIPMENT
• None

BENEFITS
• Strengthens upper body
• Increases agility
• Improves coordination

CAUTIONS
• Shoulder issues
• Wrist issues
• Lower-back issues

SIDE VIEW

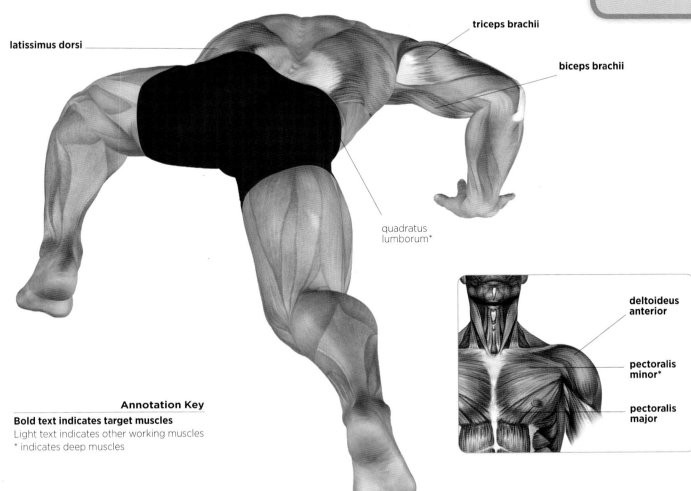

latissimus dorsi

triceps brachii

biceps brachii

quadratus lumborum*

deltoideus anterior

pectoralis minor*

pectoralis major

Annotation Key

Bold text indicates target muscles
Light text indicates other working muscles
* indicates deep muscles

Bear Crawl

A Bear Crawl is an ideal way to build upper-body strength. This is an anaerobic exercise—meaning it is an intense strength promoter.

HOW TO DO IT

- To begin, place both hands and feet on the floor. Walk your left arm and right leg forward, and then your right arm and left leg.

- Now move backward in the same way.

- Keep moving forward and backward in this position, keeping your weight evenly distributed between your arms and legs. Perform for the recommended time.

DO IT RIGHT

- Move steadily and smoothly.
- Avoid placing all of your weight on your arms and shoulders, which can stress your rotator cuffs.
- Avoid touching your knees to the floor.

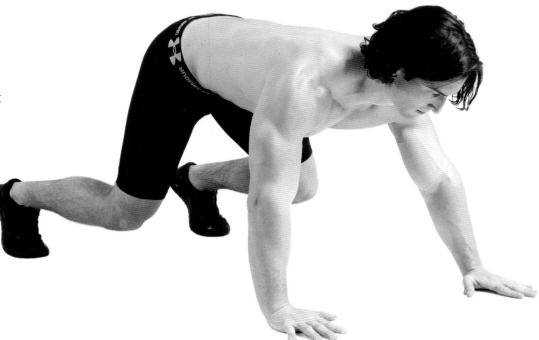

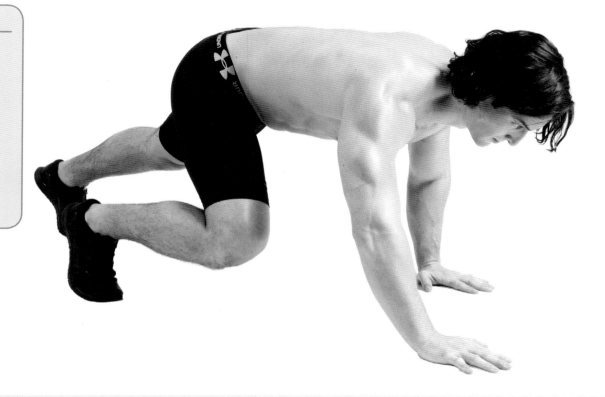

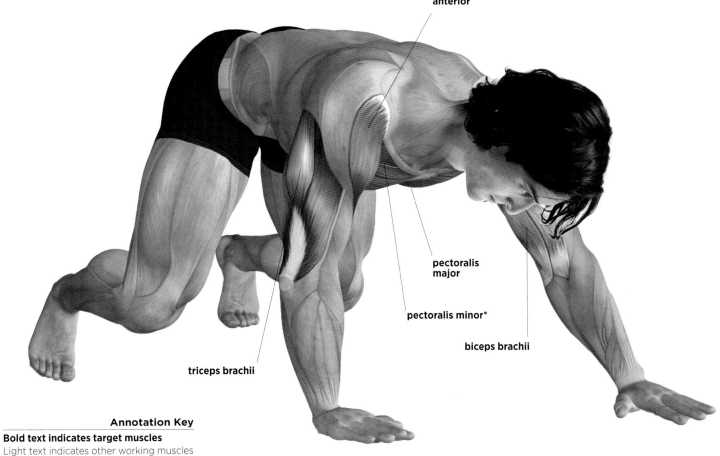

FACT FILE

TARGETS
- Pectorals
- Deltoids
- Biceps
- Triceps

EQUIPMENT
- None

BENEFITS
- Strengthens upper body
- Increases agility
- Improves coordination

CAUTIONS
- Back pain

deltoideus anterior

pectoralis major

pectoralis minor*

biceps brachii

triceps brachii

Annotation Key

Bold text indicates target muscles
Light text indicates other working muscles
* indicates deep muscles

Crab Crawl

Like its opposite, the Bear Crawl (pages 60–61), the Crab Crawl is an anaerobic strength promoter. This exercise will enhance your agility and coordination, too.

HOW TO DO IT

- Begin with both hands and feet on the floor. Lift your body slightly so that your buttocks are just above the floor.

- Walk your right foot forward one step, keeping your hands where they are.

- Now walk your left foot forward. Keeping your hands where they are, continue moving forward, taking several steps by alternating your legs.

- Next, walk alternate legs back. Alternate moving backward and forward for the recommended time.

DO IT RIGHT

- Keep your body weight evenly distributed between your arms and legs.
- Avoid letting your buttocks touch the floor.

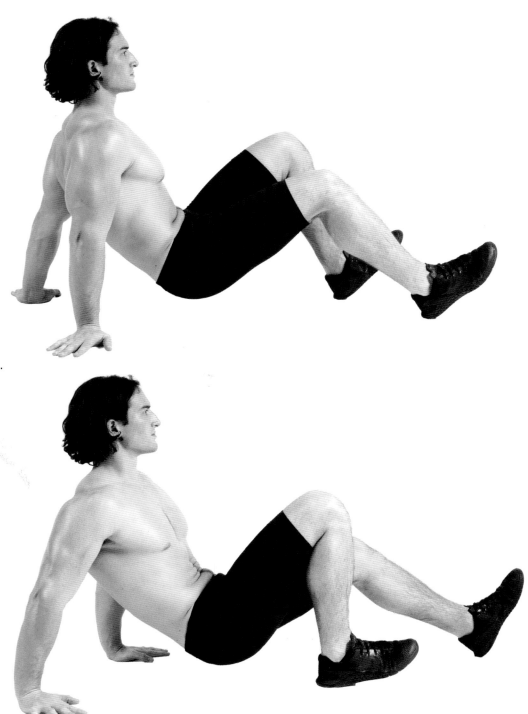

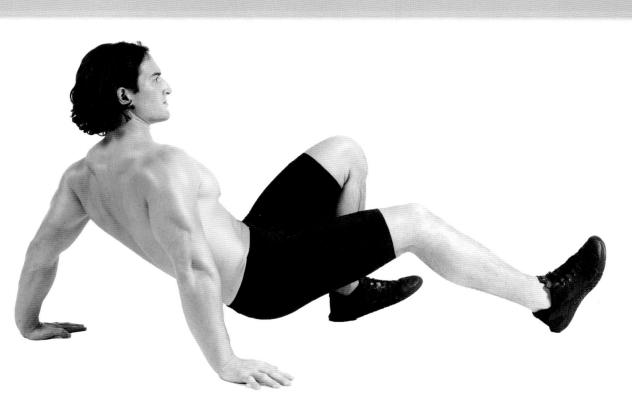

TARGETS
• Deltoids
• Triceps
• Biceps
• Thighs

EQUIPMENT
• None

BENEFITS
• Strengthens upper body
• Increases agility
• Improves coordination

CAUTIONS
• Shoulder issues
• Wrist issues
• Lower-back issues

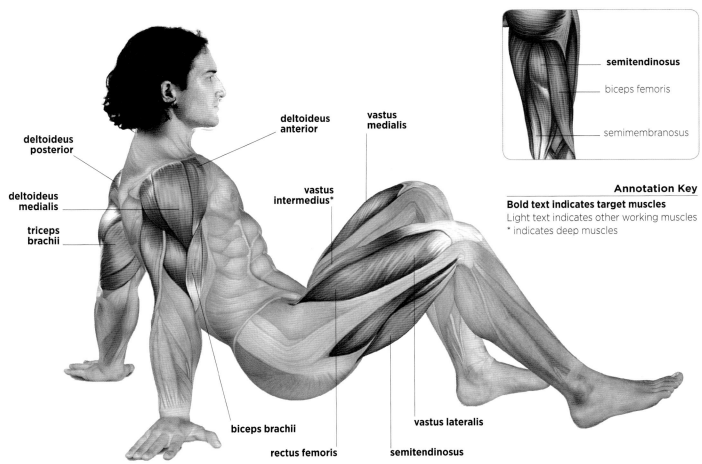

deltoideus posterior

deltoideus medialis

triceps brachii

deltoideus anterior

vastus intermedius*

biceps brachii

rectus femoris

vastus medialis

vastus lateralis

semitendinosus

semitendinosus

biceps femoris

semimembranosus

Annotation Key

Bold text indicates target muscles
Light text indicates other working muscles
* indicates deep muscles

Power Punch

The Power Punch exercise gives your upper body a great workout, strengthening and toning big muscles such as the deltoids.

HOW TO DO IT

- Stand with your feet shoulder-width apart and your left leg placed in front of your right, putting most of your weight on your back leg. Keep your elbows in, and raise both fists.

- Transferring your weight to your front leg, punch straight in front of you with your right fist as you turn your torso in to lend power to the punch.

- Punch for the recommended number of times. Switch arms and legs to repeat on the opposite side. Alternating sides, repeat for the recommended repetitions.

DO IT RIGHT

- Maintain a steady, even, but modest pace.
- Rotate your torso to drive the movement.
- Keep your fists up.
- Avoid excessive speed.
- Avoid sloppy form.

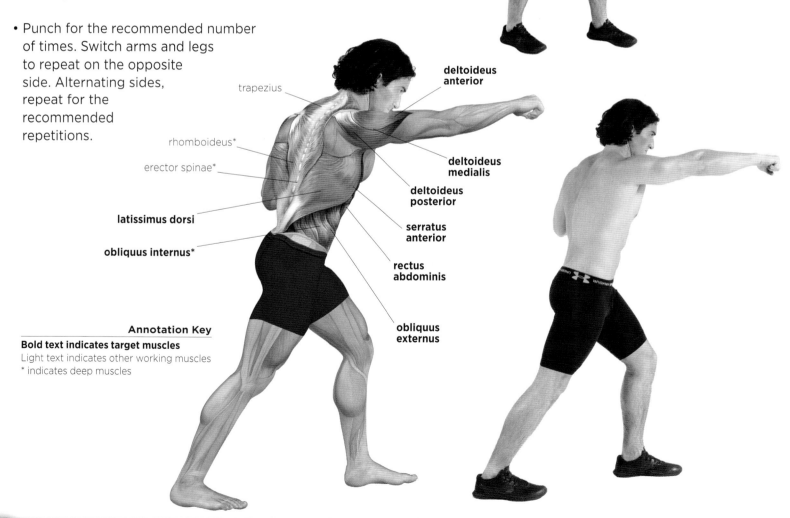

trapezius

deltoideus anterior

rhomboideus*

deltoideus medialis

erector spinae*

deltoideus posterior

latissimus dorsi

serratus anterior

obliquus internus*

rectus abdominis

obliquus externus

Annotation Key

Bold text indicates target muscles
Light text indicates other working muscles
* indicates deep muscles

Uppercut

This exercise builds upper-body strength, especially in your shoulders. It also lightly works your feet and legs, which are engaged in the upward drive.

HOW TO DO IT

- Stand with your feet shoulder-width apart and your left leg placed slightly in front of your right, putting most of your weight on your back leg. Keep your elbows in, and raise both fists.

- Keeping your elbows in and your fists raised, punch upward toward the sky with your right fist as you rotate your torso slightly toward the left and transfer most of your weight to your front foot.

- Punch for the recommended number of times, and then reverse sides, switching your legs and arm.

DO IT RIGHT

- Maintain a steady, even, but modest pace.
- Rotate your torso to drive the movement.
- Keep your fists up.
- Avoid excessive speed.
- Avoid sloppy form.

FACT FILE

TARGETS
- Back
- Shoulders
- Abdomen

EQUIPMENT
- None

BENEFITS
- Strengthens back and shoulder muscles
- Builds endurance

CAUTIONS
- Shoulder issues

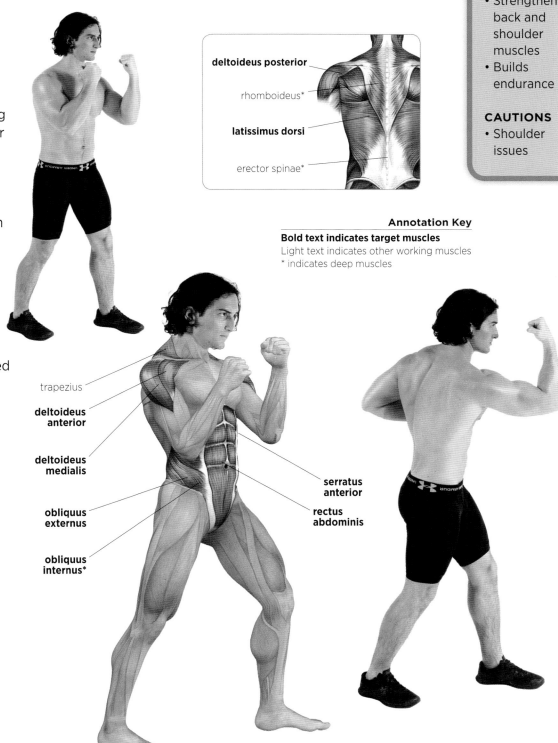

deltoideus posterior

rhomboideus*

latissimus dorsi

erector spinae*

Annotation Key
Bold text indicates target muscles
Light text indicates other working muscles
* indicates deep muscles

trapezius

deltoideus anterior

deltoideus medialis

obliquus externus

obliquus internus*

serratus anterior

rectus abdominis

Triceps Dip

You should really feel the Triceps Dip on the backs of your arms. Holding this body position works most of your other muscles, too.

HOW TO DO IT

- Sit with your knees bent. Your arms should be behind you with your elbows bent and the palms of your hands pressing into the floor, fingers facing forward. Straighten your arms as you lift your hips a few inches off the floor.

- Shift your weight back toward your arms, and, keeping your heels pressed firmly into the floor, lift your toes. Keep your chest open and your gaze diagonally upward.

- Bending your elbows gradually, lower your body down slightly, but still above the floor. Then straighten your arms to raise your body up again, keeping your toes pointed upward the whole time. Repeat the up-and-down action for the recommended repetitions.

- Release back down to your starting position and repeat for the recommended repetitions.

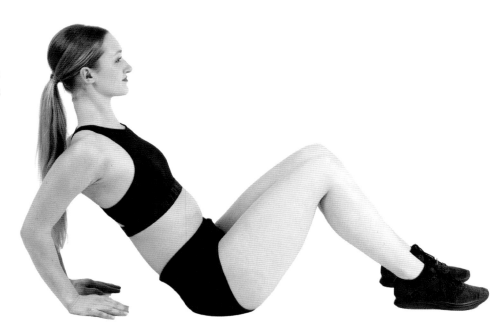

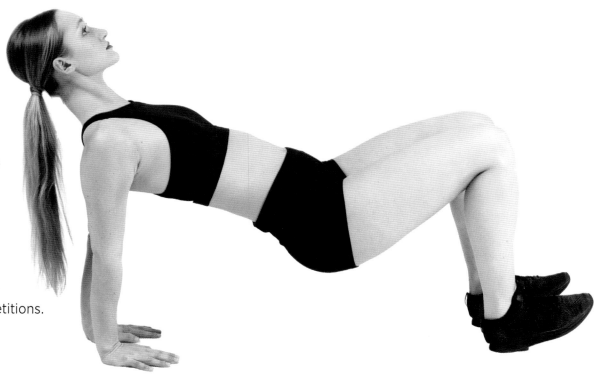

TARGETS
- Triceps
- Deltoids
- Pectorals
- Lats

EQUIPMENT
- None

BENEFITS
- Strengthens triceps, shoulders, chest, back, and core
- Tones abdominals

CAUTIONS
- Back issues
- Shoulder issues

DO IT RIGHT

- Keep your chest lifted and open.
- Hold your shoulders down.
- Avoid arching your back.
- Avoid lifting your shoulders.
- Avoid rushing through the exercise.

Annotation Key

Bold text indicates target muscles
Light text indicates other working muscles
* indicates deep muscles

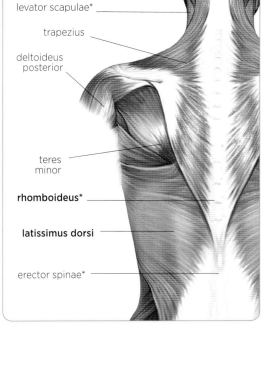

levator scapulae*
trapezius
deltoideus posterior
teres minor
rhomboideus*
latissimus dorsi
erector spinae*

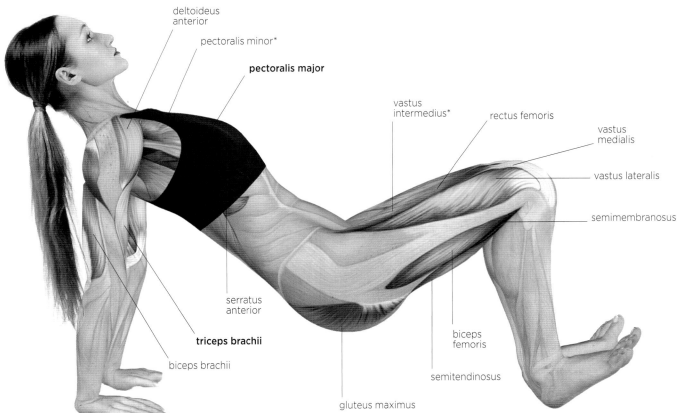

deltoideus anterior
pectoralis minor*
pectoralis major
vastus intermedius*
rectus femoris
vastus medialis
vastus lateralis
semimembranosus
serratus anterior
triceps brachii
biceps brachii
biceps femoris
semitendinosus
gluteus maximus

Push-Up

Also known as a press-up, this well-known basic exercise is popular everywhere, from military-style boot camps to Pilates studios. The reason for this is its effectiveness—it really builds power in your core and upper body.

HOW TO DO IT

- Start on your hands and knees, with your hands slightly wider apart than shoulder-width.

- Push your body up so your arms are straight, with your legs extended backward, to come into a high plank position. Keep your palms on the floor, your feet together, your back straight, and your weight on the balls of your feet. This is your starting position.

- With control, slowly bend your arms, and lower your torso toward the floor. Lower as far as you can go comfortably—which may be until your chest touches the floor.

- Straighten your arms to rise back up to your starting plank position. Repeat for the recommended repetitions.

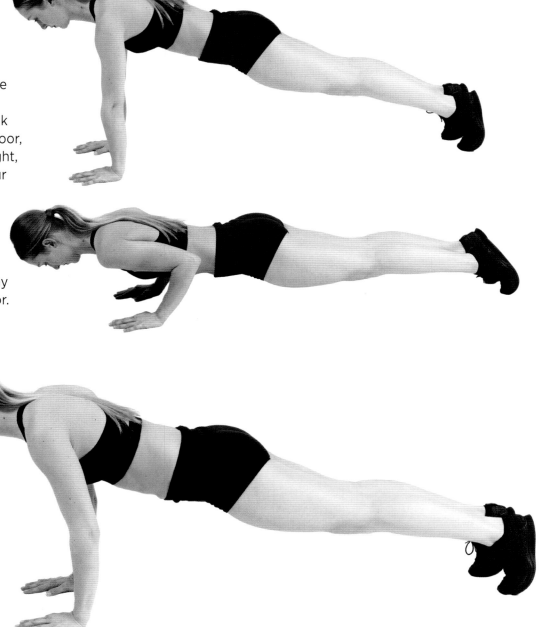

DO IT RIGHT

- Keep your shoulders pressed down your back.
- Imagine a straight line running from the top of your head to your heels.
- Avoid compromising the neutral alignment of your pelvis or spine.

TARGETS
• Core
• Shoulders
• Chest
• Arms

EQUIPMENT
• None

BENEFITS
• Strengthens biceps, shoulders, chest, back, and core
• Tones abdominals

CAUTIONS
• Shoulder issues
• Wrist pain/ issues

MODIFICATION

EASIER: Start on your hands and knees, with your hands slightly wider apart than shoulder-width. Lift your feet toward your buttocks until your calves and thighs form a 90-degree angle.

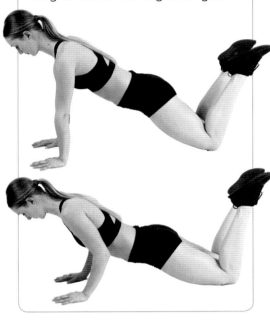

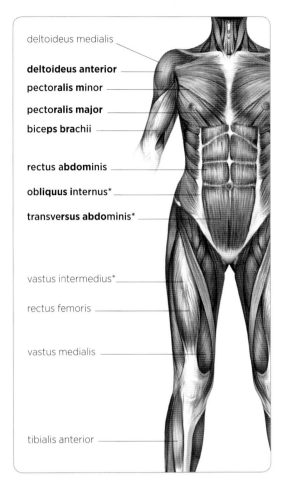

deltoideus medialis

deltoideus anterior

pectoralis minor

pectoralis major

biceps brachii

rectus abdominis

obliquus internus*

transversus abdominis*

vastus intermedius*

rectus femoris

vastus medialis

tibialis anterior

Annotation Key

Bold text indicates target muscles
Light text indicates other working muscles
* indicates deep muscles

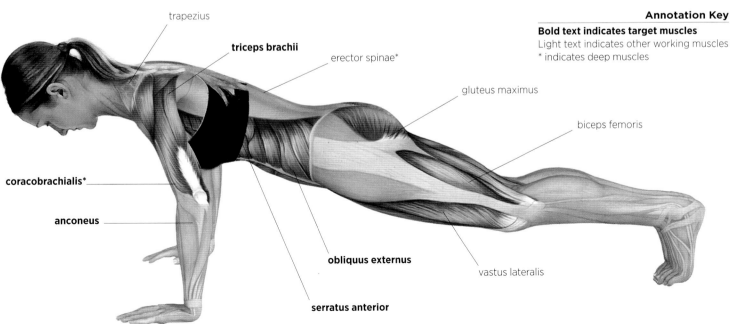

trapezius

triceps brachii

erector spinae*

gluteus maximus

biceps femoris

coracobrachialis*

anconeus

obliquus externus

vastus lateralis

serratus anterior

Wide Push-Up

This Wide Push-Up emphasizes muscles differently than the basic Push-Up (pages 68–69). It especially strengthens the front of your shoulders and chest, with other—mostly upper-body—muscles helping out.

HOW TO DO IT

- Start on your hands and knees, with your hands much wider apart than shoulder-width.

- Push your body up so your arms are straight, with your legs extended backward, to come into a high plank position. Keep your palms on the floor, your feet together, your back straight, and your weight on the balls of your feet. This is your starting position.

- With control, slowly bend your arms, and lower your torso toward the floor. Lower as far as you can go comfortably—which may be until your chest touches the floor.

- Straighten your arms to rise back up to your starting plank position. Repeat for the recommended repetitions.

DO IT RIGHT

- Slightly flare your hands outward so your elbows go toward your hips as you lower yourself to the floor. This helps prevent shoulder tendonitis.
- If you cannot keep your back straight during the entire movement or you feel back pain, start this exercise on both knees and do a modified push-up.
- Avoid pushing your hips into the air.
- Avoid pointing your elbows to the side during the down movement. This places undue stress on the front of your shoulders.

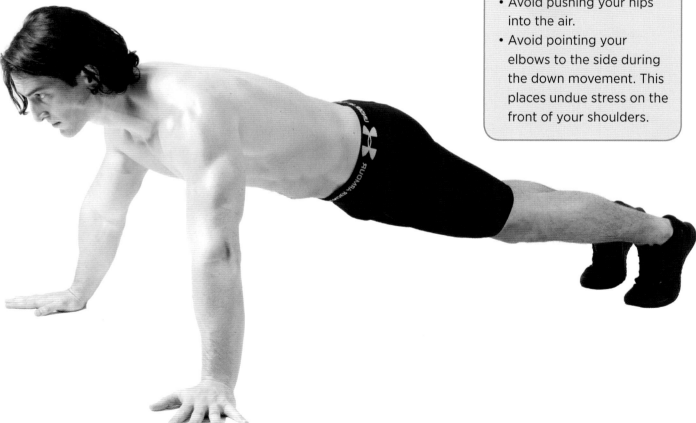

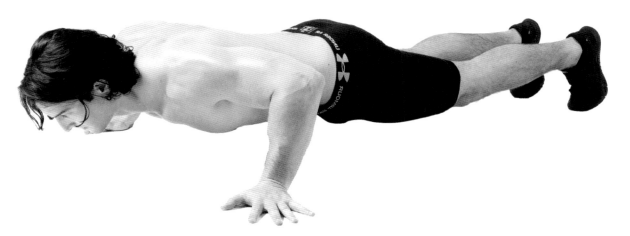

FACT FILE

TARGETS
- Chest
- Shoulders
- Abdominals
- Back
- Upper arms
- Front of thighs

EQUIPMENT
- None

BENEFITS
- Strengthens upper body
- Strengthens shoulders

CAUTIONS
- Shoulder issues
- Wrist issues
- Lower-back pain

Annotation Key

Bold text indicates target muscles
Light text indicates other working muscles
* indicates deep muscles

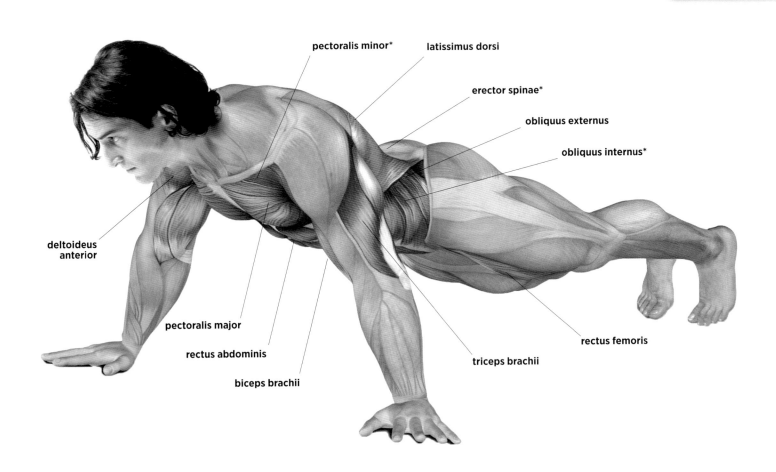

pectoralis minor*

latissimus dorsi

erector spinae*

obliquus externus

obliquus internus*

deltoideus anterior

pectoralis major

rectus abdominis

biceps brachii

triceps brachii

rectus femoris

Triceps Push-Up

Hand position really affects how your muscles are worked—and which ones.
In a basic push-up, your pectorals work especially hard. In this version, placing
your hands closer together builds strength in your shoulders and triceps.

HOW TO DO IT

- Start on your hands and knees, with your hands fairly close together, about shoulder-width apart, closer than for Push-Up (pages 68–69).

- Push your body up so your arms are straight, with your legs extended backward, to come into a high plank position. Keep your palms on the floor, your feet together, your back straight, and your weight on the balls of your feet. Your wrists should be directly beneath your shoulders, with fingers pointing forward. This is your starting position.

- With control, slowly bend your arms, and lower your torso toward the floor. Lower as far as you can go comfortably—which may be until your chest touches the floor.

- Straighten your arms to rise back to the starting position. Repeat for the recommended repetitions.

DO IT RIGHT

- Keep your elbows close to your rib cage as you lower your chest toward the floor.
- Keep your spine straight, forming a long line from your tailbone to the crown of your head.
- Avoid pushing your hips into the air.
- Avoid pointing your elbows to the side during the down movement—this places undue stress on the front of your shoulders.

FACT FILE

TARGETS
- Triceps
- Biceps
- Shoulders
- Core

EQUIPMENT
- None

BENEFITS
- Tones triceps
- Strengthens upper body and abdominals
- Stabilizes core

CAUTIONS
- Shoulder issues
- Wrist issues
- Lower-back pain

MODIFICATION

EASIER: Start on your hands and knees, with your wrists aligned beneath your shoulders. Lift your feet toward your buttocks until your calves and thighs form a 90-degree angle.

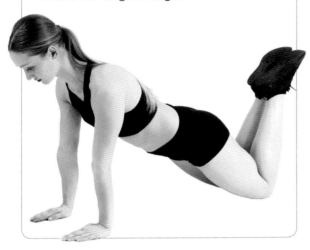

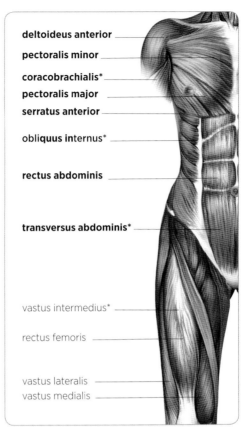

deltoideus anterior
pectoralis minor
coracobrachialis*
pectoralis major
serratus anterior
obliquus internus*
rectus abdominis
transversus abdominis*
vastus intermedius*
rectus femoris
vastus lateralis
vastus medialis

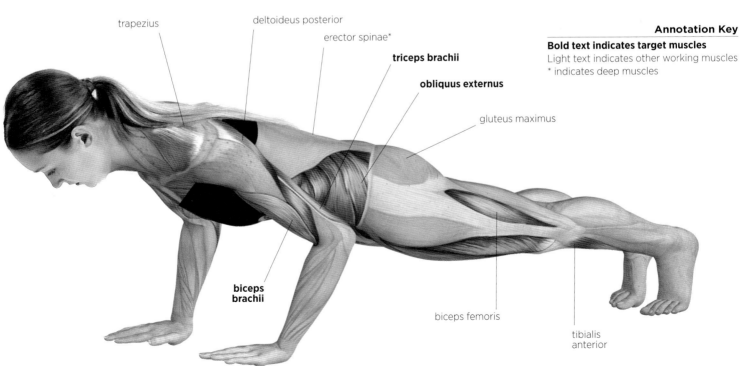

trapezius
deltoideus posterior
erector spinae*
triceps brachii
obliquus externus
gluteus maximus
biceps brachii
biceps femoris
tibialis anterior

Annotation Key

Bold text indicates target muscles
Light text indicates other working muscles
* indicates deep muscles

Diagonal Reach

This standing reach is a simple way of strengthening the torso while adding some defining tone. It eases the twisting actions that enhance general body mobility and works the shoulders, too.

HOW TO DO IT

- Stand with your feet hip-width apart and your arms at your sides.

- Raise both arms upward and to the right to form a diagonal line. Follow your hands with your gaze. Return to your starting position.

- Repeat to your left side. Repeat for the recommended repetitions.

DO IT RIGHT

- Keep your abdominal muscles engaged.
- Keep your hips facing forward.
- Press your shoulders down.
- Avoid twisting your hips.
- Avoid letting your abs bulge outward.
- Avoid hunching your shoulders.
- Avoid tensing your neck as you lift or lower your arms.

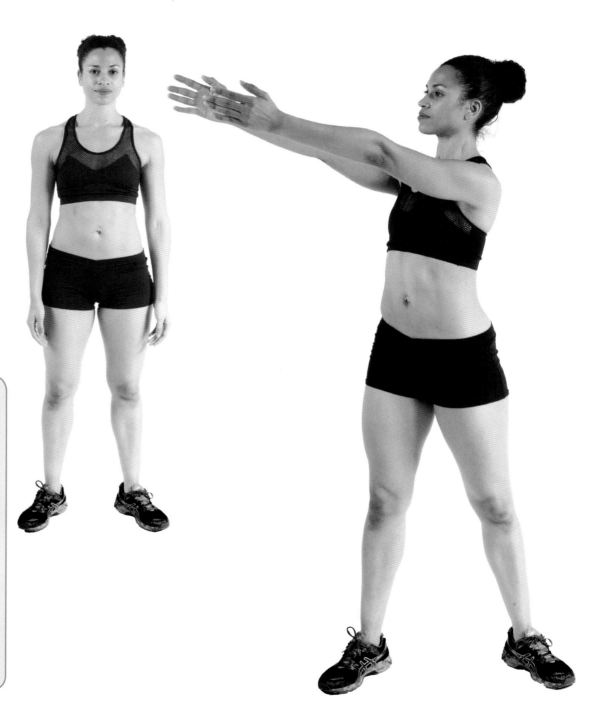

TARGETS
• Front and side abdominals

EQUIPMENT
• None

BENEFITS
• Stretches and strengthens muscles used for twisting
• Boosts performance in tennis and golf

CAUTIONS
• Severe shoulder pain

deltoideus posterior

deltoideus medialis

erector spinae*

deltoideus anterior

deltoideus medialis

deltoideus posterior

pectoralis minor*

pectoralis major

coracobrachialis*

rectus abdominis

obliquus externus

obliquus internus*

iliopsoas*

rectus femoris

MODIFICATION

HARDER: Reach farther, bringing your arms to a steeper diagonal in one direction while raising the opposite foot off the floor.

Annotation Key
Bold text indicates target muscles
Light text indicates other working muscles
* indicates deep muscles

Crunch

A straightforward lift-up Crunch is one of the best ways to tone and fire up your abdominal muscles. Doing this gives the added bonus of stabilizing your spine and so relieving backache.

HOW TO DO IT

- Lie on your back with your legs bent and your hands behind your head, elbows flared outward.

- Contracting your abdominals, raise your head and shoulders off the floor.

- Lower, and repeat for the recommended repetitions.

DO IT RIGHT

- Lead with your abs, as if a string were hoisting you up by your belly button.
- Try to keep your feet planted on the floor.
- Keep your elbows flared outward.
- Avoid using your neck to drive the movement.

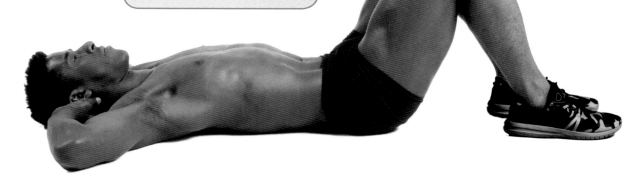

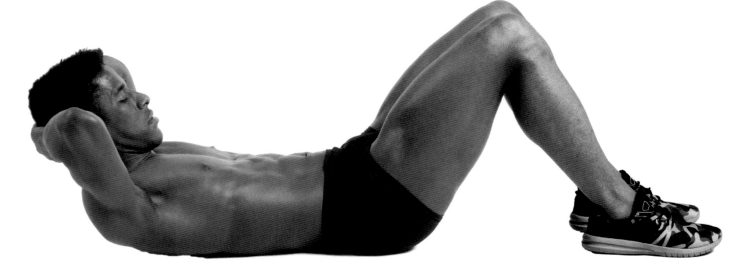

FACT FILE

TARGETS
• Front and side abdominals

EQUIPMENT
• None

BENEFITS
• Strengthens and helps to define abdominals

CAUTIONS
• Lower-back issues
• Neck pain

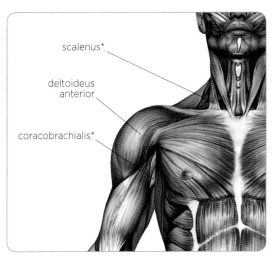

sternocleidomastoideus

splenius*

trapezius

scalenus*

deltoideus anterior

coracobrachialis*

Annotation Key
Bold text indicates target muscles
Light text indicates other working muscles
* indicates deep muscles

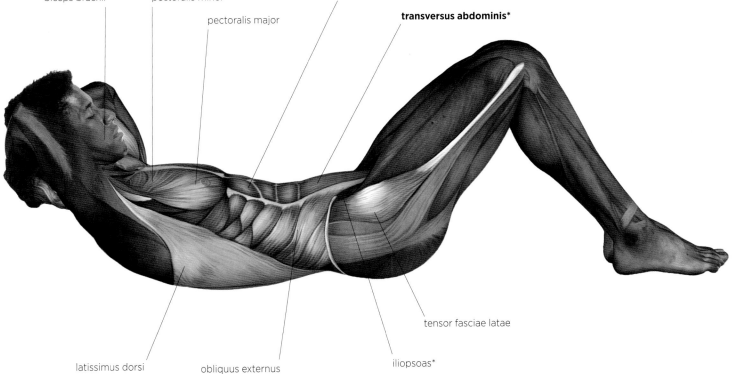

biceps brachii

pectoralis minor*

pectoralis major

rectus abdominis

transversus abdominis*

tensor fasciae latae

latissimus dorsi

obliquus externus

iliopsoas*

Reverse Crunch

The Reverse Crunch challenges your abdominals that little bit more compared to the simpler Crunch that uses an upper-body lift (pages 76–77). It works by using your lower-body weight for resistance.

HOW TO DO IT

- Lie on your back with your arms extended along your sides and your feet off the floor. Your legs should be slightly bent. This is your starting position.

- Tuck your legs in toward your body as you lift your buttocks, followed by your lower back, a few inches off the floor.

- Lower your back and buttocks down in a controlled manner, returning to the starting position. Repeat for the recommended repetitions.

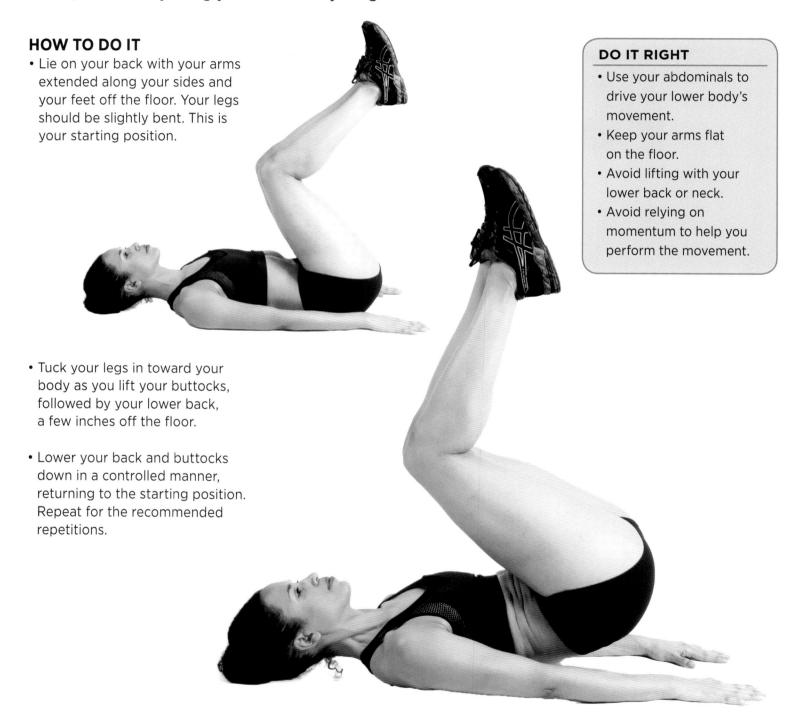

DO IT RIGHT

- Use your abdominals to drive your lower body's movement.
- Keep your arms flat on the floor.
- Avoid lifting with your lower back or neck.
- Avoid relying on momentum to help you perform the movement.

FACT FILE

TARGETS
• Abdominals: upper front and sides

EQUIPMENT
• None

BENEFITS
• Strengthens and tones abdominals

CAUTIONS
• Hip issues
• Lower-back issues

MODIFICATION

HARDER: Once you can do a controlled basic Reverse Crunch without difficulty, try lifting a little farther. Take great care with going too high, though, as the spine and neck could become very vulnerable.

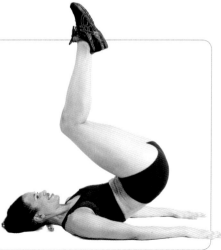

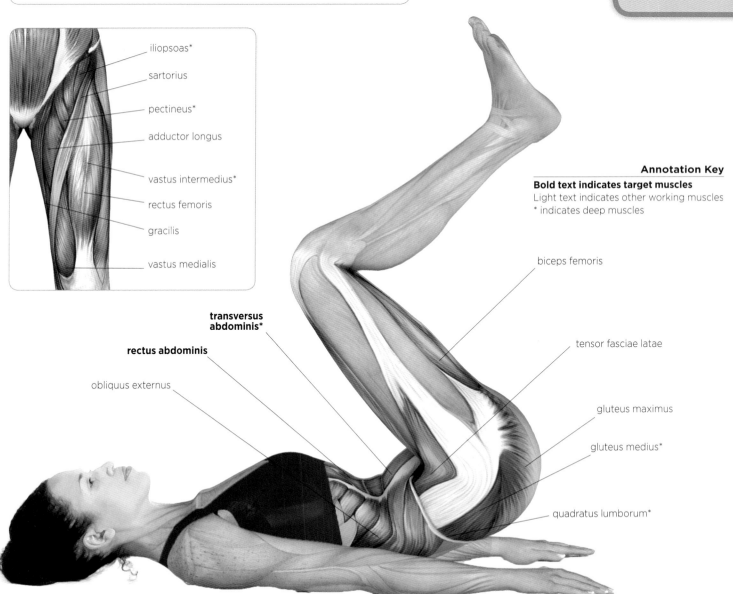

iliopsoas*

sartorius

pectineus*

adductor longus

vastus intermedius*

rectus femoris

gracilis

vastus medialis

Annotation Key

Bold text indicates target muscles
Light text indicates other working muscles
* indicates deep muscles

biceps femoris

transversus abdominis*

rectus abdominis

tensor fasciae latae

obliquus externus

gluteus maximus

gluteus medius*

quadratus lumborum*

Penguin Crunch

The Penguin Crunch really works your obliques and upper abdominals. Because it incorporates lateral movement of the abdominals, it is a great way to prepare for sports that require rotational movement, such as swimming.

HOW TO DO IT

- Lie on your back with your head elevated and your arms straight at your sides and raised off the floor. Bend your knees.

- Holding your torso in a flexed position, lean to the right, and reach your right hand forward. Hold for the recommended time, and then pull it back.

- Repeat on the opposite side. Alternate sides for the recommended repetitions.

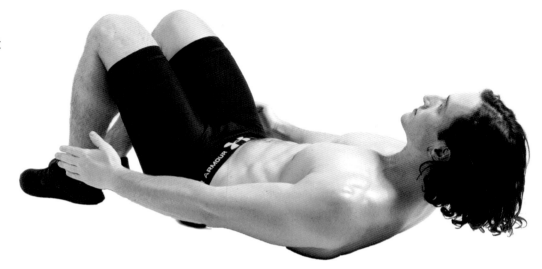

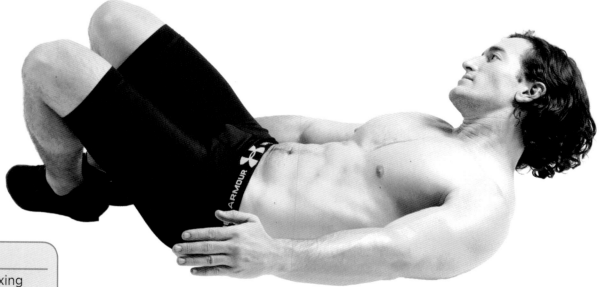

DO IT RIGHT

- Concentrate on flexing your obliques.
- As you reach, pull in using your midsection.
- Avoid overusing your neck and/or back muscles.

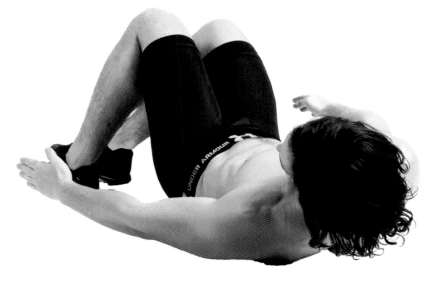

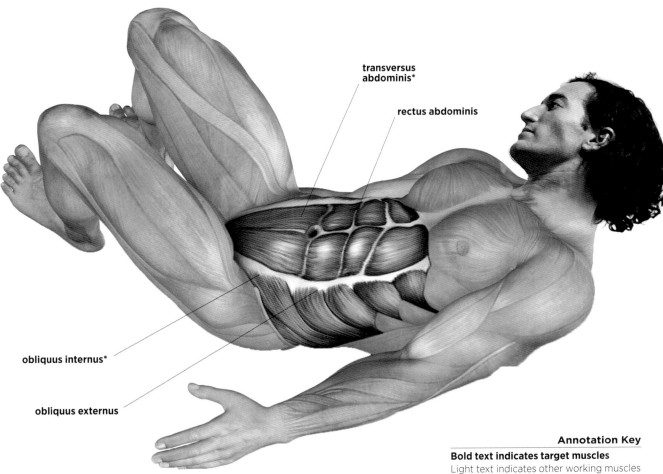

transversus
abdominis*

rectus abdominis

obliquus internus*

obliquus externus

Annotation Key

Bold text indicates target muscles
Light text indicates other working muscles
* indicates deep muscles

Bicycle Crunch

This Crunch variation really consolidates your core's power and resilience. Not only is it a great workout for your abdomen, but you'll feel and see the difference in your thighs, too.

HOW TO DO IT

- Bring your hands behind your head, lifting your legs off the floor so that your thighs are perpendicular to the floor and your shins are parallel to the floor.

- Roll up with your torso, reaching your right elbow to your left knee and extending your right leg in front of you. Imagine pulling your shoulder blades off the floor and twisting from your ribs and obliques.

- Repeat on the opposite side. Alternate sides for the recommended repetitions.

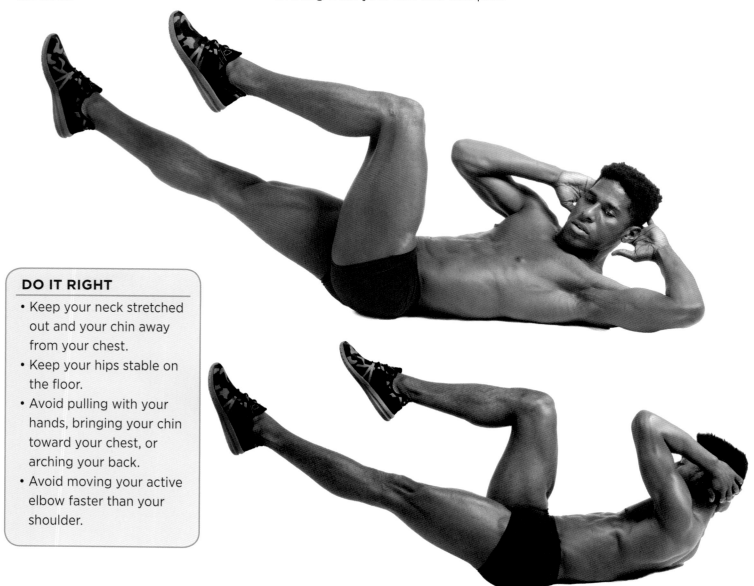

DO IT RIGHT

- Keep your neck stretched out and your chin away from your chest.
- Keep your hips stable on the floor.
- Avoid pulling with your hands, bringing your chin toward your chest, or arching your back.
- Avoid moving your active elbow faster than your shoulder.

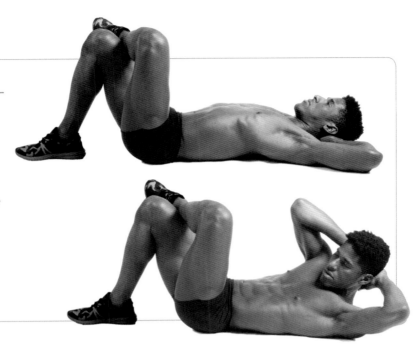

FACT FILE

TARGETS
• Abdominals
• Thighs

EQUIPMENT
• None

BENEFITS
• Stabilizes core
• Strengthens abdominals

CAUTIONS
• Neck issues
• Lower-back pain

MODIFICATION

EASIER: Begin with both feet on the floor. Place the outside of your left foot on top of your right thigh near your knee. Reach your right elbow toward the knee of your raised leg. Repeat for the recommended repetitions. Repeat on the opposite side.

Annotation Key
Bold text indicates target muscles
Light text indicates other working muscles
* indicates deep muscles

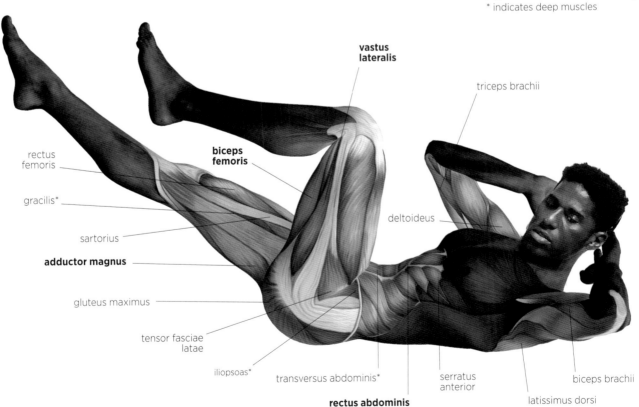

vastus lateralis

triceps brachii

rectus femoris

biceps femoris

gracilis*

deltoideus

sartorius

adductor magnus

gluteus maximus

tensor fasciae latae

iliopsoas*

transversus abdominis*

serratus anterior

biceps brachii

latissimus dorsi

rectus abdominis

Scissors

In Scissors, your legs are like scissor blades and your core like the handles. Keeping your handles stable frees your blades to cut through the air precisely. This is a great way to build up your core.

HOW TO DO IT

- Lie on your back, with your pelvis lengthened along the floor but not jammed right into it. Place your arms along your sides, and fold your knees in toward your chest.

- Curl your head and neck off the floor, extending your legs to the ceiling one at a time. Both buttocks should remain anchored to the floor throughout the exercise.

- Extend both arms toward your left leg so you can grasp it with both hands while the leg remains straight. At the same time, lower your right leg halfway to the floor.

- Start to switch legs by reaching both of them up to the ceiling so that they cross each other in midair.

- Take hold of your extended right leg, and lower your left leg halfway to the floor.

- Alternate legs for the recommended repetitions.

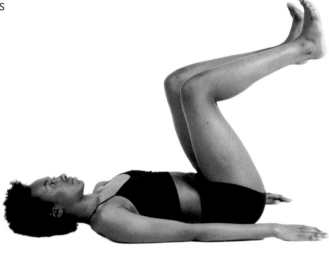

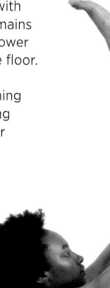

> ### DO IT RIGHT
> - Keep your core muscles engaged and active.
> - Stabilize your shoulders by pressing your shoulder blades down your back.
> - Keep your buttocks firmly planted into the floor.
> - Keep your legs lengthened.
> - Avoid pulling your shoulders forward while grasping your leg.
> - Avoid bending your knees.
> - Avoid using your arms to pull your leg toward you, rather than using your abdominal muscles to lift your upper body toward your leg.

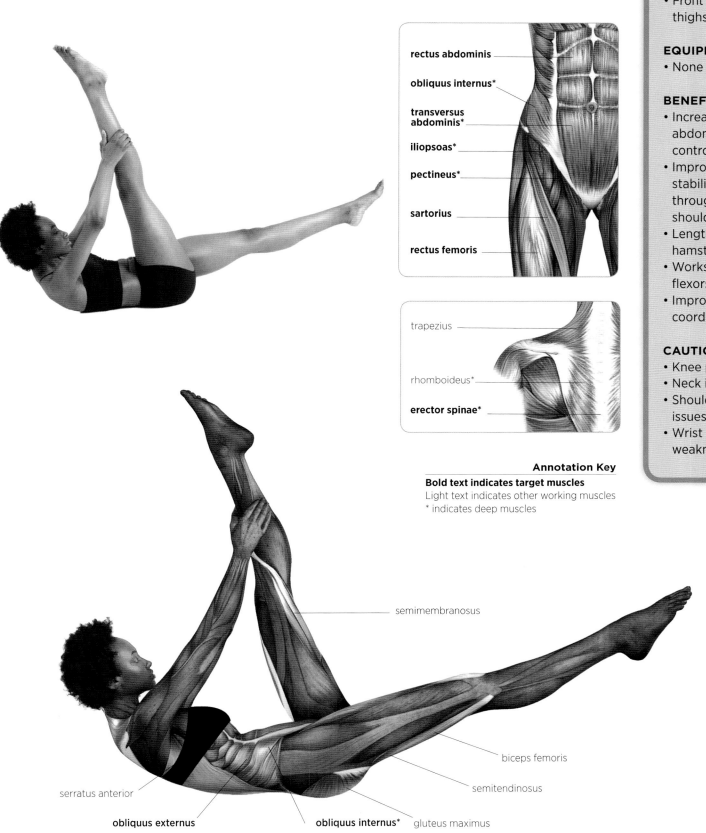

FACT FILE

TARGETS
• Abdominals
• Back
• Front of thighs

EQUIPMENT
• None

BENEFITS
• Increases abdominal control
• Improves stabilization through shoulder area
• Lengthens hamstrings
• Works hip flexors
• Improves coordination

CAUTIONS
• Knee pain
• Neck issues
• Shoulder issues
• Wrist weakness

rectus abdominis

obliquus internus*

transversus abdominis*

iliopsoas*

pectineus*

sartorius

rectus femoris

trapezius

rhomboideus*

erector spinae*

Annotation Key

Bold text indicates target muscles
Light text indicates other working muscles
* indicates deep muscles

semimembranosus

biceps femoris

semitendinosus

serratus anterior

obliquus externus

obliquus internus* gluteus maximus

Leg Levelers

Leg Levelers is a straightforward way to bring a wide range of muscles into play, from your shoulders to your thighs. This is an excellent routine for your core.

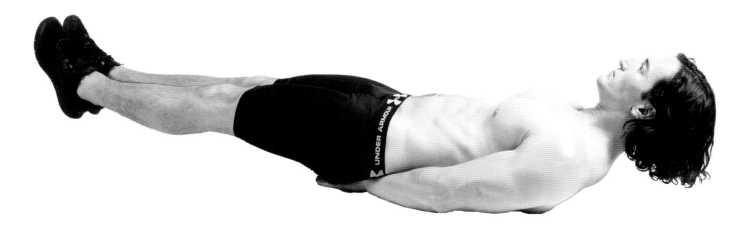

HOW TO DO IT

- Lie on your back with legs straight and your head raised off the floor. Place both hands under your buttocks to straighten the lumbar spine, and then lift both legs so that your feet are about 6 inches off the ground. Your knees should be bent slightly.

- Keeping your legs together, raise them until they form a 45-degree angle with the ground. Hold for the recommended time.

- Lower your legs back to 6 inches and hold for the recommended time. Repeat this up-and-hold and then down-and-hold sequence for the recommended repetitions.

DO IT RIGHT

- Keep your hands under your buttocks to protect your lower back from excess extension.
- Avoid resting your head on the ground.

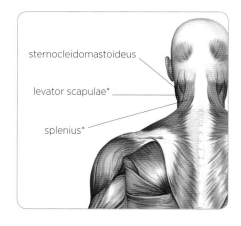

sternocleidomastoideus

levator scapulae*

splenius*

Annotation Key

Bold text indicates target muscles
Light text indicates other working muscles
* indicates deep muscles

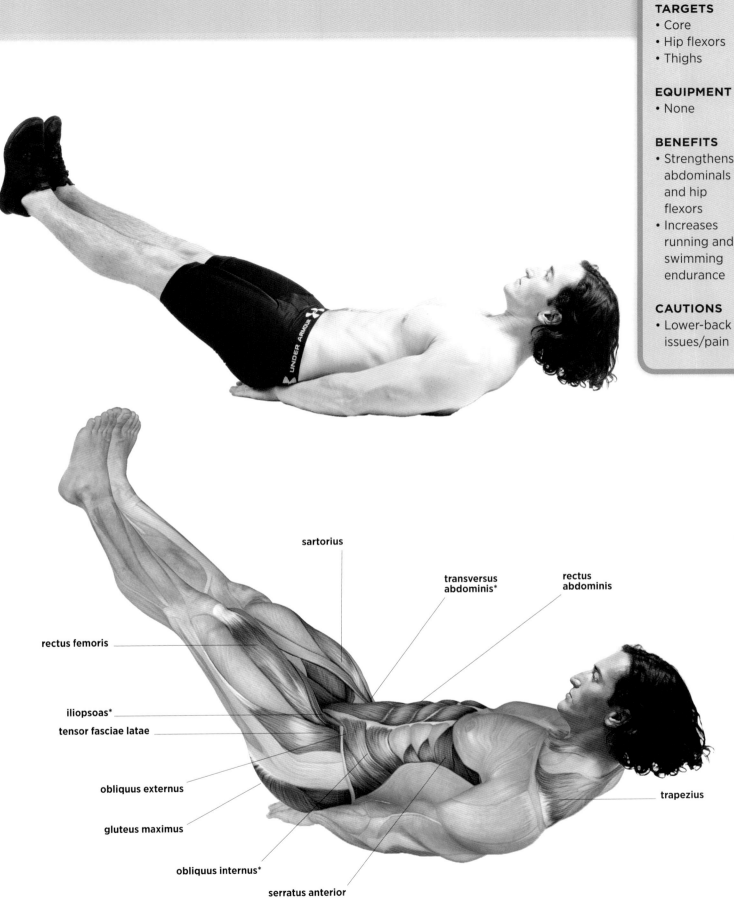

TARGETS
• Core
• Hip flexors
• Thighs

EQUIPMENT
• None

BENEFITS
• Strengthens abdominals and hip flexors
• Increases running and swimming endurance

CAUTIONS
• Lower-back issues/pain

sartorius

transversus abdominis*

rectus abdominis

rectus femoris

iliopsoas*

tensor fasciae latae

obliquus externus

gluteus maximus

trapezius

obliquus internus*

serratus anterior

Body Saw

As the name suggests, this exercise is all about moving your body back and forth like a saw. The more your body stays in a straight line, the more power you build in your abdominals and lower back.

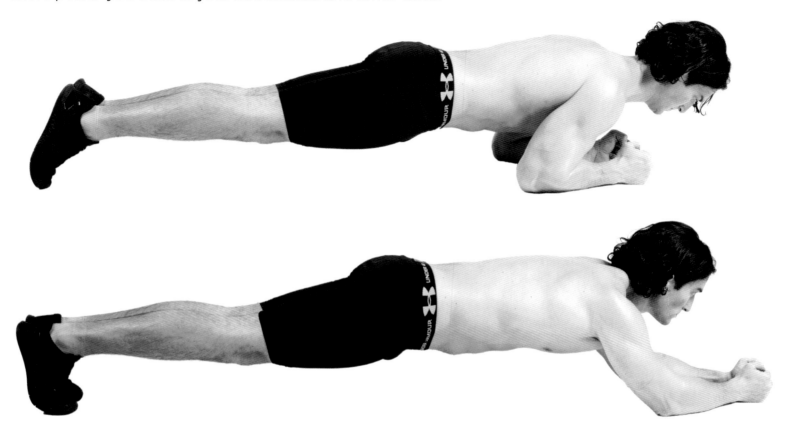

HOW TO DO IT

- Begin facedown, balancing on your toes and your forearms.

- Shift your body backward, pressing into the floor with your forearms as your feet change position.

- Shift your body forward to return to your starting position. Repeat the back-and forth sequence for the recommended repetitions.

DO IT RIGHT

- Keep your body in one straight line.
- Gaze toward the floor.
- Avoid arching your back, or curving it forward.

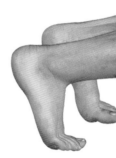

TARGETS
• Abdominals
• Back
• ITB (Iliotibial Band)

EQUIPMENT
• None

BENEFITS
• Stabilizes core
• Strengthens abdominals

CAUTIONS
• Shoulder issues
• Lower-back issues

latissimus dorsi

erector spinae*

quadratus lumborum

piriformis

gluteus maximus

tractus iliotibialis

semitendinosus

biceps femoris

semimembranosus

Annotation Key

Bold text indicates target muscles
Light text indicates other working muscles
* indicates deep muscles

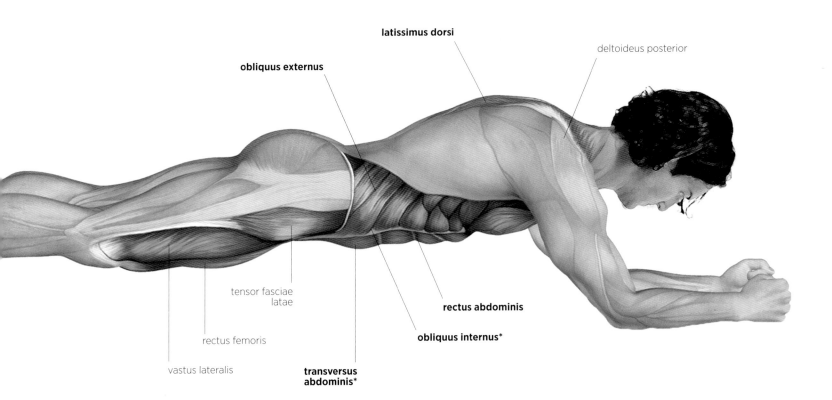

latissimus dorsi

deltoideus posterior

obliquus externus

tensor fasciae latae

rectus femoris

vastus lateralis

transversus abdominis*

obliquus internus*

rectus abdominis

Thigh Rock-Back

The Thigh Rock-Back drives through the thighs and core. It builds particular strength in the quads center-front of your thighs and the central abdominals. Keeping your body straight teaches stability and focus.

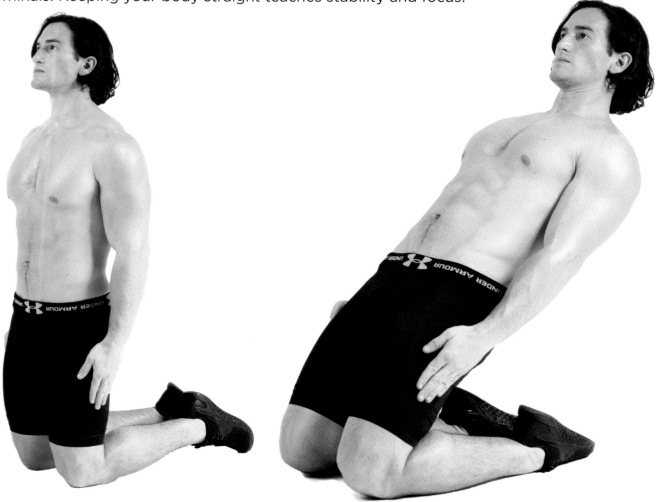

HOW TO DO IT

- Kneel on the floor with your back straight and your knees slightly apart, your arms by your sides. Pull in your abdominals, drawing your navel toward your spine.

- Lean back, keeping your hips open and aligned with your shoulders, stretching the front of your thighs.

- Once you have leaned back as far as you can, squeeze your glutes and slowly bring your body back to the upright position. Repeat for the recommended repetitions.

DO IT RIGHT

- Keep a straight line between your torso and your knees.
- Ensure your abdominals are controlling the movement.
- Keep your glutes tight.
- Avoid rocking so far back that you cannot return to the starting position.
- Avoid bending in your hips.

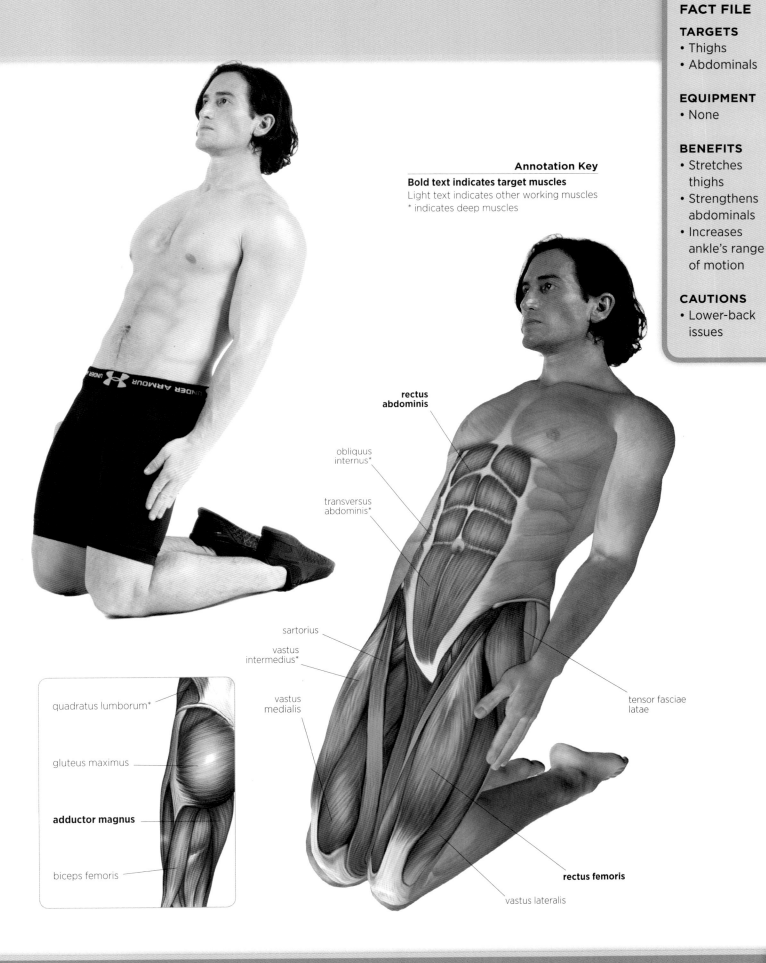

FACT FILE

TARGETS
- Thighs
- Abdominals

EQUIPMENT
- None

BENEFITS
- Stretches thighs
- Strengthens abdominals
- Increases ankle's range of motion

CAUTIONS
- Lower-back issues

Annotation Key

Bold text indicates target muscles
Light text indicates other working muscles
* indicates deep muscles

rectus abdominis

obliquus internus*

transversus abdominis*

sartorius

vastus intermedius*

quadratus lumborum*

gluteus maximus

adductor magnus

biceps femoris

vastus medialis

tensor fasciae latae

rectus femoris

vastus lateralis

Single-Leg V-Up

Regular practice of Single-Leg V-Up will make your abdominal muscles stronger, which it turn makes the exercise's upward motion smoother and easier. This is a great way to prepare your core muscles for all kinds of workouts.

HOW TO DO IT

- Lie on your back, with your arms extended over your head, hovering just above the floor behind you, palms up. Bend your knees and press them together. Anchor your feet into the floor.

- Slowly and with control, extend your right leg, straightening it from your hip and out through your foot.

- Initiating the movement from your lower abdomen, raise your torso to form a 45-degree angle with the floor as you bring your arms up and over your head to reach forward.

- With control, curl your spine down to the floor as you bring your arms up overhead and behind you again, keeping your knees pressed together.

- Repeat for the recommended repetitions. Repeat on the opposite side.

DO IT RIGHT

- Keep your neck stretched out.
- Maintain a tight core and a level pelvis.
- When balancing, your arms should be parallel to your extended leg.
- Avoid arching your back or rolling your shoulders forward.
- Avoid relying on momentum to propel you up or down.
- Avoid allowing your stomach to bulge outward.

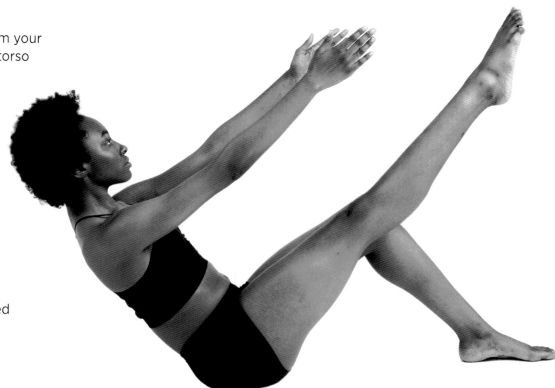

TARGETS
• Abdominals
• Thighs
• Hip flexors

EQUIPMENT
• None

BENEFITS
• Strengthens
  and tones
  abdominals
• Mobilizes
  spine

CAUTIONS
• Herniated disc
• Lower-back
  issues
• Osteoporosis

MODIFICATION

HARDER: For a really tough workout for your core, try raising both legs at the same time. Proceed carefully so that this doesn't cause any back issues.

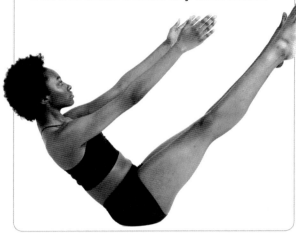

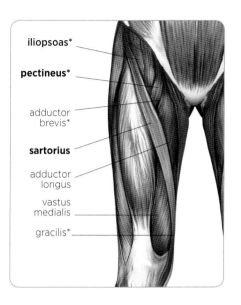

iliopsoas*
pectineus*
adductor brevis*
sartorius
adductor longus
vastus medialis
gracilis*

Annotation Key

Bold text indicates target muscles
Light text indicates other working muscles
* indicates deep muscles

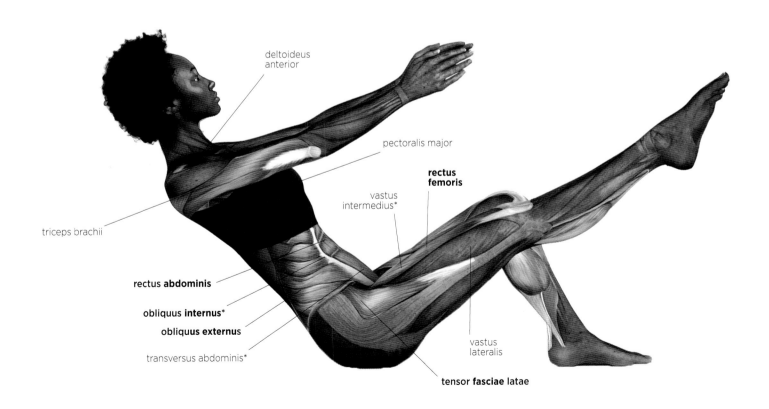

deltoideus anterior

pectoralis major

rectus femoris

vastus intermedius*

triceps brachii

rectus **abdominis**

obliquus **internus***

obliquus **externus**

transversus abdominis*

vastus lateralis

tensor **fasciae** latae

Fire-Hydrant In-Out

Fire Hydrant In-Out is a hardworking core-stabilizing exercise, as well as a great abdominal strengthener. It targets your glutes, with assistance from your abdominal muscles. It also powers up your inner thighs and hamstrings.

HOW TO DO IT

- Begin on your hands and knees, with your palms on the floor and spaced shoulder-width apart. Your spine should be in a neutral position: straight but relaxed.

- Keeping your right leg bent at a 90-degree angle, raise it laterally (to the side).

- Now straighten your right leg until it is fully extended behind you.

- Bend your right knee and bring your leg back into its 90-degree position, and then lower it to meet your left leg. Repeat for the recommended repetitions. Repeat on the opposite side.

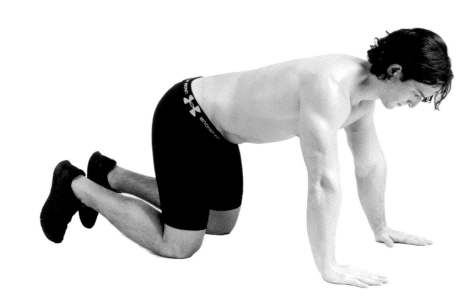

DO IT RIGHT

- Press your hands into the floor to keep your shoulders from sinking.
- Squeeze your glutes with your leg fully extended.
- Avoid lifting your hip as you lift your bent leg to the side.
- Avoid rushing; make sure you feel each part of the repetition.

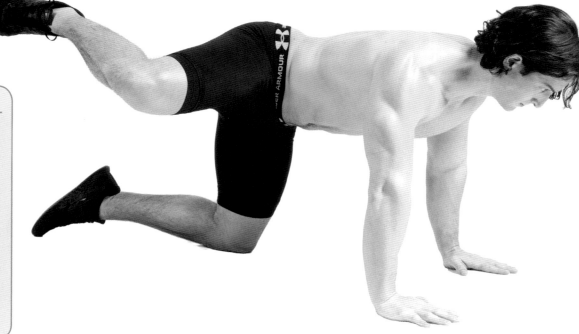

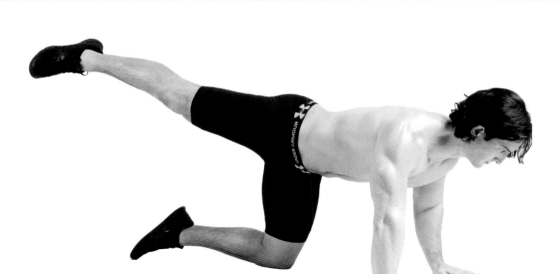

FACT FILE

TARGETS
• Core
• Abdominals
• Glutes

EQUIPMENT
• None

BENEFITS
• Stabilizes pelvis
• Strengthens glutes

CAUTIONS
• Wrist pain
• Knee issues

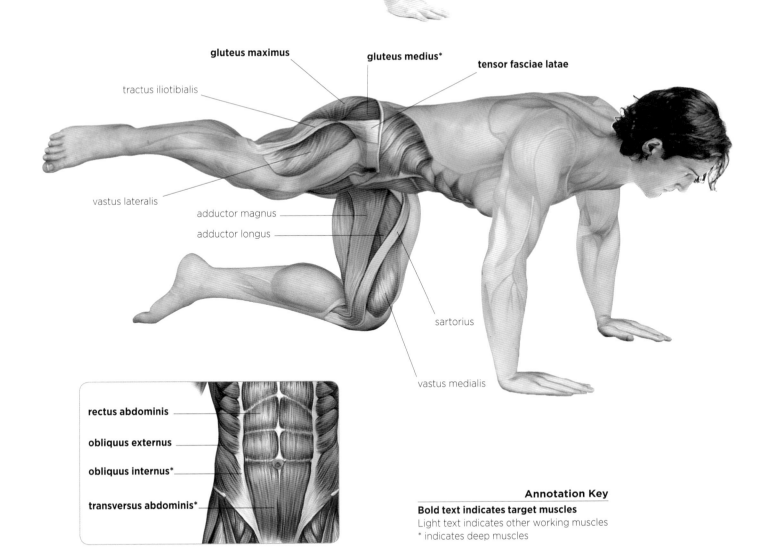

gluteus maximus

gluteus medius*

tensor fasciae latae

tractus iliotibialis

vastus lateralis

adductor magnus

adductor longus

sartorius

vastus medialis

rectus abdominis

obliquus externus

obliquus internus*

transversus abdominis*

Annotation Key

Bold text indicates target muscles
Light text indicates other working muscles
* indicates deep muscles

Bridge

Bridge pose is a favorite of all kinds of exercise programs—because it opens up and strengthens so effectively. This is a great exercise for the upper body, while also putting your legs through their paces.

HOW TO DO IT

- Lie on your back, with your pelvis and spine aligned but feeling natural and not pressed flat to the floor. Your legs should be bent with feet on the floor, and your knees aligned with your hips and feet. Your feet shouldn't be too far away from your buttocks, and firmly planted on the floor. Extend your arms along your sides, palms downward, and press your shoulders down your back to stabilize your shoulder blades.

- Curl your hips upward from the floor, creating a stable bridge position from your shoulders to your parallel knees. Hold this position for the recommended time.

- Curl your spine back toward the floor, starting with your cervical vertebrae and rolling down your thoracic vertebrae and farther down to your lumbar vertebrae.

- Repeat for the recommended repetitions.

DO IT RIGHT

- Maintain strongly engaged lower abdominals.
- Keep your inner thighs active to maintain parallel legs.
- Keep your hips level.
- Avoid jamming your chin into your chest.
- Avoid letting your rib cage "pop" forward and upward.
- Avoid arching, and pushing into, your lower back while in the bridge.

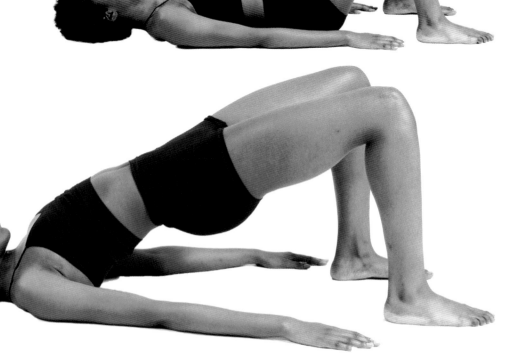

MODIFICATION

HARDER: Place a small medicine ball between your knees, squeezing it as you perform the Bridge. This increases lower-body resistance and enhances your awareness of the physical interconnections involved in the movement.

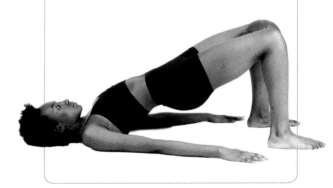

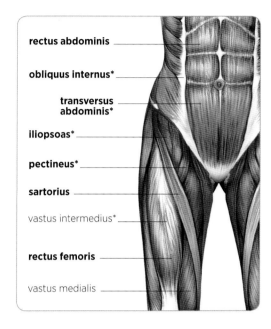

rectus abdominis

obliquus internus*

transversus abdominis*

iliopsoas*

pectineus*

sartorius

vastus intermedius*

rectus femoris

vastus medialis

Annotation Key
Bold text indicates target muscles
Light text indicates other working muscles
* indicates deep muscles

FACT FILE
TARGETS
- Abdominals
- Hip flexors
- Chest
- Thighs
- Glutes
- Back
- Neck

EQUIPMENT
- None/small medicine ball for modification

BENEFITS
- Increases shoulder stability
- Strengthens powerhouse muscles
- Opens chest and pelvic area
- Works legs

CAUTIONS
- Back injury
- Neck issues
- Shoulder issues

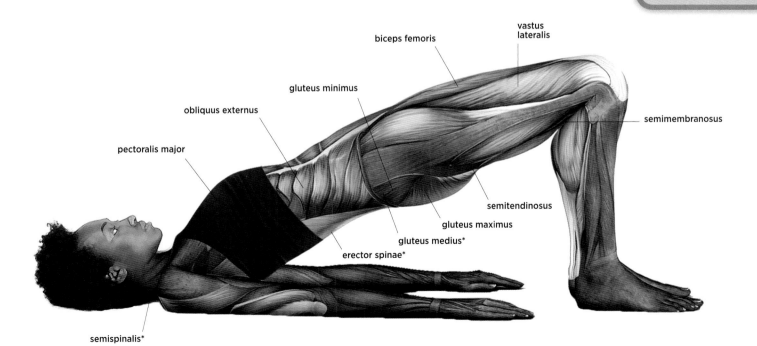

vastus lateralis

biceps femoris

gluteus minimus

obliquus externus

pectoralis major

semimembranosus

semitendinosus

gluteus maximus

gluteus medius*

erector spinae*

semispinalis*

Extension Heel Beats

This exercise is especially effective for your glutes and inner-thigh adductors, but it also works much of your core and upper legs. As with all exercises performed in a prone position, keep your abdominals fully engaged.

HOW TO DO IT

- Lie on your stomach, resting your forehead on the back of your stacked hands. Slightly rotate your legs from the hip joints outward and press the inner sides of your legs and your heels together.

- Fully engage your glutes. Slightly lift your extended legs up from the floor.

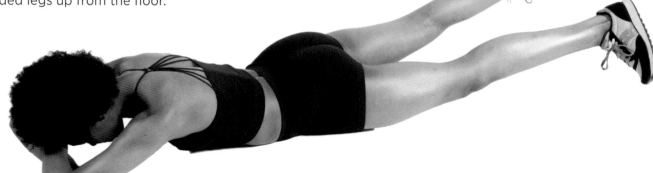

- With your feet fairly pointed, lightly beat your heels together for the recommended number of times.

- Flex your feet (that is, not pointed), and move your legs to hip-distance apart. Hold for the recommended time.

- Now stretch out your feet again and press your legs and heels together to begin another set of heel beats. Repeat for the recommended repetitions.

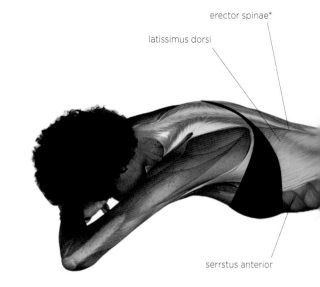

erector spinae*

latissimus dorsi

serrstus anterior

TARGETS
- Adductors
- Glutes

EQUIPMENT
- None

BENEFITS
- Strengthens and stretches leg muscles
- Increases hip-joint mobility
- Facilitates proper alignment

CAUTIONS
- Lower-back issues

DO IT RIGHT
- Stabilize your shoulder girdle.
- Keep your neck extended.
- Keep your hips firmly pressed into the floor as you press your navel toward your spine.
- Stretch your legs fully without locking your knees.
- Avoid lifting your legs so high that you feel tension in your lower back.
- Avoid altering the slightly turned-out position of your legs.

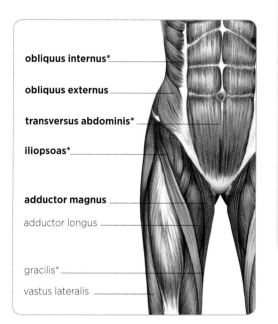

obliquus internus*

obliquus externus

transversus abdominis*

iliopsoas*

adductor magnus

adductor longus

gracilis*

vastus lateralis

Annotation Key
Bold text indicates target muscles
Light text indicates other working muscles
* indicates deep muscles

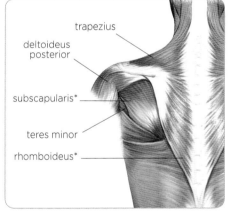

trapezius

deltoideus posterior

subscapularis*

teres minor

rhomboideus*

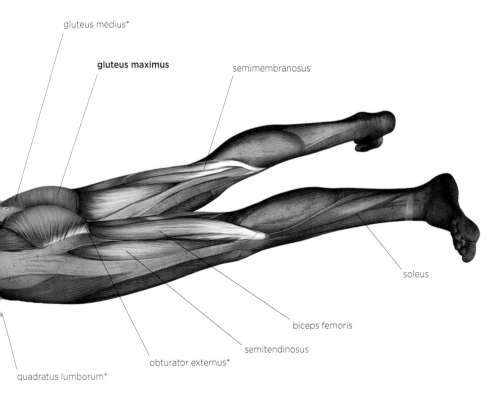

gluteus medius*

gluteus maximus

semimembranosus

soleus

biceps femoris

semitendinosus

obturator externus*

quadratus lumborum*

Lunge

The Lunge strengthens your hamstrings, thighs, and glutes, but also does so much more. This exercise is a dynamic stretch for your hip flexors and also stabilizes your hips, knees, and ankles.

HOW TO DO IT

- Stand with your feet a little way apart, up to hip-width, and your arms at the sides of your body or with your hands on your hips.

- Step your left leg forward. Keep a slight bend in your left knee.

- Bend both knees as you move into a lunge position. Lower your body, flexing your left knee and hip until your right leg is in light contact with the floor.

- Return to the starting position by straightening out your right leg and bringing your left leg back to meet your right.

- Switch legs and repeat on the opposite side. Alternate sides for the recommended repetitions.

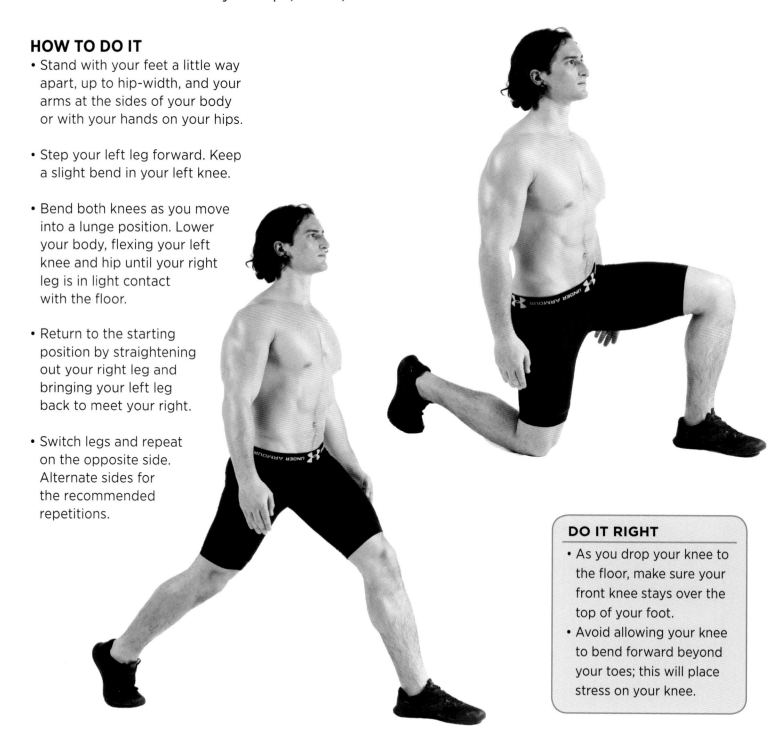

DO IT RIGHT

- As you drop your knee to the floor, make sure your front knee stays over the top of your foot.
- Avoid allowing your knee to bend forward beyond your toes; this will place stress on your knee.

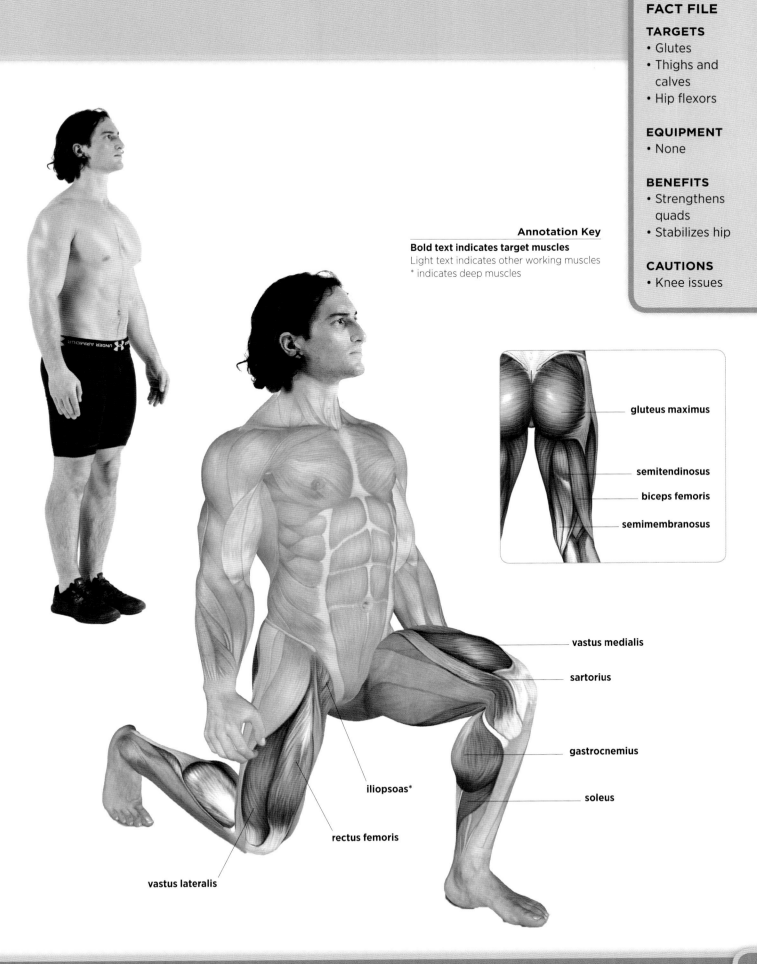

FACT FILE

TARGETS
- Glutes
- Thighs and calves
- Hip flexors

EQUIPMENT
- None

BENEFITS
- Strengthens quads
- Stabilizes hip

CAUTIONS
- Knee issues

Annotation Key

Bold text indicates target muscles
Light text indicates other working muscles
* indicates deep muscles

gluteus maximus

semitendinosus

biceps femoris

semimembranosus

vastus medialis

sartorius

gastrocnemius

soleus

iliopsoas*

rectus femoris

vastus lateralis

Lateral-Extension Reverse Lunge

Backward lunges can be easier than forward ones because your knees take less strain, plus keeping your weight on your forward leg stabilizes the pose. This exercise is certainly great for the glutes, quads, and hamstrings.

HOW TO DO IT

• Stand with your feet a little way apart, up to hip-width, and your arms at the sides of your body or with your hands on your hips.

• Step your right leg backward. Keep a slight bend in your right knee and rest the ball of your foot on the floor.

• Bend both knees as you move into a lunge position. Lower your body, flexing your left knee and hip until your right leg is almost in contact with the floor. Raise your arms to the sides until they are level with your shoulders.

• Return to the starting position by straightening out your left leg and bringing your right leg forward to meet your left.

• Switch legs and repeat on the opposite side. Alternate sides for the recommended repetitions.

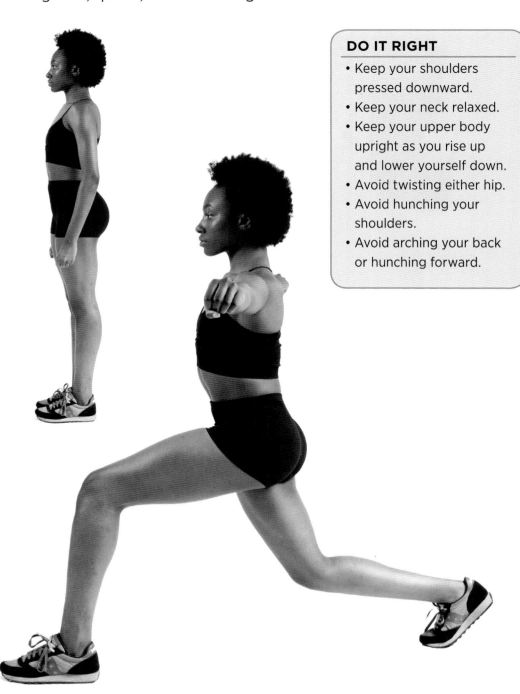

DO IT RIGHT

• Keep your shoulders pressed downward.
• Keep your neck relaxed.
• Keep your upper body upright as you rise up and lower yourself down.
• Avoid twisting either hip.
• Avoid hunching your shoulders.
• Avoid arching your back or hunching forward.

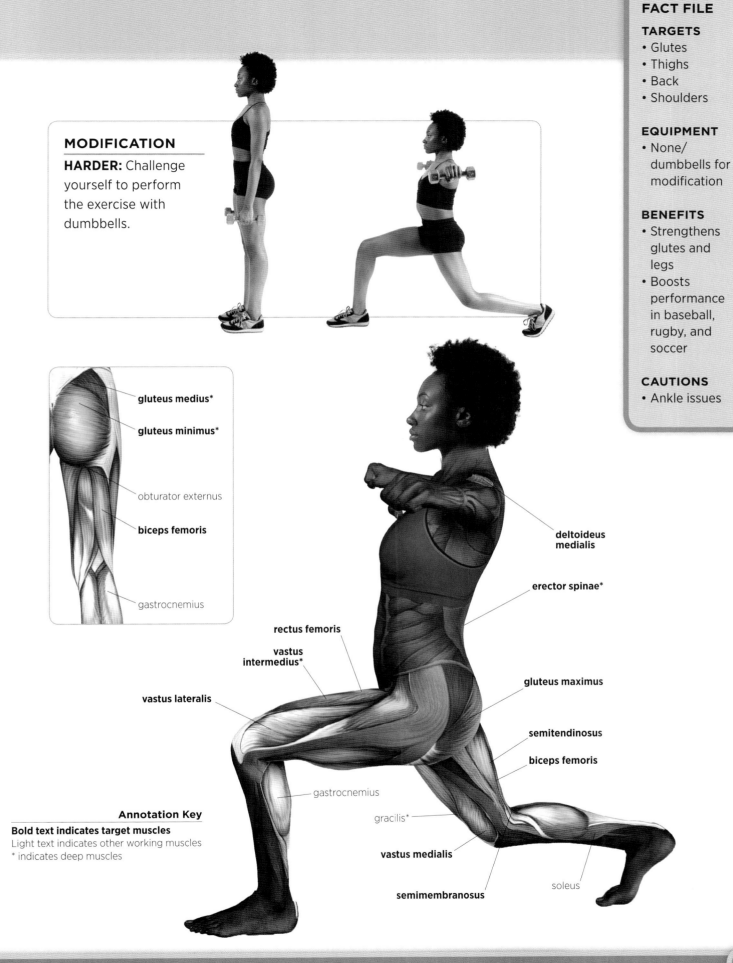

TARGETS
- Glutes
- Thighs
- Back
- Shoulders

EQUIPMENT
- None/ dumbbells for modification

BENEFITS
- Strengthens glutes and legs
- Boosts performance in baseball, rugby, and soccer

CAUTIONS
- Ankle issues

MODIFICATION

HARDER: Challenge yourself to perform the exercise with dumbbells.

gluteus medius*

gluteus minimus*

obturator externus

biceps femoris

gastrocnemius

deltoideus medialis

erector spinae*

rectus femoris

vastus intermedius*

gluteus maximus

vastus lateralis

semitendinosus

biceps femoris

gastrocnemius

gracilis*

vastus medialis

soleus

semimembranosus

Annotation Key

Bold text indicates target muscles
Light text indicates other working muscles
* indicates deep muscles

Skater's Lunge

If you want to strengthen your glutes and quads, then look no further than this simple exercise. Skater's Lunge will also give a thorough workout to your hamstrings.

HOW TO DO IT

- Stand with your legs wider than shoulder-width apart and your toes pointing forward.

- Slide to your left side into a side lunge as you bend forward slightly, with your hands placed on your left thigh, and your right leg straight.

- Repeat on the opposite side. Alternate sides for the recommended time.

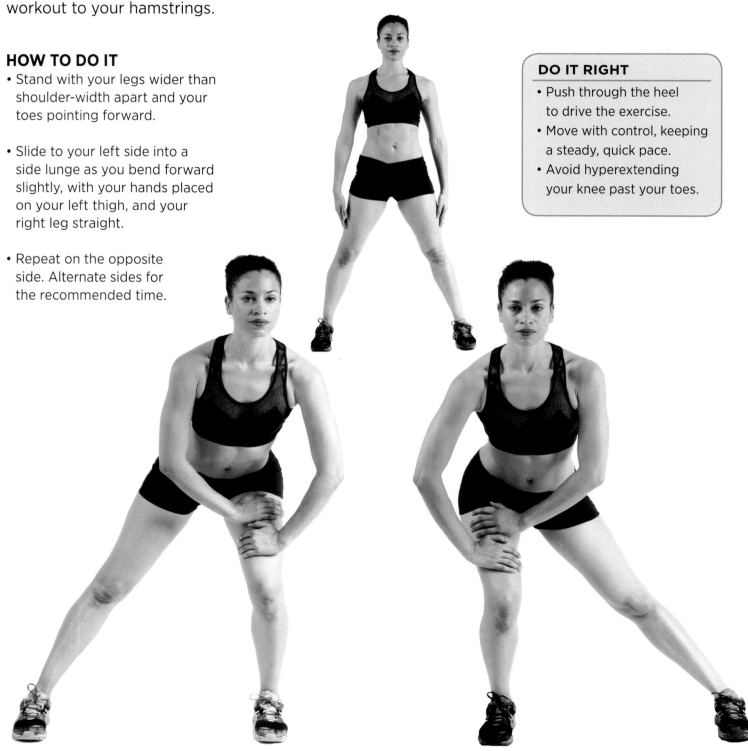

DO IT RIGHT

- Push through the heel to drive the exercise.
- Move with control, keeping a steady, quick pace.
- Avoid hyperextending your knee past your toes.

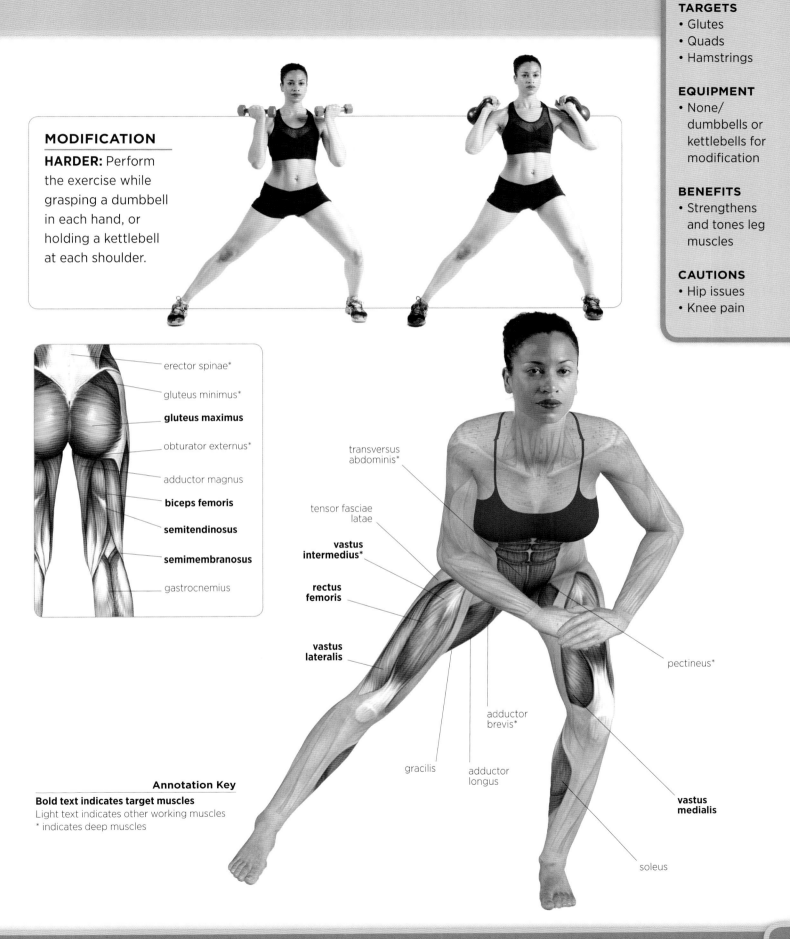

MODIFICATION

HARDER: Perform the exercise while grasping a dumbbell in each hand, or holding a kettlebell at each shoulder.

FACT FILE

TARGETS
• Glutes
• Quads
• Hamstrings

EQUIPMENT
• None/ dumbbells or kettlebells for modification

BENEFITS
• Strengthens and tones leg muscles

CAUTIONS
• Hip issues
• Knee pain

erector spinae*

gluteus minimus*

gluteus maximus

obturator externus*

adductor magnus

biceps femoris

semitendinosus

semimembranosus

gastrocnemius

transversus abdominis*

tensor fasciae latae

vastus intermedius*

rectus femoris

vastus lateralis

pectineus*

adductor brevis*

gracilis

adductor longus

vastus medialis

soleus

Annotation Key
Bold text indicates target muscles
Light text indicates other working muscles
* indicates deep muscles

Squat

Another very simple exercise that really delivers for your buttocks and legs. The Squat works your abdominals, too, which means that it helps to stabilize your core. Plus the pose promotes better balance.

HOW TO DO IT

- Stand with your feet shoulder-width apart, your toes pointed slightly outwards and your arms extended in front of you.

- Bend your knees, while keeping your back flat. Lower yourself toward the floor until your thighs are parallel to it.

- Push through your heels to stand erect. Repeat for the recommended repetitions.

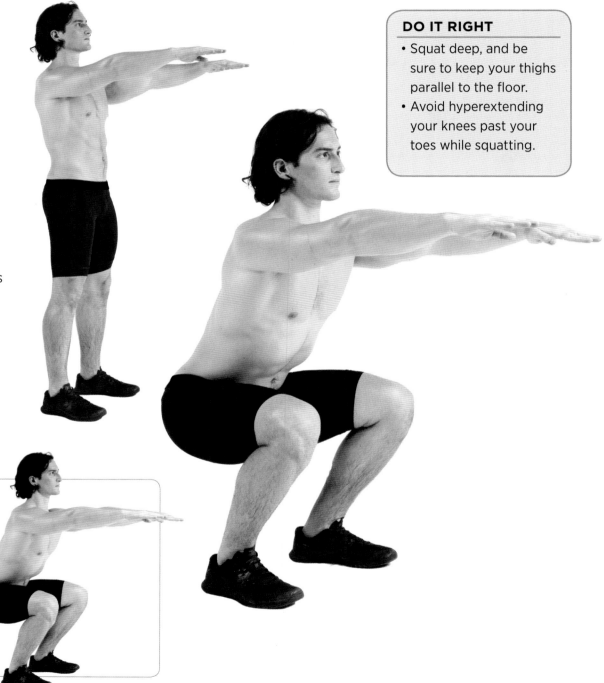

DO IT RIGHT

- Squat deep, and be sure to keep your thighs parallel to the floor.
- Avoid hyperextending your knees past your toes while squatting.

MODIFICATION

HARDER: Bringing your feet closer together increases the effort required.

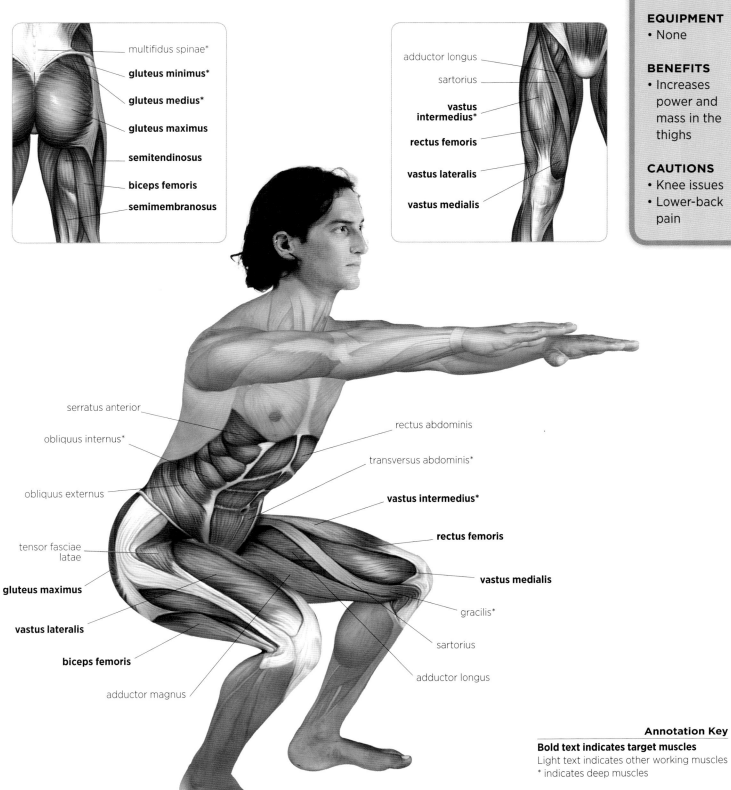

FACT FILE

TARGETS
• Quads
• Hamstrings
• Glutes

EQUIPMENT
• None

BENEFITS
• Increases power and mass in the thighs

CAUTIONS
• Knee issues
• Lower-back pain

multifidus spinae*
gluteus minimus*
gluteus medius*
gluteus maximus
semitendinosus
biceps femoris
semimembranosus

adductor longus
sartorius
vastus intermedius*
rectus femoris
vastus lateralis
vastus medialis

serratus anterior
obliquus internus*
obliquus externus
tensor fasciae latae
gluteus maximus
vastus lateralis
biceps femoris
adductor magnus

rectus abdominis
transversus abdominis*
vastus intermedius*
rectus femoris
vastus medialis
gracilis*
sartorius
adductor longus

Annotation Key

Bold text indicates target muscles
Light text indicates other working muscles
* indicates deep muscles

Single-Leg Gluteal Lift

The Single-Leg Gluteal Lift develops tight, strong glutes while working many other major muscles. A key to safe success here is to use your abdominals to lift your body.

HOW TO DO IT

- Lie on your back with your arms along your sides and legs bent with your feet directly under your knees. Extend your left leg upward, pointing through your foot.

- Engage your abdominals to pop up to a one-legged, stable Bridge pose (pages 96–97). Raise your body only as high as you can go while maintaining correct alignment.

- Maintain this position, focusing on keeping your hips level, navel pressing to spine, and your raised leg extending from the hip joint.

- Lower your body back down to the floor, keeping your left leg extended.

- Repeat the bridge, with the same leg raised, for the recommended repetitions. Switch legs and repeat on the opposite side for the recommended repetitions.

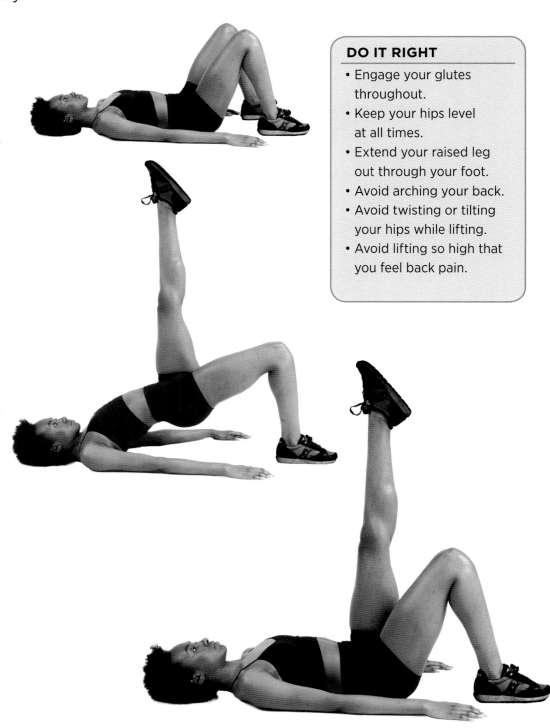

DO IT RIGHT

- Engage your glutes throughout.
- Keep your hips level at all times.
- Extend your raised leg out through your foot.
- Avoid arching your back.
- Avoid twisting or tilting your hips while lifting.
- Avoid lifting so high that you feel back pain.

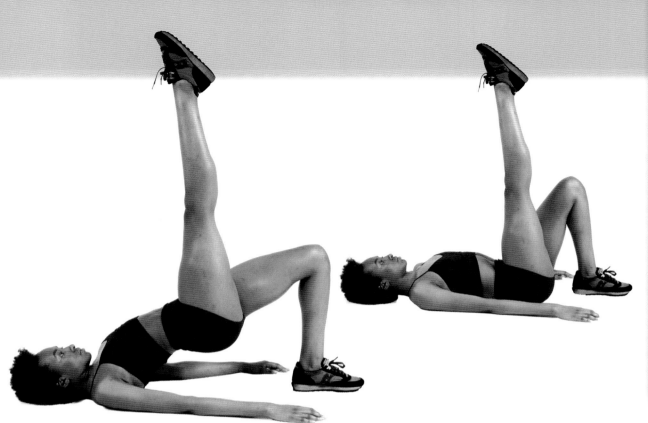

FACT FILE

TARGETS
- Glutes
- Hip flexors
- Legs
- Abdominals
- Neck, shoulders, and back

EQUIPMENT
- None

BENEFITS
- Strengthens and tones glutes and abdominals

CAUTIONS
- Back pain/ issues

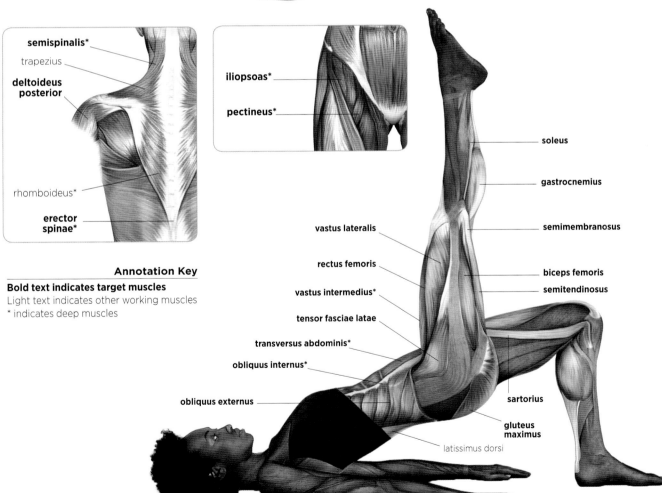

semispinalis*

trapezius

deltoideus posterior

rhomboideus*

erector spinae*

iliopsoas*

pectineus*

soleus

gastrocnemius

semimembranosus

vastus lateralis

rectus femoris

biceps femoris

vastus intermedius*

semitendinosus

tensor fasciae latae

transversus abdominis*

obliquus internus*

obliquus externus

sartorius

gluteus maximus

latissimus dorsi

Annotation Key

Bold text indicates target muscles
Light text indicates other working muscles
* indicates deep muscles

Butt Kick

Doing the Butt Kick regularly will make those often-problematic hamstrings much stronger—which helps with so many types of exercise and sports. It should also give your cardiovascular system a mild workout.

HOW TO DO IT

- Begin in a standing position, and then jog in place.

- Kick your heels up high toward your buttocks.

- Continue jogging in place, lifting your heels high, for the recommended time while increasing your speed as you go.

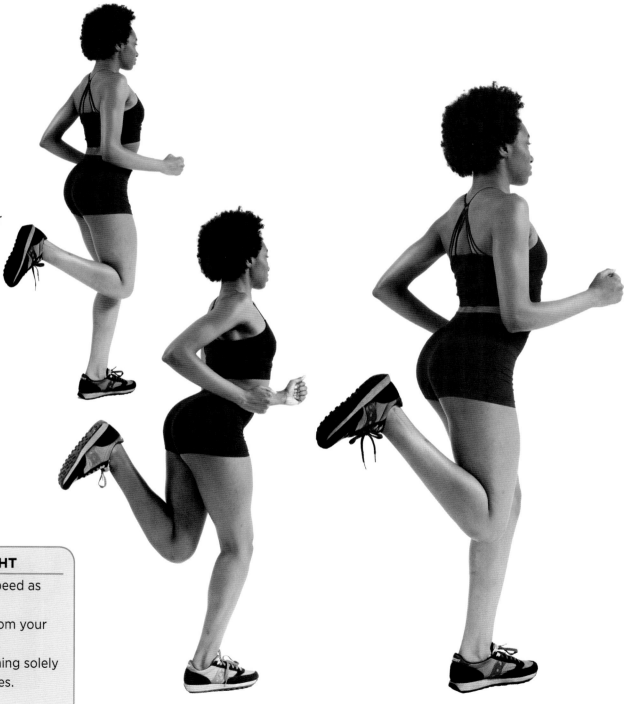

DO IT RIGHT

- Build up speed as you go.
- Push off from your entire foot.
- Avoid pushing solely off your toes.

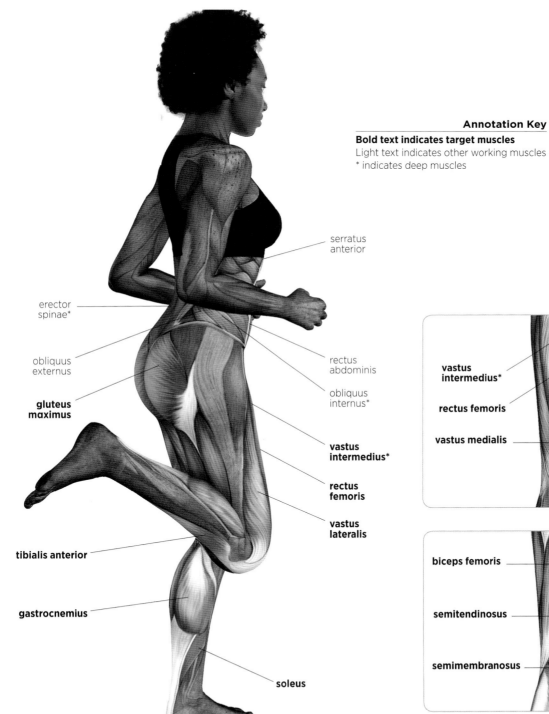

FACT FILE

TARGETS
- Glutes
- Quads
- Hamstrings
- Calves

EQUIPMENT
- None

BENEFITS
- Strengthens lower body
- Serves as a warm-up for other exercise
- Builds endurance

CAUTIONS
- Knee issues
- Ankle pain

Annotation Key

Bold text indicates target muscles
Light text indicates other working muscles
* indicates deep muscles

serratus anterior

erector spinae*

obliquus externus

gluteus maximus

rectus abdominis

obliquus internus*

vastus intermedius*

rectus femoris

vastus lateralis

tibialis anterior

gastrocnemius

soleus

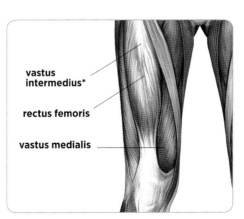

vastus intermedius*

rectus femoris

vastus medialis

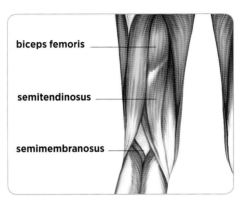

biceps femoris

semitendinosus

semimembranosus

Forearm Plank

This form of the Plank (pages 114–115) is a classic choice for the core, strengthening and stabilizing all of its muscles. It also builds extra strength into your lower back.

HOW TO DO IT

- Lie on your stomach on the floor, with your legs extended behind you and your torso raised off the floor. Bend your arms so that your forearms and palms rest flat on the floor.

- Bend your knees, supporting your weight between your knees and your forearms, and then push through with your forearms to bring your shoulders up toward the ceiling as you straighten your legs. Your toes are curled under.

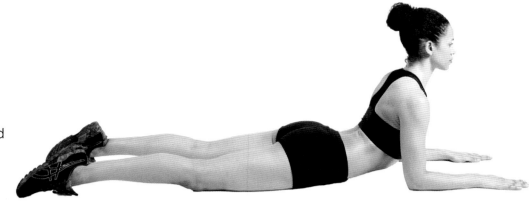

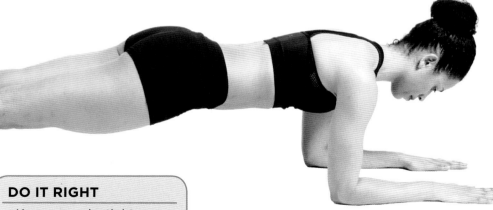

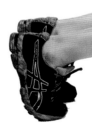

- With control, lower your shoulders until you feel them coming together at your back. Hold your raise for the recommended time.

DO IT RIGHT

- Keep your abs tight.
- Keep your body in a straight line.
- Keep your neck lengthened.
- Avoid allowing your shoulders to collapse into your shoulder joints.
- Avoid arching your neck.
- Avoid allowing your back to sag.

FACT FILE

TARGETS
- Abdominals
- Core
- Back

EQUIPMENT
- None

BENEFITS
- Strengthens and stabilizes core

CAUTIONS
- Shoulder injury
- Severe back pain

MODIFICATION

HARDER: While in the plank position, lift and lower your legs one at a time. Keep the rest of your body still and your abs engaged throughout.

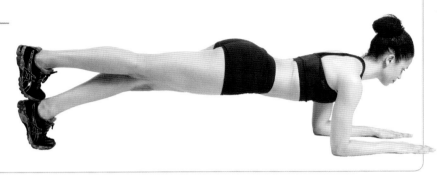

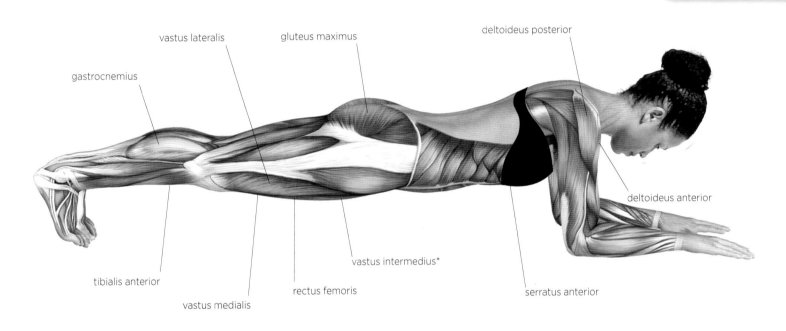

gastrocnemius

vastus lateralis

gluteus maximus

deltoideus posterior

deltoideus anterior

tibialis anterior

vastus medialis

rectus femoris

vastus intermedius*

serratus anterior

Annotation Key

Bold text indicates target muscles
Light text indicates other working muscles
* indicates deep muscles

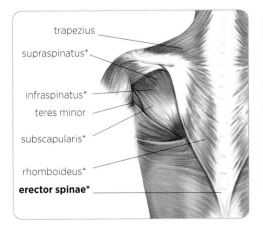

trapezius

supraspinatus*

infraspinatus*

teres minor

subscapularis*

rhomboideus*

erector spinae*

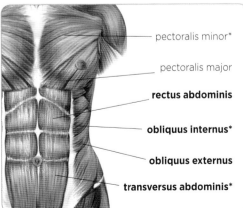

pectoralis minor*

pectoralis major

rectus abdominis

obliquus internus*

obliquus externus

transversus abdominis*

Plank

The Plank is an amazing upper-body stabilizer that teaches you to keep your body firm and steady. Promoting strength and stability in your upper back and shoulders, this is an important exercise for preventing injuries.

HOW TO DO IT

- Start on your hands and knees, with your hands shoulder-width apart.

- Push your body up so your arms are straight, with your legs extended backward, to come into a high plank position. Keep your palms on the floor, your feet together, your back straight, and your weight on the balls of your feet.

- Hold your raise for the recommended time.

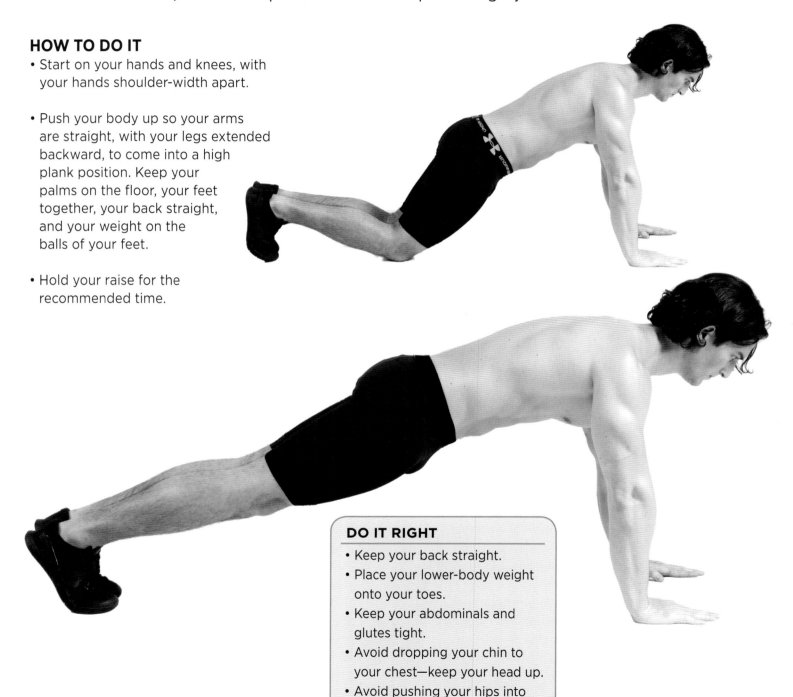

DO IT RIGHT
- Keep your back straight.
- Place your lower-body weight onto your toes.
- Keep your abdominals and glutes tight.
- Avoid dropping your chin to your chest—keep your head up.
- Avoid pushing your hips into the air.

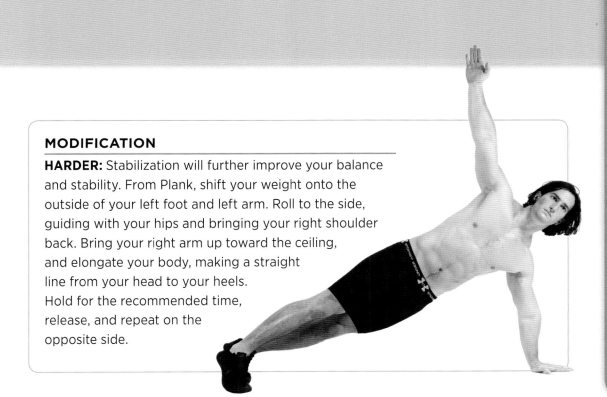

FACT FILE

TARGETS
- Shoulders
- Chest
- Legs
- Glutes
- Triceps

EQUIPMENT
- None

BENEFITS
- Strengthens and stabilizes core

CAUTIONS
- Shoulder issues
- Lower-back issues
- Wrist issues

MODIFICATION

HARDER: Stabilization will further improve your balance and stability. From Plank, shift your weight onto the outside of your left foot and left arm. Roll to the side, guiding with your hips and bringing your right shoulder back. Bring your right arm up toward the ceiling, and elongate your body, making a straight line from your head to your heels. Hold for the recommended time, release, and repeat on the opposite side.

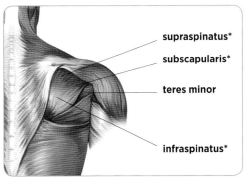

supraspinatus*

subscapularis*

teres minor

infraspinatus*

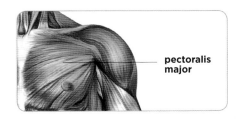

pectoralis major

Annotation Key
Bold text indicates target muscles
Light text indicates other working muscles
* indicates deep muscles

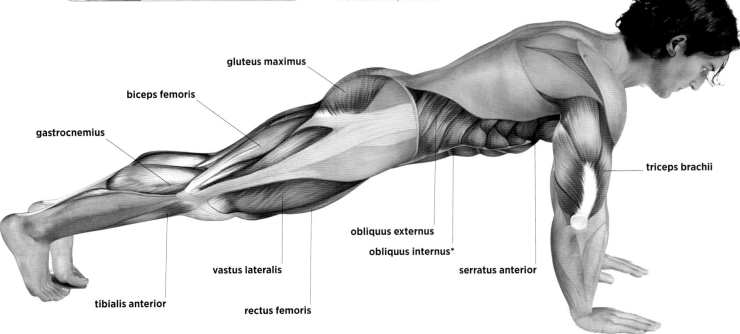

gluteus maximus

biceps femoris

gastrocnemius

triceps brachii

obliquus externus

obliquus internus*

serratus anterior

vastus lateralis

tibialis anterior

rectus femoris

Plank-Up

Plank-Up is an effective exercise to build power into your abdominals and arms. Make sure that you focus on keeping your core fully engaged as you move from low to high and back again.

HOW TO DO IT

- Start in a Forearm Plank position (pages 112–113) with your weight evenly distributed on your forearms and the balls of your feet. Take a moment to stabilize your hips and fully engage your abdominals.

- Reposition your left arm and then the right so that your hands are planted beneath your shoulders, lifting your body into a high Plank position.

- Return to the Forearm Plank, repositioning your left arm and then the right.

- Alternate leading with one arm and then the other for the recommended repetitions.

DO IT RIGHT

- Pull your navel in toward your spine to engage your abdominals.
- Avoid letting your stomach or rib cage sag.
- Avoid lifting your shoulders up or forward.
- Avoid shifting your weight when you change levels.

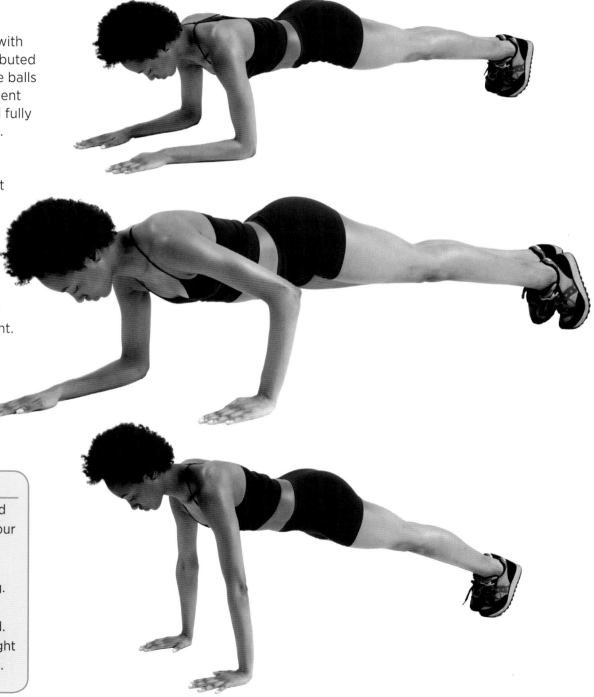

TARGETS
- Triceps
- Abdominals
- Shoulders

EQUIPMENT
- None

BENEFITS
- Stabilizes core
- Strengthens abdominals
- Strengthens triceps

CAUTIONS
- Shoulder issues
- Back issues
- Wrist issues

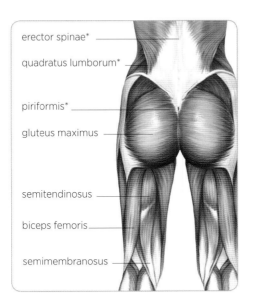

erector spinae*

quadratus lumborum*

piriformis*

gluteus maximus

semitendinosus

biceps femoris

semimembranosus

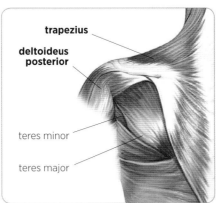

trapezius

deltoideus posterior

teres minor

teres major

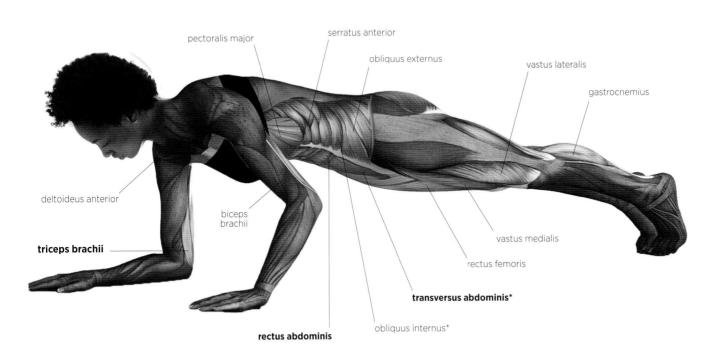

pectoralis major

serratus anterior

obliquus externus

vastus lateralis

gastrocnemius

deltoideus anterior

biceps brachii

triceps brachii

vastus medialis

rectus femoris

transversus abdominis*

obliquus internus*

rectus abdominis

Annotation Key

Bold text indicates target muscles
Light text indicates other working muscles
* indicates deep muscles

Arm-Reach Plank

As well as building durability and tone into your torso, legs, and arms, this Arm-Reach form of the Plank works wonders in improving your overall balance.

HOW TO DO IT

- Begin facedown, resting on your forearms and knees.

- One at a time, step your feet back into a Forearm Plank (pages 112–113). Engage your abdominal muscles and find a straight but relaxed spine. This is your starting position.

- Maintaining a proper Plank form, slowly lift your right arm off the floor. Hold for the recommended time. Release, return to your starting position, and repeat on the opposite side.

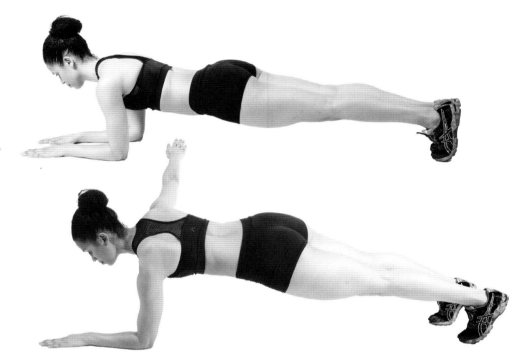

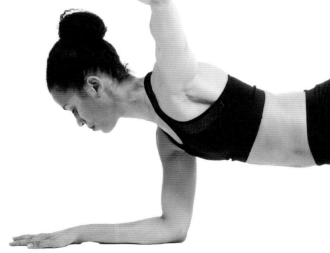

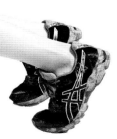

DO IT RIGHT

- Contract your abdominal muscles.
- Keep your spine parallel to the floor.
- Avoid allowing your hips to sink or tilt upward.
- Avoid letting your abs bulge outward.

FACT FILE
- Abdominals
- Back
- Quads
- ITB
- Elbow flexors

BENEFITS
- Improves balance
- Strengthens and tones arms, legs, and abdominals
- Boosts performance in swimming, gymnastics, and dance

MODIFICATION

EASIER: To make the exercise less strenuous, lie on your front in a Forearm Plank with your legs bent up behind you. And instead of raising each arm fully off the floor to the side, lift only your forearm, to the front.

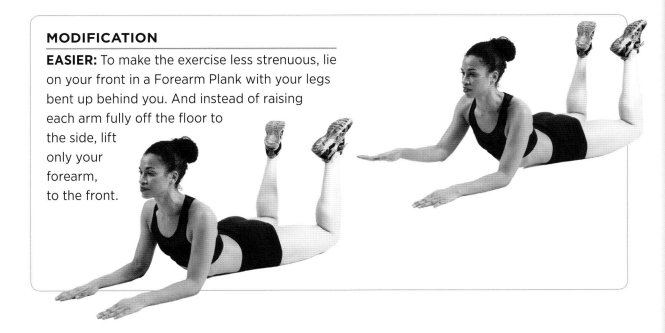

Annotation Key
Bold text indicates target muscles
Light text indicates other working muscles
* indicates deep muscles

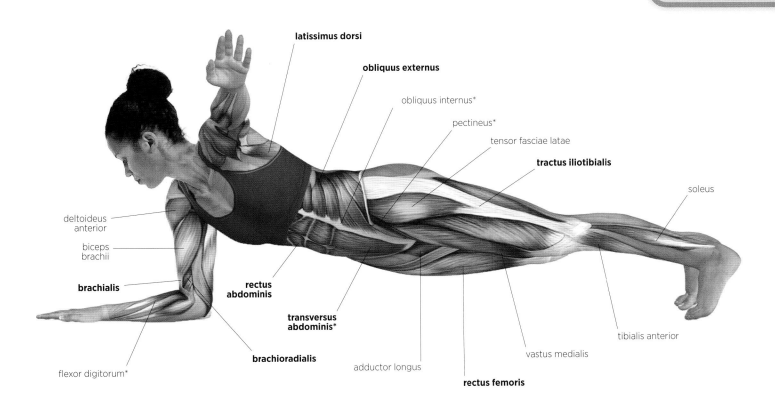

latissimus dorsi

obliquus externus

obliquus internus*

pectineus*

tensor fasciae latae

tractus iliotibialis

soleus

deltoideus anterior

biceps brachii

brachialis

rectus abdominis

transversus abdominis*

brachioradialis

adductor longus

rectus femoris

vastus medialis

tibialis anterior

flexor digitorum*

Side Plank

Side Plank builds durability into your abdominal muscles, especially your obliques. This, in turn, will help to stabilize your spine and so make back problems less likely to occur.

HOW TO DO IT

- Lie on your right side, with your legs extended and your left leg stacked on top of your right.

- Bend your right arm to a 90-degree angle with your forearm on the floor, fingers facing forward. Rest your left arm along the side of your body.

- Push into the floor with your right hand and forearm, and raise your hips off the floor until your body forms a straight line.

- Hold for the recommended time, lower your body, and repeat on the opposite side.

DO IT RIGHT

- Push equally from your forearm and hip as you raise your body.
- Keep your body as stable and aligned as possible.
- Keep your feet flexed and stacked.
- Avoid arching your back.
- Avoid allowing your hips to sink.
- Avoid arching your neck.
- Avoid hunching your shoulders.

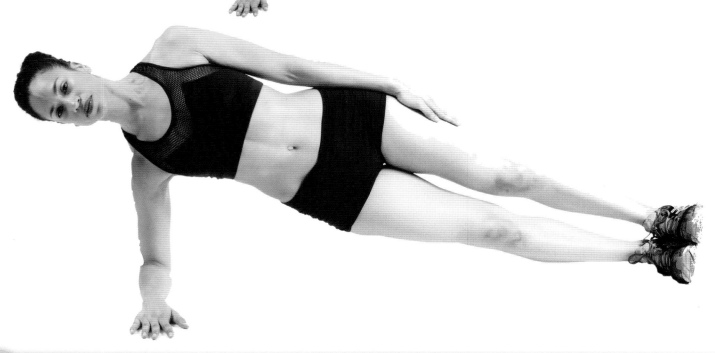

TARGETS
- Abdominals, especially obliques
- Glutes
- Chest
- Inner thighs
- Shoulders

EQUIPMENT
- None

BENEFITS
- Strengthens upper body, glutes, core, and thighs
- Stabilizes trunk

CAUTIONS
- Rotator cuff injury
- Neck issues
- Lower-back pain

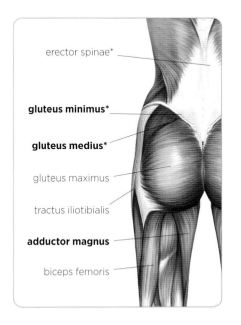

erector spinae*

gluteus minimus*

gluteus medius*

gluteus maximus

tractus iliotibialis

adductor magnus

biceps femoris

MODIFICATION

SIMILAR DIFFICULTY: Cross your legs at the ankles instead of stacking your feet.

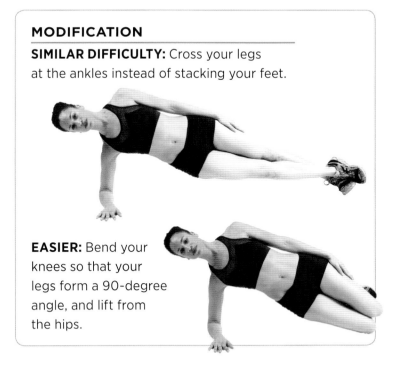

EASIER: Bend your knees so that your legs form a 90-degree angle, and lift from the hips.

Annotation Key
Bold text indicates target muscles
Light text indicates other working muscles
* indicates deep muscles

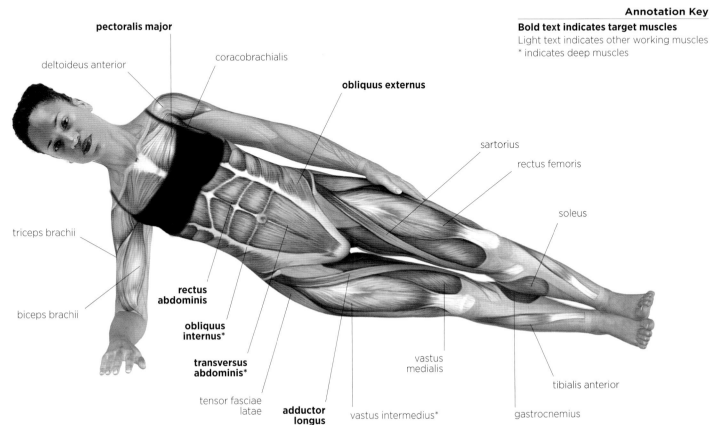

pectoralis major

deltoideus anterior

coracobrachialis

obliquus externus

sartorius

rectus femoris

soleus

triceps brachii

biceps brachii

rectus abdominis

obliquus internus*

transversus abdominis*

tensor fasciae latae

adductor longus

vastus intermedius*

vastus medialis

tibialis anterior

gastrocnemius

Side Plank with Reach-Under

In Side Plank with Reach-Under, strength lies in stillness rather than in motion. As you maintain the static position of your torso and legs while moving one of your arms, you are effectively strengthening your abs, lower back, and shoulders.

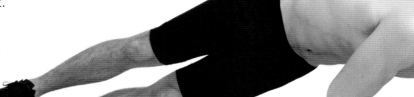

HOW TO DO IT

- Lie on your left side, with your legs extended and your right leg stacked on top of your left.

- Bend your left arm to a 90-degree angle with your fist on the floor, knuckles pointing forward. Rest your right arm along the side of your body or put your right hand on your waist.

- Push into the floor with your left hand and forearm, and raise your hips off the floor until your body orms a straight line.

- Twist your upper torso toward the floor as you reach your right arm under your chest as far as you can stretch.

- Twist your upper torso back to the front as you extend your right arm toward the ceiling.

- Repeat for the recommended repetitions, and then repeat on the opposite side for the recommended repetitions.

DO IT RIGHT

- Push equally from your forearm and hip as you raise your body.
- Allow your head and neck to follow the movement of your torso, so you look toward the floor during the reach-under and straight ahead in the finished position with your top arm extended.
- Keep your feet flexed and stacked.
- Avoid placing too much strain on your shoulders.
- Avoid losing your alignment when your top arm is extended.

FACT FILE

TARGETS
• Abdominals
• Back
• ITB
• Elbow flexors

EQUIPMENT
• None

BENEFITS
• Strengthens and stabilizes core
• Builds endurance
• Strengthens shoulders

CAUTIONS
• Neck issues
• Rotator cuff injury

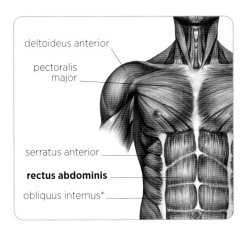

deltoideus anterior

pectoralis major

serratus anterior

rectus abdominis

obliquus internus*

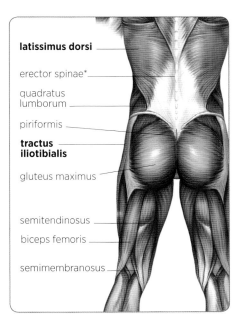

latissimus dorsi

erector spinae*

quadratus lumborum

piriformis

tractus iliotibialis

gluteus maximus

semitendinosus

biceps femoris

semimembranosus

Annotation Key

Bold text indicates target muscles
Light text indicates other working muscles
* indicates deep muscles

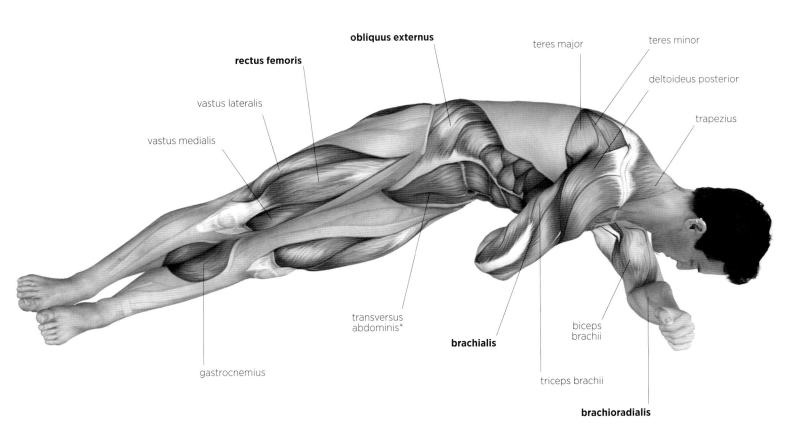

obliquus externus

rectus femoris

vastus lateralis

vastus medialis

teres major

teres minor

deltoideus posterior

trapezius

transversus abdominis*

brachialis

biceps brachii

gastrocnemius

triceps brachii

brachioradialis

T-Stabilization

T-Stabilization, another advanced variation on the traditional Plank, is a proven exercise for targeting your abdominals, including your obliques, as well as your hips and lower back.

HOW TO DO IT

- Begin in a raised Plank position (pages 114–115). Your hands should be shoulder-width apart, palms on the floor with fingers pointing forward, feet together with toes tucked under, and your back straight.

- Turn your right-hand hips to one side, stacking your right foot on top of the left and raising your right arm across your body until you are pointing toward the ceiling. If you feel stable, look up toward your raised hand.

- Hold for the recommended time. Lower, returning to your raised plank, and repeat on the opposite side for the recommended repetitions.

DO IT RIGHT

- Keep your body in one straight line.
- Avoid arching or bridging your back.

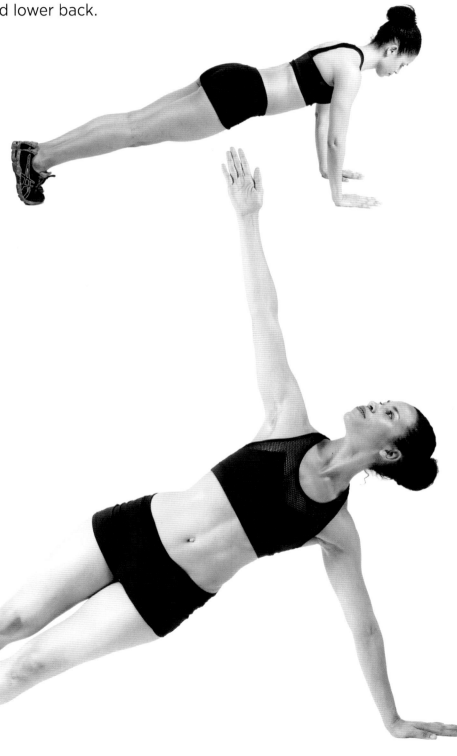

FACT FILE

TARGETS
- Shoulders and chest
- Triceps and elbow flexors
- Back
- Abdominals
- Glutes
- Legs

EQUIPMENT
- None

BENEFITS
- Stabilizes spine and core
- Strengthens leg abductors and adductors
- Strengthens back

CAUTIONS
- Shoulder issues
- Neck issues
- Wrist pain

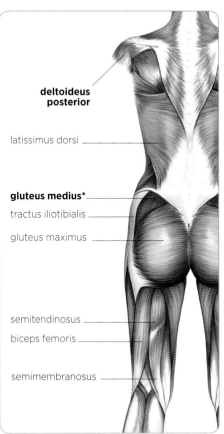

deltoideus posterior

latissimus dorsi

gluteus medius*

tractus iliotibialis

gluteus maximus

semitendinosus

biceps femoris

semimembranosus

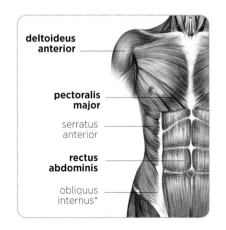

deltoideus anterior

pectoralis major

serratus anterior

rectus abdominis

obliquus internus*

Annotation Key
Bold text indicates target muscles
Light text indicates other working muscles
* indicates deep muscles

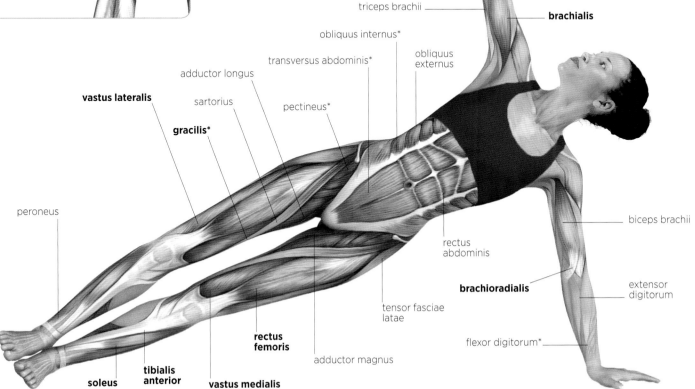

triceps brachii

obliquus internus*

transversus abdominis*

adductor longus

vastus lateralis

sartorius

pectineus*

gracilis*

brachialis

obliquus externus

biceps brachii

rectus abdominis

brachioradialis

extensor digitorum

peroneus

tensor fasciae latae

flexor digitorum*

rectus femoris

tibialis anterior

adductor magnus

soleus

vastus medialis

Mountain Climber

The explosive Mountain Climber builds upper-body strength while giving your cardiovascular system an intense workout. It also helps hone your balance, coordination, and agility.

HOW TO DO IT

- Begin in a raised Plank position (pages 114–115). Your hands should be shoulder-width apart, palms on the floor with fingers pointing forward, feet together with toes tucked under, and your back straight.

- Bring your right knee in toward your chest, resting the ball of that foot on the floor.

- Jump to switch your feet in the air, bringing your left foot in and your right foot back.

- Continue alternating your feet as fast as you can safely go for the recommended time.

> ### DO IT RIGHT
> - Keep your back straight.
> - Flare your hands out to ease shoulder stress.
> - Avoid small leg movements; try to bring your knee straight toward your upper body in one clean move.

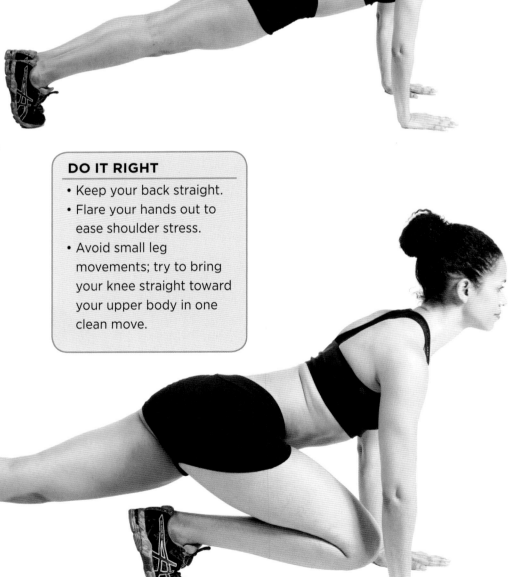

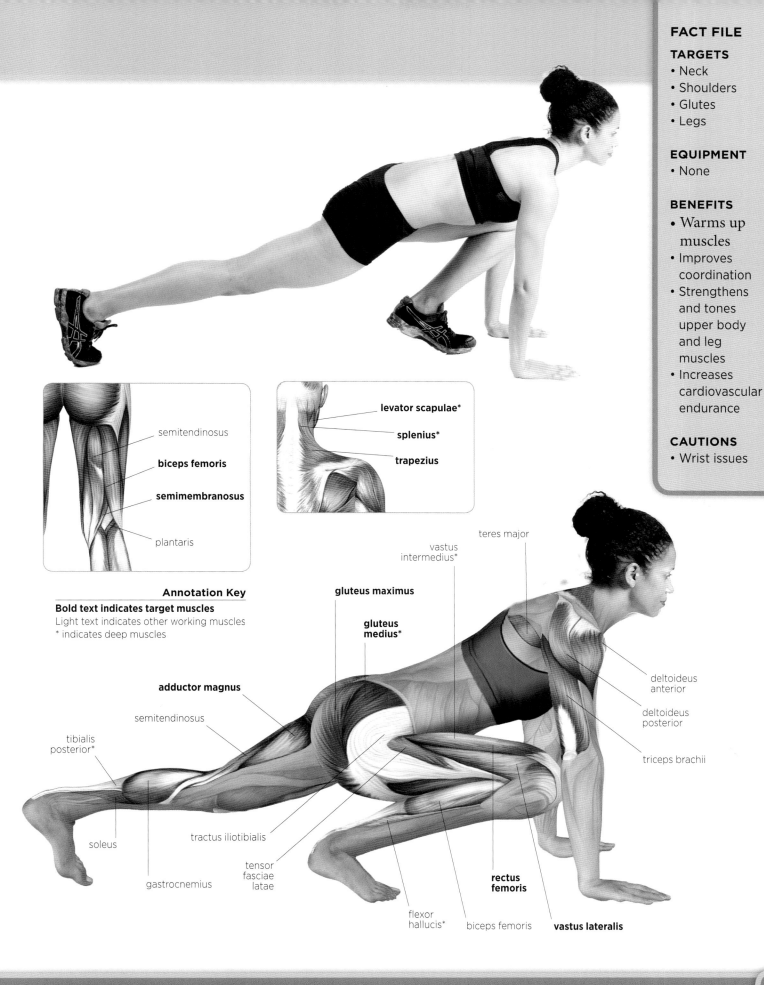

TARGETS
- Neck
- Shoulders
- Glutes
- Legs

EQUIPMENT
- None

BENEFITS
- Warms up muscles
- Improves coordination
- Strengthens and tones upper body and leg muscles
- Increases cardiovascular endurance

CAUTIONS
- Wrist issues

semitendinosus

biceps femoris

semimembranosus

plantaris

levator scapulae*

splenius*

trapezius

Annotation Key

Bold text indicates target muscles
Light text indicates other working muscles
* indicates deep muscles

teres major

vastus intermedius*

gluteus maximus

gluteus medius*

adductor magnus

semitendinosus

tibialis posterior*

soleus

tractus iliotibialis

gastrocnemius

tensor fasciae latae

flexor hallucis*

biceps femoris

rectus femoris

vastus lateralis

deltoideus anterior

deltoideus posterior

triceps brachii

Up-Down

The Up-Down is a multiphase exercise designed to tax your cardiovascular system by using almost all of your muscles. It has the added benefit of increasing your coordination and agility.

HOW TO DO IT

- Run in place, bringing your knees waist-high with each step.

- Drop down and touch your chest to the floor.

- Immediately stand back up and continue running with high knees as quickly as possible.

- Repeat for the recommended repetitions.

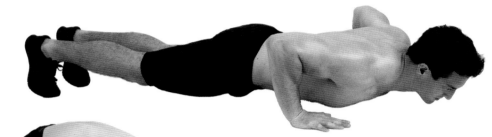

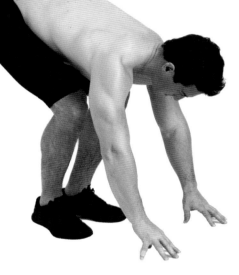

DO IT RIGHT

- Keep your knees at waist level while running in place.
- Avoid landing on your chest—allow your hands to contact the floor first, and then lower onto your chest.
- Avoid flopping onto the ground—move with control.

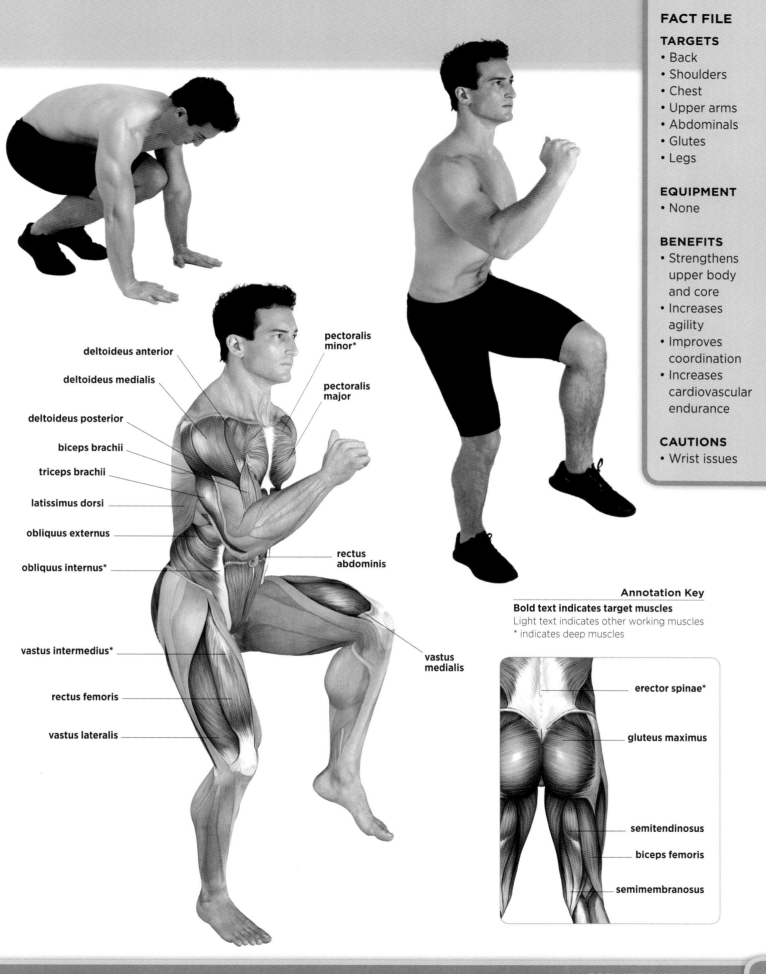

TARGETS
- Back
- Shoulders
- Chest
- Upper arms
- Abdominals
- Glutes
- Legs

EQUIPMENT
- None

BENEFITS
- Strengthens upper body and core
- Increases agility
- Improves coordination
- Increases cardiovascular endurance

CAUTIONS
- Wrist issues

deltoideus anterior

deltoideus medialis

deltoideus posterior

biceps brachii

triceps brachii

latissimus dorsi

obliquus externus

obliquus internus*

vastus intermedius*

rectus femoris

vastus lateralis

pectoralis minor*

pectoralis major

rectus abdominis

vastus medialis

Annotation Key

Bold text indicates target muscles
Light text indicates other working muscles
* indicates deep muscles

erector spinae*

gluteus maximus

semitendinosus

biceps femoris

semimembranosus

Burpee

The names Burpee and Squat Thrust are often used interchangeably, but a Burpee takes you through the same moves as a Squat Thrust but adds a jump at the end. This added boost takes the exercise to the next cardio and strength level.

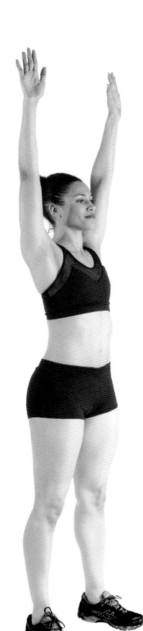

HOW TO DO IT

- Stand with your feet a little way apart and your arms above your head.

- Drop into a squat position, placing your hands on the floor.

- In one quick, explosive motion, kick your feet back to assume a raised plank position and perform a push-up.

- In another quick motion, jump into the air, and return to the starting position. Repeat for as many repetitions as possible within the recommended time.

DO IT RIGHT

- Make sure your chest touches the floor in the push-up.
- Jump as high as you can as you rise from the squat.
- Avoid moving with floppy or jerky motions—your movements should be smooth and controlled.

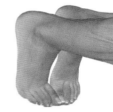

Annotation Key

Bold text indicates target muscles
Light text indicates other working muscles
* indicates deep muscles

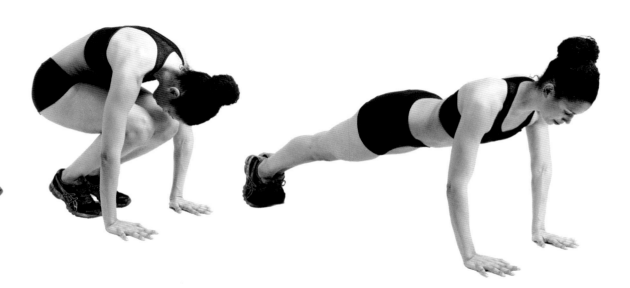

TARGETS
- Abdominals
- Shoulders
- Chest
- Triceps and elbow flexor

EQUIPMENT
- None

BENEFITS
- Improves cardio fitness
- Strengthens multiple muscle groups

CAUTIONS
- Wrist issues

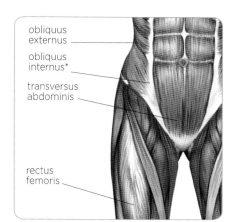

obliquus externus
obliquus internus*
transversus abdominis
rectus femoris

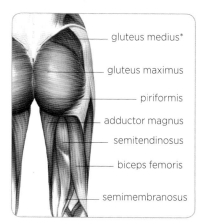

gluteus medius*
gluteus maximus
piriformis
adductor magnus
semitendinosus
biceps femoris
semimembranosus

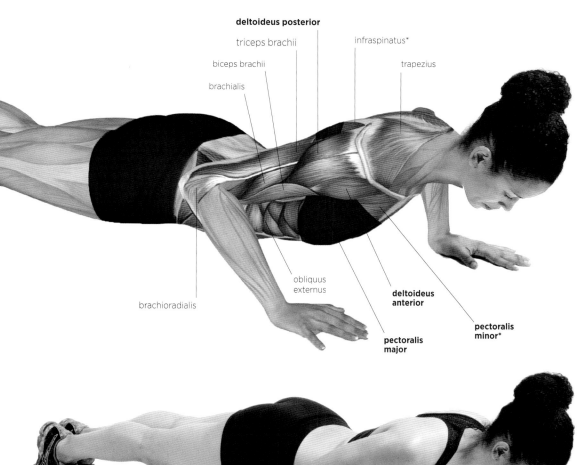

deltoideus posterior
triceps brachii
biceps brachii
brachialis
infraspinatus*
trapezius
brachioradialis
obliquus externus
deltoideus anterior
pectoralis major
pectoralis minor*

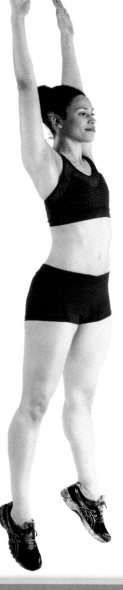

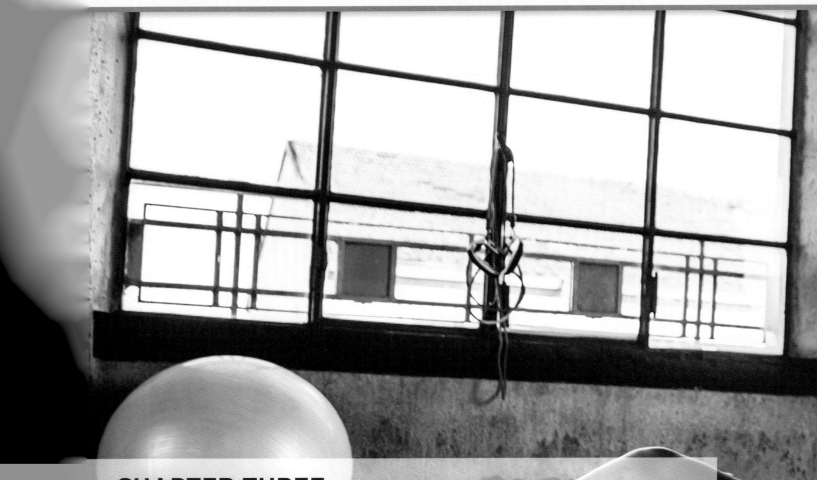

CHAPTER THREE

WEIGHTED EXERCISES

There are many good reasons for exercising with weights, and developing your strength is an obvious one. For example, weight-work can really strengthen your core to support a healthier, less problem-prone back. As a bonus, evidence suggests it may improve your overall metabolism and heart health, aid osteoporosis, and develop coordination. Depending on your exercise goals, remember that weights don't have to be huge—just enough to provide some resistance.

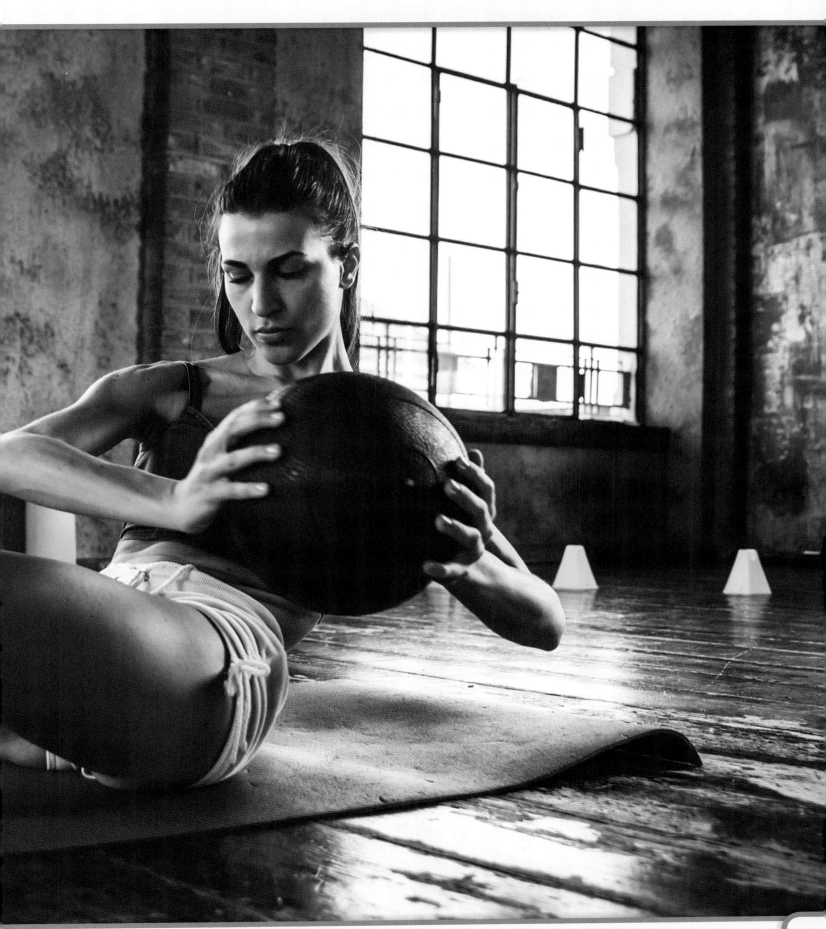

Dumbbell Shrug

Your back health should improve from using weights. This exercise strengthens your back's large trapezius muscle—as well as other muscles of the back, neck, and shoulder girdle—to ease tightness in your upper back.

HOW TO DO IT

- Stand with your arms by your sides, holding a dumbbell in each hand. Your feet should be about shoulder-width apart and your knees slightly bent.

- Lift your shoulders straight up toward your ears.

- Slowly and deliberately lower your shoulders to your starting position. Repeat for the recommended repetitions.

DO IT RIGHT

- Keep your chest lifted during the upward movement.
- Keep your jaw relaxed throughout.
- Keep your elbows pointing out behind you.
- Avoid bending your elbows—lift your shoulders up toward your ears.
- Avoid using your back to lower the dumbbells when you finish—bend and use your knees instead.

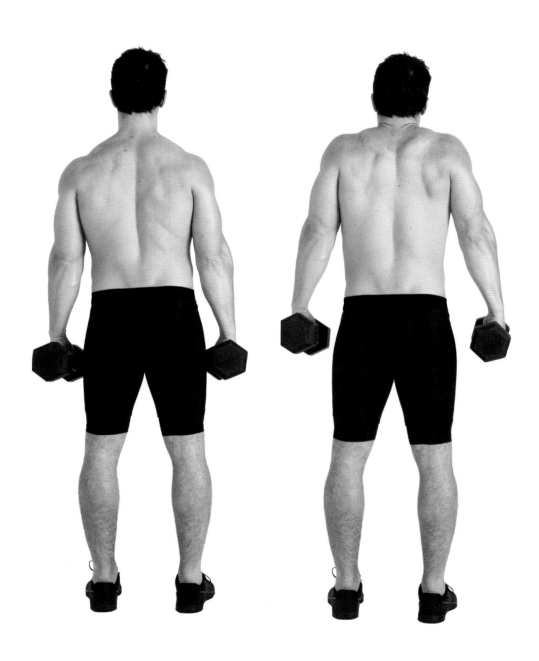

TARGETS
• Upper back

EQUIPMENT
• Dumbbells

BENEFITS
• Strengthens the upper back
• Works the whole upper body, neck, and arms

CAUTIONS
• Back issues
• Shoulder issues

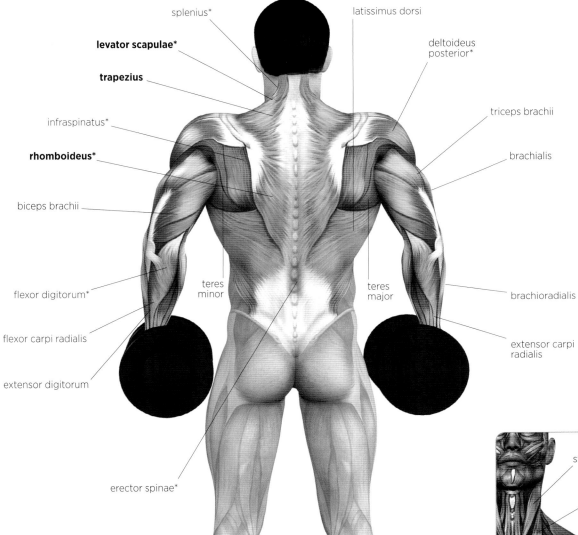

splenius*

levator scapulae*

trapezius

infraspinatus*

rhomboideus*

biceps brachii

flexor digitorum*

flexor carpi radialis

extensor digitorum

teres minor

erector spinae*

latissimus dorsi

deltoideus posterior*

triceps brachii

brachialis

teres major

brachioradialis

extensor carpi radialis

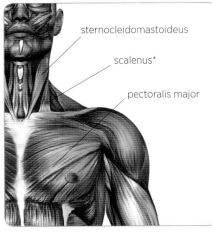

sternocleidomastoideus

scalenus*

pectoralis major

Annotation Key
Bold text indicates target muscles
Light text indicates other working muscles
* indicates deep muscles

Stiff-Legged Dumbbell Deadlift

The Deadlift is a classic back-strengthener. This Stiff-Legged version targets the erector muscles in your back—which keep your spine straight and mobile—while also working your glutes and hamstrings.

HOW TO DO IT

- Hold a pair of dumbbells in front of your thighs, with your feet about shoulder-width apart, your knees bent, and your buttocks pushed out slightly.

- Keeping your back flat, lower your dumbbells toward the floor.

- Raise your torso as you bring the dumbbells slightly above your knees. Repeat for the recommended repetitions.

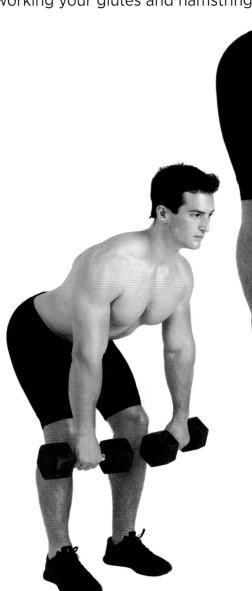

DO IT RIGHT

- Keep your back flat throughout the exercise.
- Gaze forward.
- Avoid arching or rounding your back.
- Avoid standing up completely on your torso-raise, to keep the tension on your hamstrings and glutes.

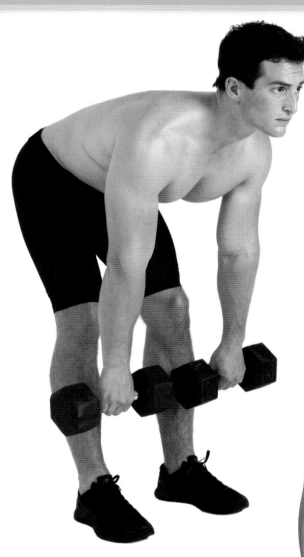

FACT FILE

TARGETS
• Spinal erectors
• Glutes
• Hamstrings

EQUIPMENT
• Dumbbells

BENEFITS
• Stretches and strengthens back
• Works hamstrings and glutes
• Improves lower-body flexibility

CAUTIONS
• Lower-back issues

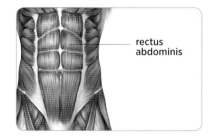

rectus abdominis

Annotation Key

Bold text indicates target muscles
Light text indicates other working muscles
* indicates deep muscles

gluteus medius*

obliquus externus

rhomboideus*

trapezius

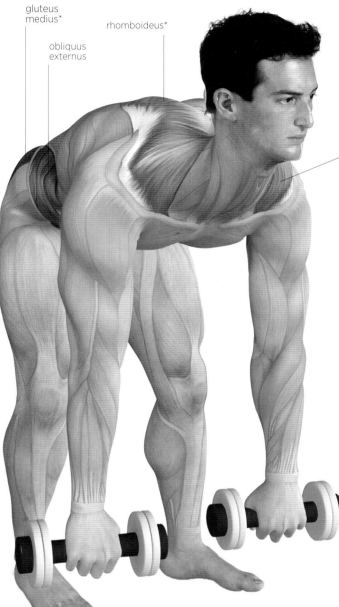

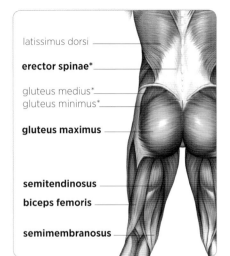

latissimus dorsi

erector spinae*

gluteus medius*
gluteus minimus*

gluteus maximus

semitendinosus

biceps femoris

semimembranosus

Dumbbell Upright Row

This exercise is another good one for the trapezius. Its "rowing" action—as if pulling oars—also strengthens deeper back muscles, your deltoids, and your biceps.

HOW TO DO IT

• Stand, holding a pair of dumbbells in front of your thighs, with your feet about shoulder-width apart.

• Bend your elbows to the side as you raise your weights, aiming for shoulder height.

• Lower the dumbbells to your starting position. Repeat for the recommended repetitions.

DO IT RIGHT

• Keep your torso stable, your back straight, and your abs engaged.
• Lead with your elbows.
• Avoid swinging your weights; instead, move slowly and with control.
• Avoid arching your back or slumping forward.

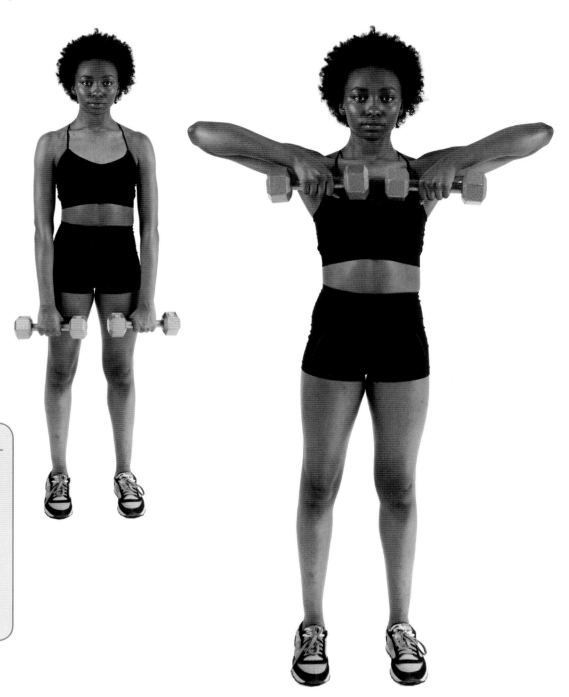

FACT FILE

TARGETS
- Upper back
- Shoulders

EQUIPMENT
- Dumbbells

BENEFITS
- Strengthens muscles in upper back and shoulders

CAUTIONS
- Shoulder issues

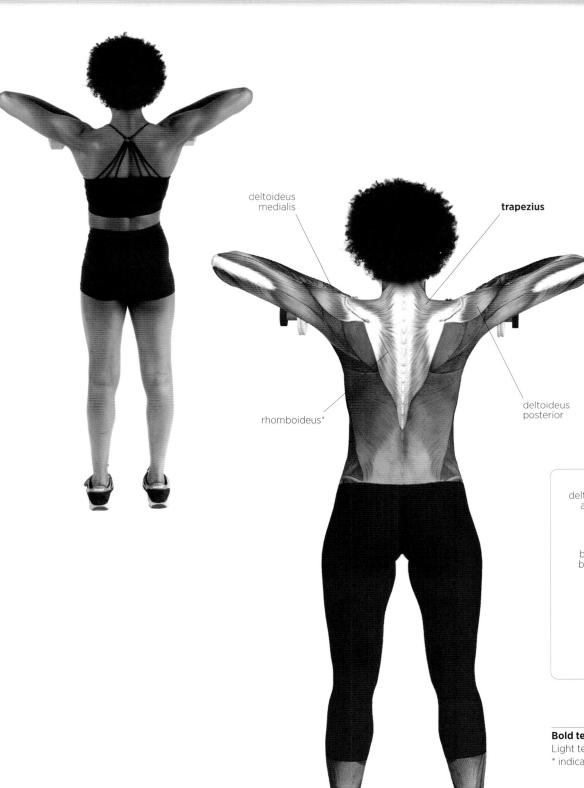

deltoideus medialis

trapezius

rhomboideus*

deltoideus posterior

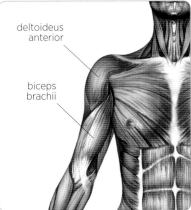

deltoideus anterior

biceps brachii

Annotation Key

Bold text indicates target muscles
Light text indicates other working muscles
* indicates deep muscles

Standing Single-Leg Row

Standing Single-Leg Rows work the latissimus dorsi—the major muscle that crosses your back—and so bring huge benefits to that part of your body. They also stabilize your shoulder joints, which in turn helps your back.

HOW TO DO IT

• Stand, holding a dumbbell in your right hand, with your feet about shoulder-width apart.

• Extend your right leg behind you. At the same time, lean forward, extending your left arm in front of you for balance. Try to bend your left leg slightly, or if it's straighter make sure it's not stiffly locked out.

• Bend your right elbow as you lift your weight upward into the row (pull-back) position.

• Lower and extend your right arm down again. Repeat the up-down rowing (pulling) arm movement for the recommended repetitions.

• Return to your upright starting position and repeat on the opposite side. Repeat for the recommended repetitions on each arm.

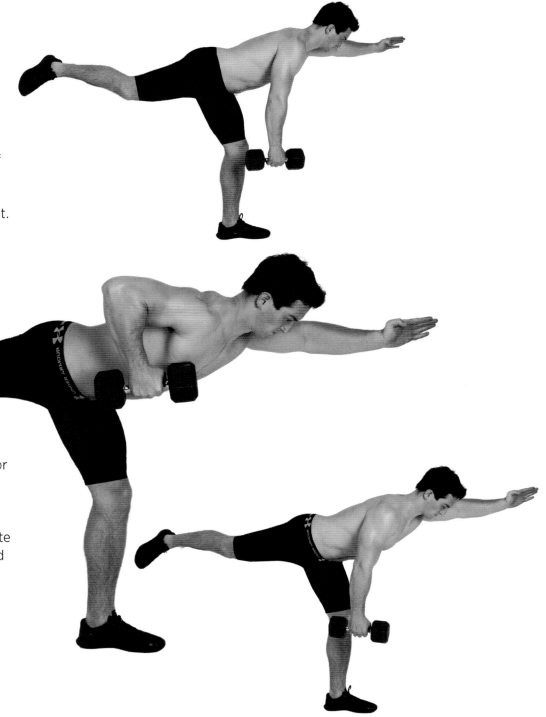

TARGETS
- Latissimus muscle of the back
- Rotator cuff muscles
- Elbow flexors

EQUIPMENT
- Dumbbells/ Swiss ball for modification

BENEFITS
- Strengthens back
- Stabilizes and strengthens shoulders, torso, and arms
- Improves balance

CAUTIONS
- Lower-back issues

DO IT RIGHT
- Keep your back flat.
- Move smoothly and with control.
- Gaze toward the floor.
- Contract your arm muscles when in the row position with your weight lifted.
- Keep your standing foot anchored into the floor.
- Avoid arching your back, or curving it forward.
- Avoid losing your balance.
- Avoid straining your neck by trying to look forward.

MODIFICATION
EASIER: For help with balance, rest one arm on top of a Swiss ball as you carry out the row.

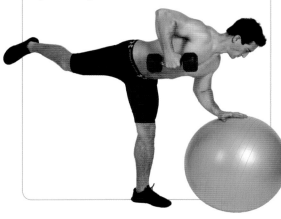

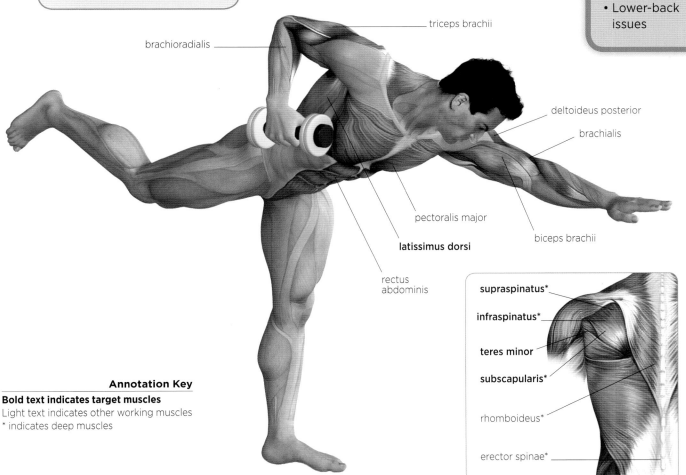

brachioradialis

triceps brachii

deltoideus posterior

brachialis

pectoralis major

biceps brachii

latissimus dorsi

rectus abdominis

supraspinatus*

infraspinatus*

teres minor

subscapularis*

rhomboideus*

erector spinae*

Annotation Key
Bold text indicates target muscles
Light text indicates other working muscles
* indicates deep muscles

Alternating Floor Row

Keep your focus and balance steady as you work this floor-row exercise. Designed to target the middle of your back, it works major interconnected muscles so that it also delivers for your shoulders and core.

HOW TO DO IT

• Begin in Plank position (pages 114–115), with a dumbbell in each hand. Your hands should be planted shoulder-width apart, palms facing each other.

• Using a "rowing" pull-back motion, pull your right-hand dumbbell into your chest.

• Lower and repeat with the opposite arm. Repeat the recommended repetitions on each arm.

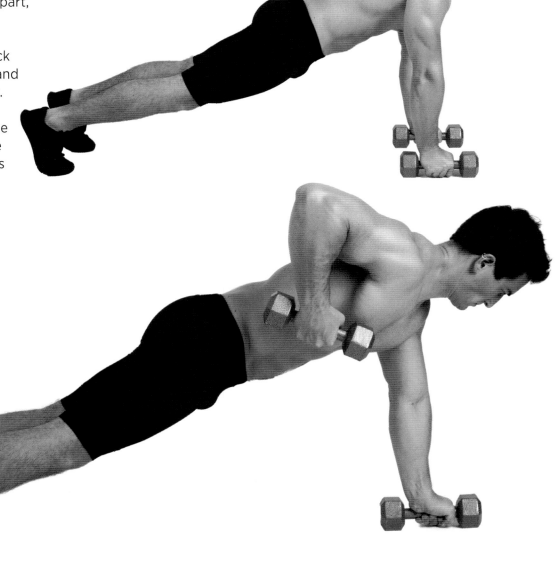

DO IT RIGHT

- Keep your core straight.
- Move your arms smoothly and with control.
- Engage your abs and keep your torso stable.
- Keep your neck elongated and your gaze downward.
- Avoid rushing the exercise.
- Avoid using momentum to drive the movement.
- Avoid allowing your lower back to sag.

FACT FILE

TARGETS
- Mid-back
- Core
- Shoulders

EQUIPMENT
- Dumbbells

BENEFITS
- Strengthens middle part of back
- Strengthens shoulders
- Stabilizes core

CAUTIONS
- Lower-back issues

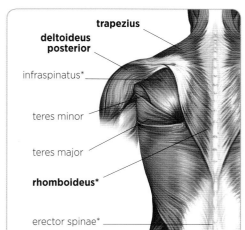

trapezius
deltoideus posterior
infraspinatus*
teres minor
teres major
rhomboideus*
erector spinae*

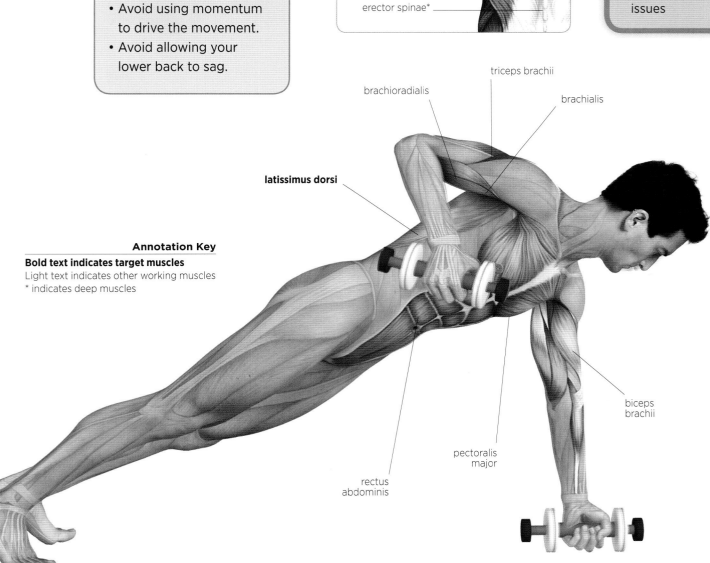

triceps brachii
brachioradialis
brachialis
latissimus dorsi
biceps brachii
pectoralis major
rectus abdominis

Annotation Key
Bold text indicates target muscles
Light text indicates other working muscles
* indicates deep muscles

Swiss Ball Pullover

Pullovers are great for your back, shoulders, chest, and arms, and this version really builds durability into your upper back, targeting its latissimus muscle. Using a Swiss ball adds some instability, forcing you to keep everything engaged and steady.

HOW TO DO IT

• Lie faceup on your Swiss ball, with your upper back, neck, and head supported. Your torso should be stretched out, and your knees bent to as near a 90-degree angle as possible. Plant your feet a little wider than shoulder-width apart.

• Grasp a dumbbell in each hand and extend your arms behind you as far as is comfortable. Do not extend your arms past the point at which they are level with your shoulders, with your body forming a straight line from knees to hands.

• Keeping the rest of your body stable and your arms as straight as possible, raise your arms upward so that they are perpendicular to your body.

• Return your arms to your starting position. Repeat for the recommended repetitions.

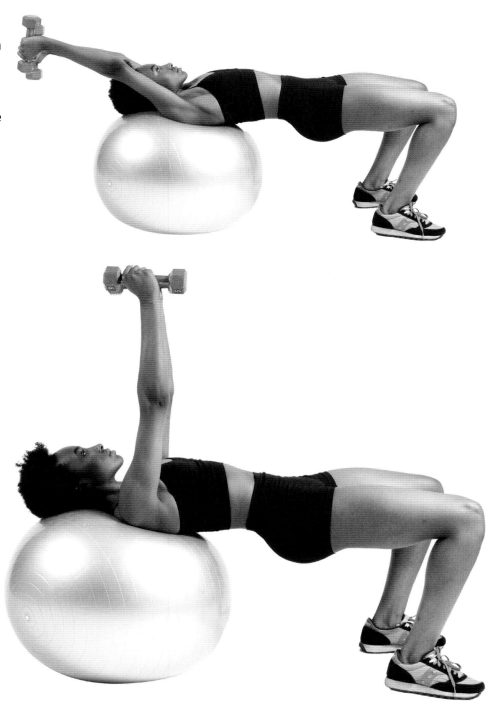

DO IT RIGHT

- Ease into the movement.
- Keep your arms directly above your shoulders when lifting the weights overhead.
- Keep your torso stable and feet planted throughout the exercise.
- Engage your abs.
- Keep your buttocks and pelvis lifted so that your upper legs, torso, and neck form a straight line.
- Move your arms smoothly and with control.
- Avoid locking your arms when they are extended behind your head.
- Avoid arching your back.
- Avoid rushing the exercise.

Annotation Key
Bold text indicates target muscles
Light text indicates other working muscles
* indicates deep muscles

MODIFICATION

SIMILAR DIFFICULTY: Instead of using dumbbells, grasp a medicine ball in your hands as you perform the exercise.

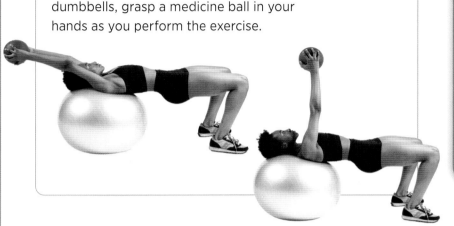

TARGETS
- Upper back
- Core

EQUIPMENT
- Dumbbells
- Swiss ball
- Medicine ball for modification

BENEFITS
- Strengthens upper back
- Stabilizes core

CAUTIONS
- Shoulder issues

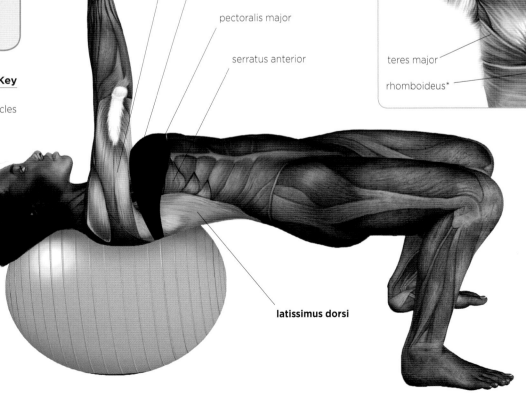

triceps brachii

pectoralis minor*

pectoralis major

serratus anterior

levator scapulae*

deltoideus posterior

teres major

rhomboideus*

latissimus dorsi

Alternating Kettlebell Row

Also known as Bent-Over Row, Kettlebell Alternating Row, and Alternating Bent-Over Row, this exercise targets your back—especially the middle—while building up strength in your core, shoulders, arms, and thighs.

HOW TO DO IT

- Stand, holding a pair of kettlebells, with your feet shoulder-width apart. Bend forward slightly at the waist, maintaining a flat back.

- Bend your arm at the elbow, pull your right hand up toward your abdomen, then lower it again.

- Pull your left hand up, then lower it. Continue alternating sides for the recommended repetitions.

DO IT RIGHT

- Maintain a flat back during the exercise.
- Avoid rotating your core.

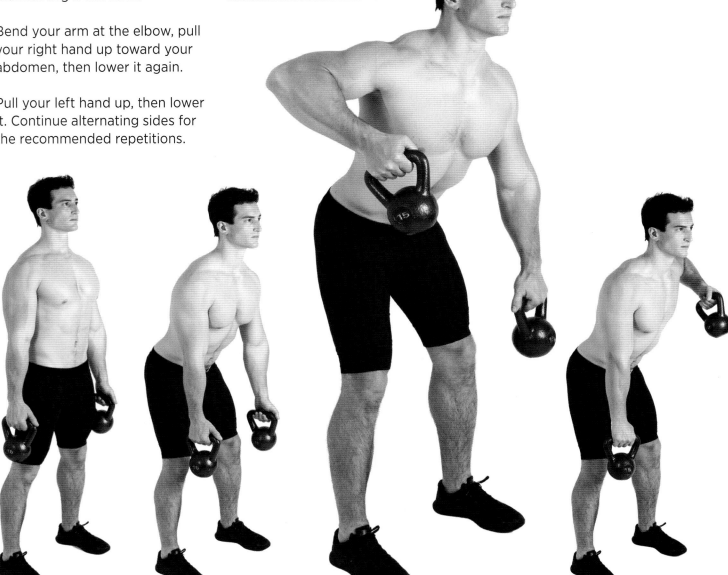

FACT FILE

TARGETS
- Middle back
- Latissimus dorsi

EQUIPMENT
- Kettlebells

BENEFITS
- Strengthens middle back

CAUTIONS
- If you're new to kettlebell exercises, seek advice from a fitness professional

MODIFICATION

EASIER: Lift with both arms at the same time (below).

HARDER: Raise one leg off the floor.

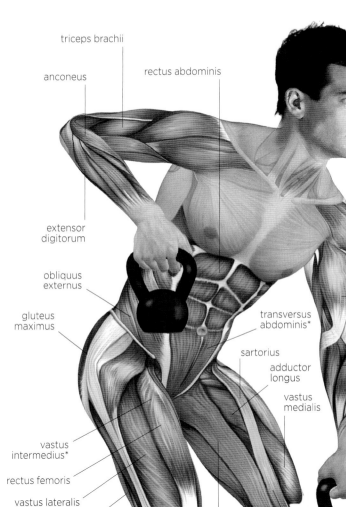

triceps brachii

anconeus

rectus abdominis

extensor digitorum

obliquus externus

gluteus maximus

transversus abdominis*

sartorius

adductor longus

vastus medialis

deltoideus medialis

deltoideus anterior

biceps brachii

palmaris longus

flexor digitorum*

vastus intermedius*

rectus femoris

vastus lateralis

biceps femoris

gracilis*

adductor magnus

semitendinosus

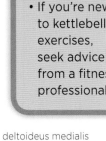

trapezius

rhomboideus*

latissimus dorsi

erector spinae*

multifidus spinae*

Annotation Key

Bold text indicates target muscles
Light text indicates other working muscles
* indicates deep muscles

Barbell Deadlift

This deadlift homes in on the deep erector muscles that move and straighten your spine. You'll find it also benefits much of the rest of your body, from your glutes, quads, and hamstrings to your core and arms.

HOW TO DO IT

- Stand behind a barbell with your feet shoulder-width apart. Looking straight ahead, squat down and grab the barbell with a wide overhand grip. Your legs must be close to the bar.

- Push through your heels as you stand upright while holding the barbell below you, at arms' length. Keep your back as straight as possible throughout this movement.

- Stand fully upright while holding the completed movement, then carefully lower the barbell to the ground. Repeat for the recommended repetitions.

DO IT RIGHT

- Use your glutes to help with the movement.
- Avoid overarching your back.

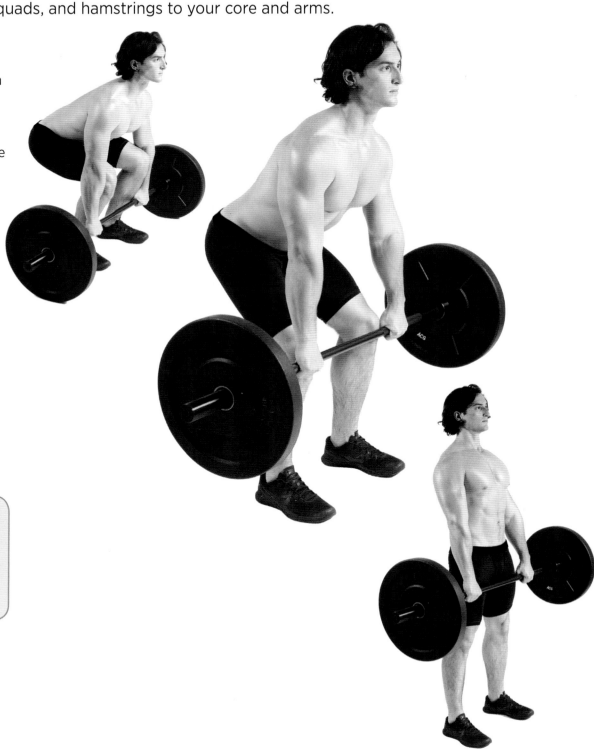

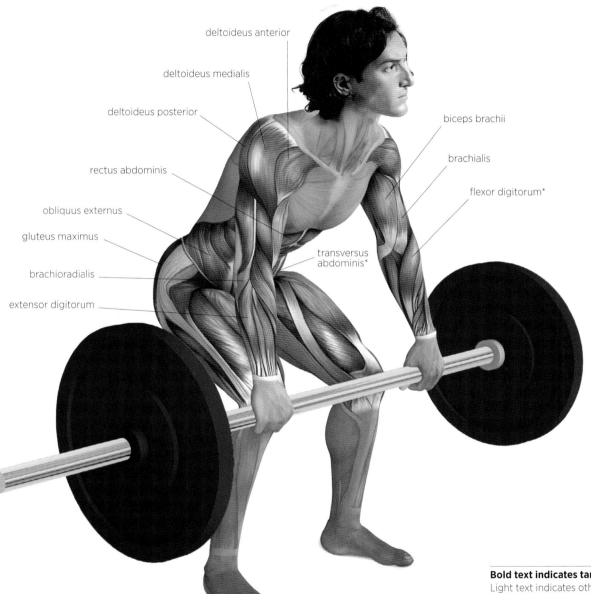

deltoideus anterior

deltoideus medialis

deltoideus posterior

rectus abdominis

obliquus externus

gluteus maximus

brachioradialis

extensor digitorum

biceps brachii

brachialis

flexor digitorum*

transversus
abdominis*

FACT FILE

TARGETS
• Spinal erector
muscles

EQUIPMENT
• Barbell

BENEFITS
• Increases
strength,
power, and
mass in back
and torso

CAUTIONS
• Important:
Check with
your doctor
before
performing
this exercise
• Any back
issues
• Take care
to build up
gradually
from lesser
to greater
weights

Annotation Key

Bold text indicates target muscles
Light text indicates other working muscles
* indicates deep muscles

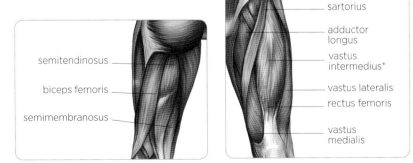

semitendinosus

biceps femoris

semimembranosus

sartorius

adductor
longus

vastus
intermedius*

vastus lateralis

rectus femoris

vastus
medialis

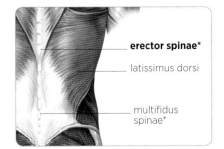

erector spinae*

latissimus dorsi

multifidus
spinae*

Lower-Back Extension

Lumbar problems are common when exercising, so it's smart to include a lower-back-isolation exercise in your fitness routine. The Lower-Back Extension eases lumbar issues by strengthening your lower back and glutes. It also works other areas that support back health.

HOW TO DO IT

- Stand with your arms by your sides, holding a dumbbell in each hand.

- While keeping your legs straight, lean forward and reach toward your toes. Try to touch the dumbbells to the floor with your legs straight.

- Stand back up to your starting position. Repeat for the recommended repetitions.

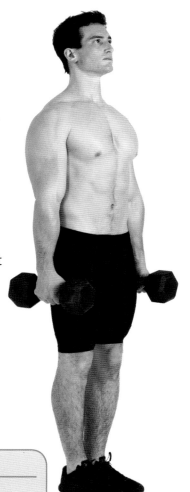

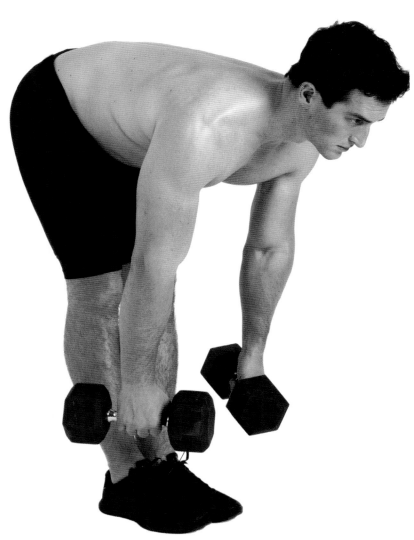

DO IT RIGHT
- As you lean forward, shift your weight to your heels.
- Contract your abdominal muscles as you bend forward and rise back up.
- Avoid jerky movements— keep your movements smooth and controlled.

TARGETS
- Lower back
- Glutes
- Hamstrings
- Upper body and core
- Calves

EQUIPMENT
- Dumbbells

BENEFITS
- Strengthens lower-back muscles
- Strengthens glutes
- Increases hamstring flexibility

CAUTIONS
- Any lower-back issues
- Important: Check with your doctor before performing this exercise

MODIFICATION

EASIER: Perform the exercise without dumbbells, trying to touch your fingers to the floor instead—or as far as you can go.

obliquus externus

erector spinae*

rhomboideus*

obliquus internus*

deltoideus anterior

gastrocnemius

soleus

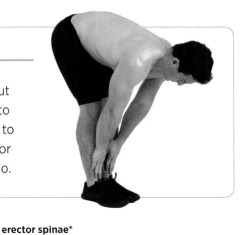

gluteus minimus*

gluteus medius*

gluteus maximus

semitendinosus

biceps femoris

semimembranosus

Annotation Key

Bold text indicates target muscles
Light text indicates other working muscles
* indicates deep muscles

Shoulder Press

The Shoulder Press effectively focuses on your deltoids and triceps. It is also an excellent general strengthener for the top part of your arms and upper body.

HOW TO DO IT

- Stand with your arms by your sides, holding a dumbbell in each hand. Your legs and feet should be together, with your spine and pelvis in a neutral position—relaxed but upright and not slouching.

- Extend your arms out to your sides at shoulder level.

- Bend your elbows so that your arms form roughly 90-degree angles, with palms facing forward. This is your starting position.

- Keeping your shoulder blades pressed firmly down your back, raise your arms overhead so that the weights meet.

- Open and lower your arms back to your starting position. Repeat for the recommended repetitions.

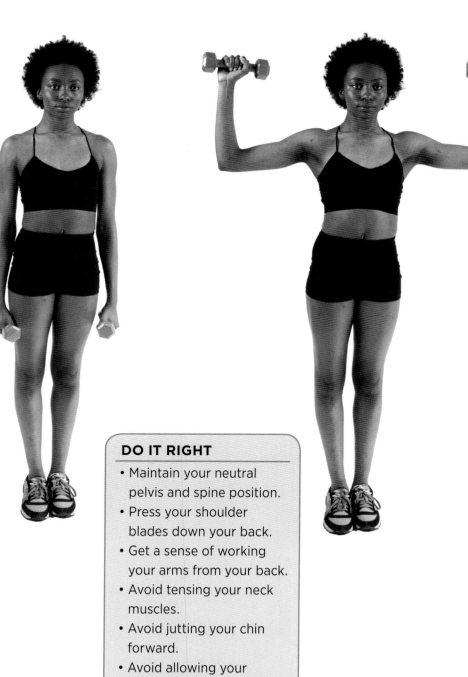

DO IT RIGHT

- Maintain your neutral pelvis and spine position.
- Press your shoulder blades down your back.
- Get a sense of working your arms from your back.
- Avoid tensing your neck muscles.
- Avoid jutting your chin forward.
- Avoid allowing your elbows to sink below shoulder height.

FACT FILE

TARGETS
- Deltoids
- Triceps
- Chest

EQUIPMENT
- Dumbbells

BENEFITS
- Strengthens arms
- Develops shoulder muscles
- Opens and stretches chest

CAUTIONS
- Elbow issues
- Shoulder injury

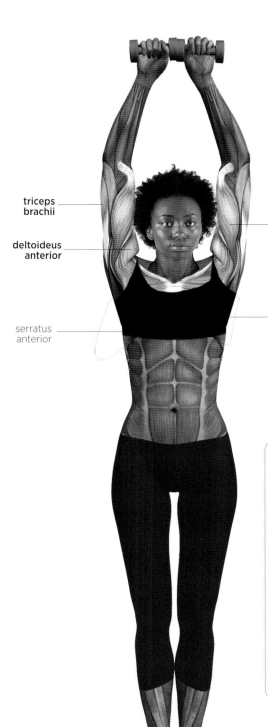

triceps brachii

deltoideus anterior

serratus anterior

biceps brachii

pectoralis major

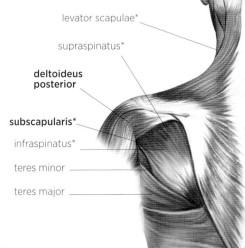

levator scapulae*

supraspinatus*

deltoideus posterior

subscapularis*

infraspinatus*

teres minor

teres major

Annotation Key

Bold text indicates target muscles
Light text indicates other working muscles
* indicates deep muscles

Shoulder Flexing

Shoulder flexion means moving your arms up and in front of you as you bend your shoulder joint. Shoulder Flexing is a resistance exercise that strengthens your shoulders while increasing their range of motion.

HOW TO DO IT

- Stand with your legs and feet together. Hold a dumbbell in each hand, with your arms down in front of your body.

- Keeping your arms straight, lift both arms up in front of you, to around shoulder height.

- Lower both arms slowly back down to your starting position. Repeat for the recommended repetitions.

DO IT RIGHT

- Bring the dumbbells down close to your body, but do not rest them against it between repetitions.
- Avoid jerking your lower back to get the weights to shoulder height.

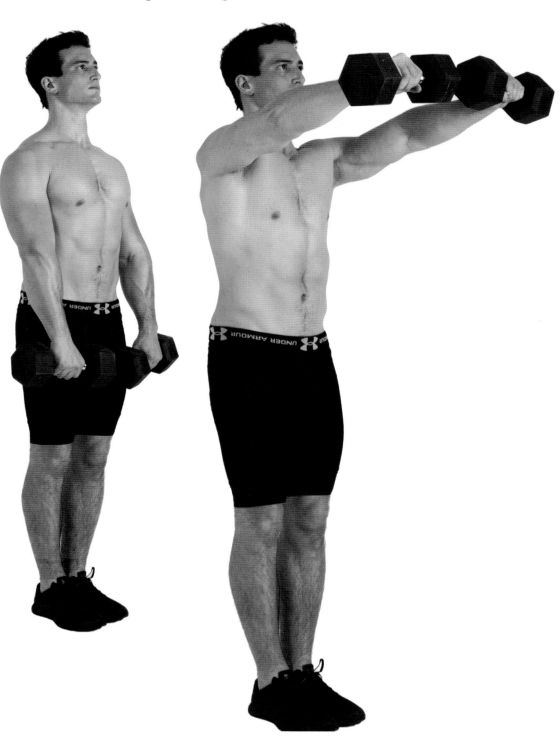

FACT FILE

TARGETS
- Deltoids
- Upper back

EQUIPMENT
- Dumbbells

BENEFITS
- Stabilizes and strengthens shoulder muscles
- Stabilizes upper-back muscles
- Increases Push-Up strength

CAUTIONS
- Lower-back issues

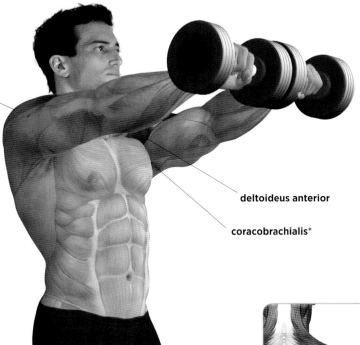

deltoideus medialis

deltoideus anterior

coracobrachialis*

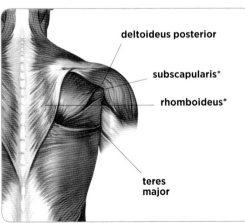

deltoideus posterior

subscapularis*

rhomboideus*

teres major

Annotation Key

Bold text indicates target muscles
Light text indicates other working muscles
* indicates deep muscles

Lateral Shoulder Raise

Here you are primarily targeting the lateral, or side, part of your deltoids. As the name suggests, the lateral deltoid—scientific term, deltoideus medialis—lets you move your shoulder out to the side.

HOW TO DO IT

• Stand with your arms by your sides, holding a dumbbell in each hand. Your feet should be shoulder-width apart.

• Extend your arms out to your sides at shoulder level, elbows very slightly bent. Your arms must be in line with your shoulders, elbows not dropped too far, so that you work your lateral deltoids more than your anterior (front) deltoids.

• Slowly lower the dumbbells back to your starting position. Repeat for the recommended repetitions.

DO IT RIGHT

• Keep your elbows in a fixed and slightly bent position throughout.
• Make sure your elbows are in line with your shoulders in the raised position.
• Keep your chest elevated and your shoulders down and back away from your ears.
• Avoid using momentum to lift the dumbbells.
• Avoid letting your elbows drop much lower than your wrists in the raised position.

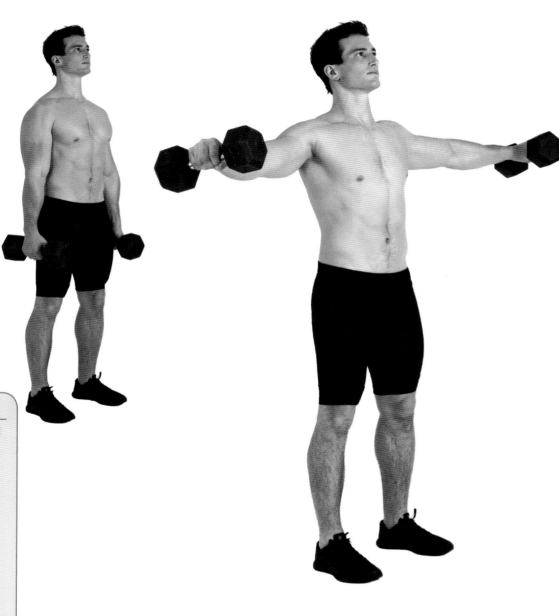

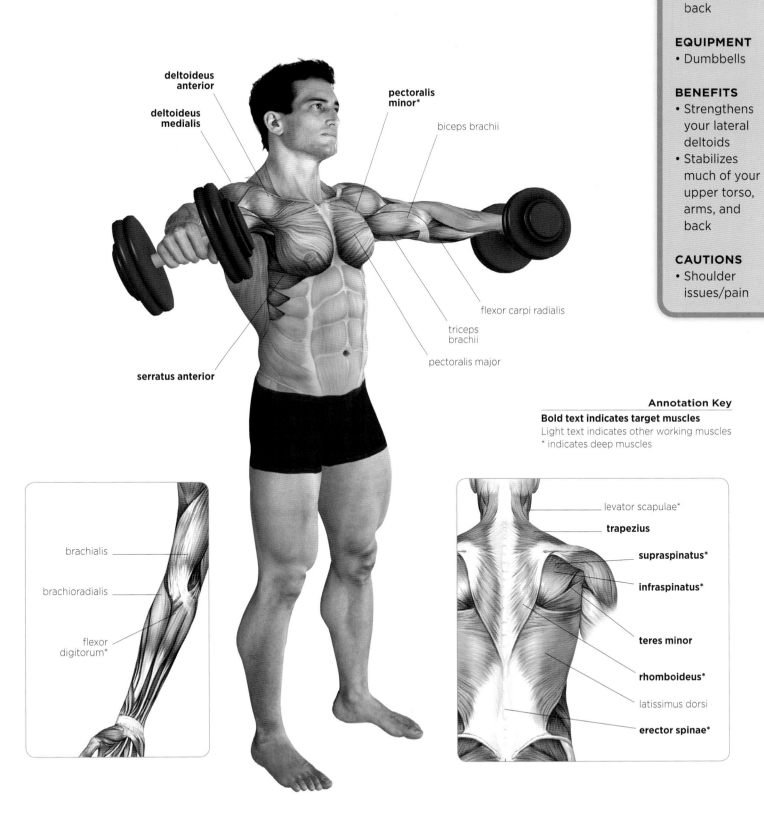

deltoideus anterior

deltoideus medialis

pectoralis minor*

biceps brachii

serratus anterior

flexor carpi radialis

triceps brachii

pectoralis major

brachialis

brachioradialis

flexor digitorum*

FACT FILE

TARGETS
• Lateral deltoids
• Shoulders in general, chest, back

EQUIPMENT
• Dumbbells

BENEFITS
• Strengthens your lateral deltoids
• Stabilizes much of your upper torso, arms, and back

CAUTIONS
• Shoulder issues/pain

Annotation Key

Bold text indicates target muscles
Light text indicates other working muscles
* indicates deep muscles

levator scapulae*

trapezius

supraspinatus*

infraspinatus*

teres minor

rhomboideus*

latissimus dorsi

erector spinae*

Ballet Biceps

Ballet Biceps is a variation on the Shoulder Press (pages 152–153). This time, you use rounded arms to curve up, instead of angular ones that press up. Your upward position should resemble the fifth position in ballet.

HOW TO DO IT

• Stand with your arms by your sides, holding a dumbbell in each hand. Your legs and feet should be together, with your spine and pelvis in a neutral position—relaxed but upright and not slouching.

• Extend your arms out to your sides at shoulder level, palms facing up. This is your starting position. Relax your elbows slightly so your arms form gentle, though strong, curves.

• Keep your shoulder blades pressed firmly down your back. Raise your arms up and around in smooth arcs until they frame your head and the weights meet overhead, palms facing down.

• Open and lower your arms back to your starting position. Repeat for the recommended repetitions.

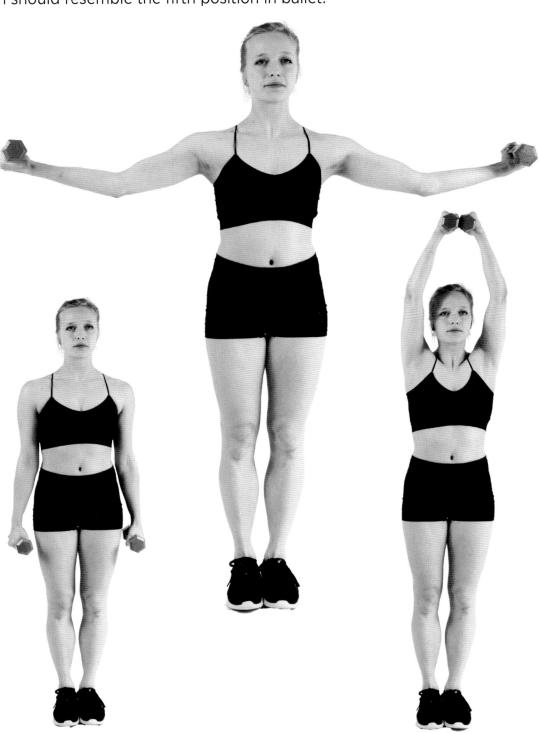

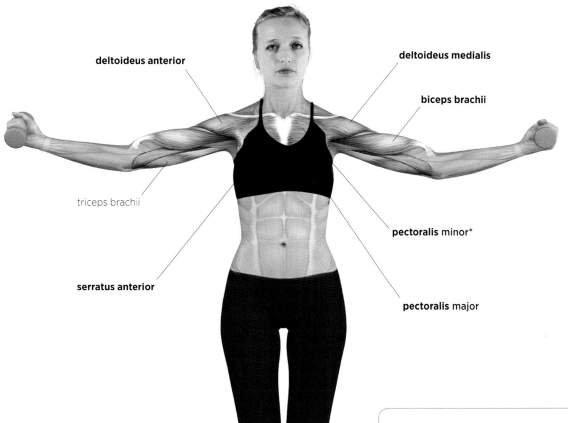

deltoideus anterior

deltoideus medialis

biceps brachii

triceps brachii

pectoralis minor*

serratus anterior

pectoralis major

DO IT RIGHT

• Maintain your neutral pelvis and spine position.
• Stabilize your shoulders down your back.
• Hold the shape of your arms strongly.
• Avoid tensing your neck muscles.
• Avoid lifting your shoulders.
• Avoid rolling your shoulders forward.

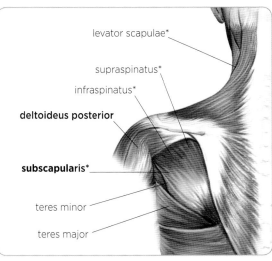

levator scapulae*

supraspinatus*

infraspinatus*

deltoideus posterior

subscapularis*

teres minor

teres major

Annotation Key

Bold text indicates target muscles
Light text indicates other working muscles
* indicates deep muscles

Alternating Hammer Curl

Hammer exercises are named for the working grip they use. This is a neutral grip, palms facing, that's rather like grasping a hammer's handle—as opposed to an underhand grip. Hammer curls work your arms differently than underhand curls.

HOW TO DO IT

- Stand with your arms by your sides, holding a dumbbell in each hand. Your feet should be shoulder-width apart and your pelvis slightly tucked in. Ideally, bend your knees very slightly.

- Check you're holding your dumbbells with a hammer-grip grasp, palms facing inward. Your elbows should be close to your torso.

- With your upper arms remaining stationary, flex from the elbow to curl the right dumbbell toward your upper chest.

- Slowly lower the weight back to your starting position, and repeat on the opposite side. Alternate sides for the recommended repetitions.

DO IT RIGHT
- Ensure your biceps are fully contracted at the top of the raise.
- Avoid using momentum to lift the weight—keep your torso upright and focus on isolating and engaging the biceps.
- Avoid bending at the wrists—keep them aligned with your forearms.

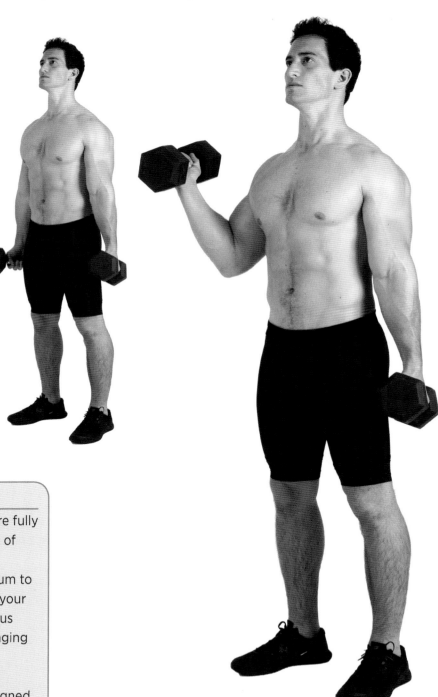

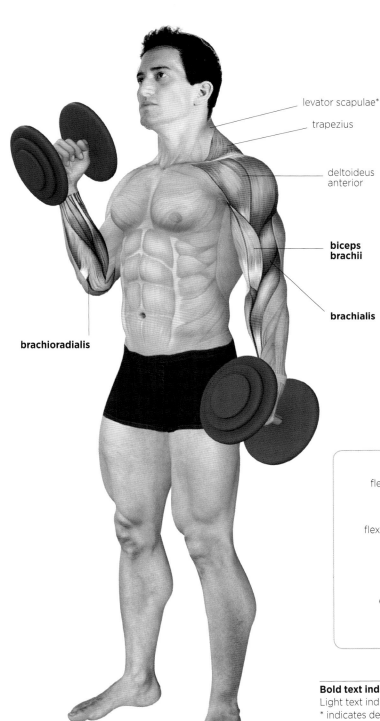

FACT FILE

TARGETS
- Biceps
- Elbow flexors

EQUIPMENT
- Dumbbells

BENEFITS
- Strengthens biceps and elbow flexors
- Stabilizes shoulders and wrist flexors

CAUTIONS
- Elbow injury/ issues
- Arm, wrist, or shoulder issues/pain

levator scapulae*

trapezius

deltoideus anterior

biceps brachii

brachialis

brachioradialis

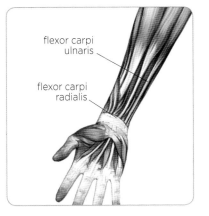

flexor carpi ulnaris

flexor carpi radialis

Annotation Key

Bold text indicates target muscles
Light text indicates other working muscles
* indicates deep muscles

Single-Arm Concentration Curl

The brachialis and brachioradialis—of your upper arm and forearm respectively—are flexors that play a major role when you bend your arm at the elbow. So, too, does the biceps, although this curl is especially effective for the brachialis.

HOW TO DO IT

- Sit facing forward on a bench with your legs spread generously, wider than shoulder width. Hold a dumbbell down in front of you in your right hand, between your legs.

- Rest the back of your right upper arm on your inner right thigh.

- With your right palm facing upward and your upper right arm stationary, curl the dumbbell forward and up toward your face, stopping at shoulder height. Pause slightly at the top and focus on contracting your biceps.

- Slowly lower the weight back to your starting position, and repeat for the recommended repetitions. Repeat on the opposite side for the recommended repetitions.

DO IT RIGHT

- When the arm is extended down in the starting position, the dumbbell should be a few inches from the floor.
- Keep your pinky finger higher than your thumb and squeeze your pinky—this ensures everything works properly.
- Avoid swinging motions during this exercise.
- Avoid bending your wrist—keep it aligned with your forearm.
- Avoid rolling your shoulder inward.

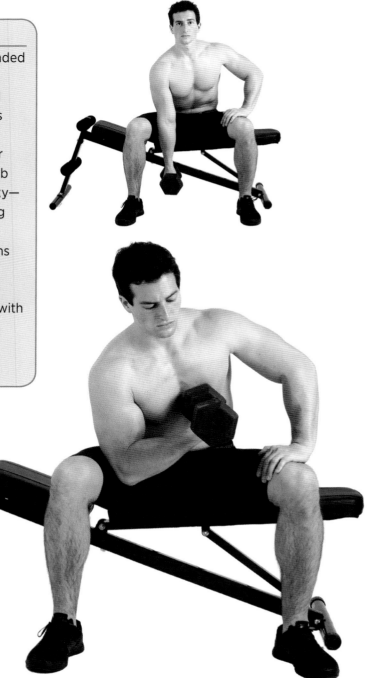

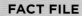

FACT FILE

TARGETS
- Elbow flexors
- Biceps

EQUIPMENT
- Dumbbells
- Bench/seat

BENEFITS
- Strengthens elbow flexors and biceps
- Stabilizes shoulders, back, obliques, and wrists

CAUTIONS
- Elbow injury/issues
- Wrist issues

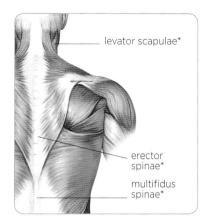

levator scapulae*

erector spinae*

multifidus spinae*

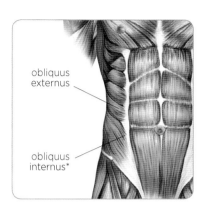

obliquus externus

obliquus internus*

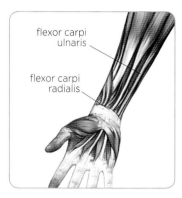

flexor carpi ulnaris

flexor carpi radialis

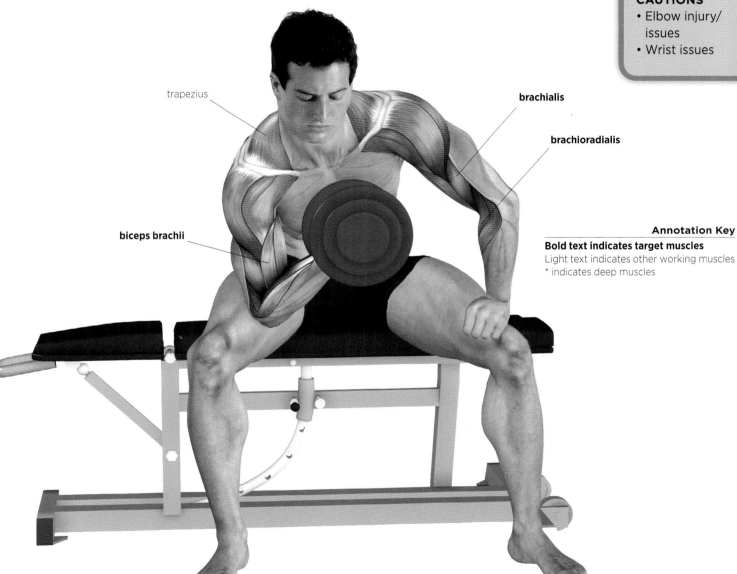

trapezius

brachialis

brachioradialis

biceps brachii

Annotation Key

Bold text indicates target muscles
Light text indicates other working muscles
* indicates deep muscles

Dumbbell Triceps Kickback

This Dumbbell Triceps Kickback is an excellent, simple exercise that strengthens and tones your triceps. Focus on keeping your core strong and your whole body stable, even while you're balanced on two legs and just one arm.

HOW TO DO IT

- Kneel on all fours, with your hands below your shoulders, fingers pointing forwards, and knees aligned under your hips. Your hips and spine should be in a neutral position, the tops of your feet on the floor, and your gaze toward the floor.

- Holding a dumbbell in your right hand, flex your elbow tightly into your side. Keep pressing your shoulder blades down your back.

- Slowly straighten your right arm out behind you, as if pulling on an elastic attached to the wall in front of you.

- Slowly flex your elbow forward again, controlling the movement all the way, and repeat for the recommended repetitions. Repeat on the opposite side for the recommended repetitions.

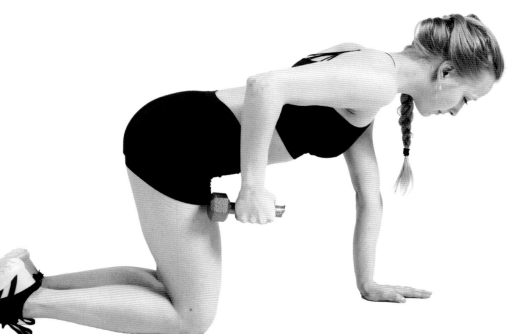

DO IT RIGHT

- Keep your pelvis and spine in a neutral position.
- Keep your line of sight toward the floor, so you don't shorten your cervical vertebrae.
- Hold your weight directly under your shoulder.
- Avoid swinging your arm to move from one position to the next.
- Avoid overextending your arm by locking your elbow.
- Avoid relaxing your abdominals.

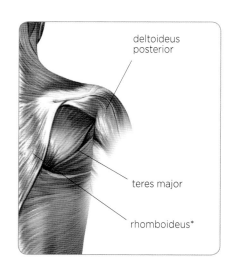

deltoideus posterior

teres major

rhomboideus*

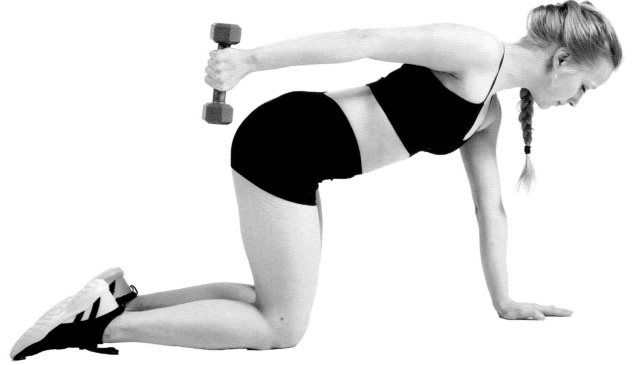

FACT FILE

TARGETS
• Triceps

EQUIPMENT
• Dumbbell

BENEFITS
• Strengthens triceps
• Develops control of upper body

CAUTIONS
• Elbow injury/ issues
• Lower-back issues

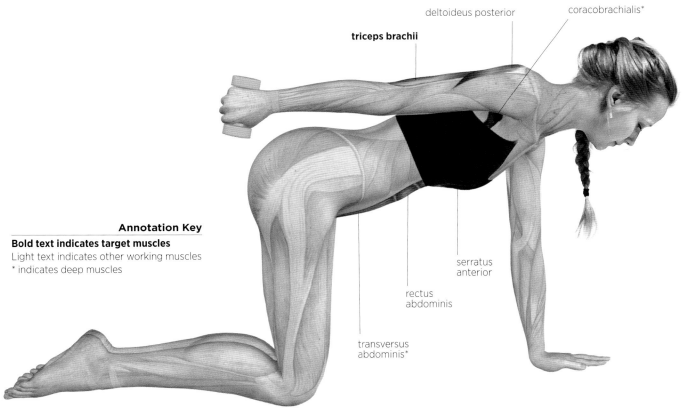

deltoideus posterior

coracobrachialis*

triceps brachii

serratus anterior

rectus abdominis

transversus abdominis*

Annotation Key
Bold text indicates target muscles
Light text indicates other working muscles
* indicates deep muscles

Alternating Kettlebell Press

Work your shoulders, back, and arms with Alternating Kettlebell Press. This exercise, also known as Kettlebell Shoulder Press and Kettlebell Alternating Military Press, offers an effective shoulder stability workout, as well as a cardio boost.

HOW TO DO IT

- Stand with your feet about shoulder-width apart, your knees slightly bent, and a pair of kettlebells on the floor in front of you. Reach down and pick them up.

- In a smooth, decisive motion, extend through your legs and hips as you lift the kettlebells up until they are cleaned to the sides of your shoulders.

- Raise the left kettlebell directly overhead until your arm locks out. Your wrist should be rotated so that your palm faces forward. Keep the other kettlebell as still as possible.

- Lower your left arm, turning your palm toward you, and repeat on the opposite side. Continue alternating sides for the recommended repetitions.

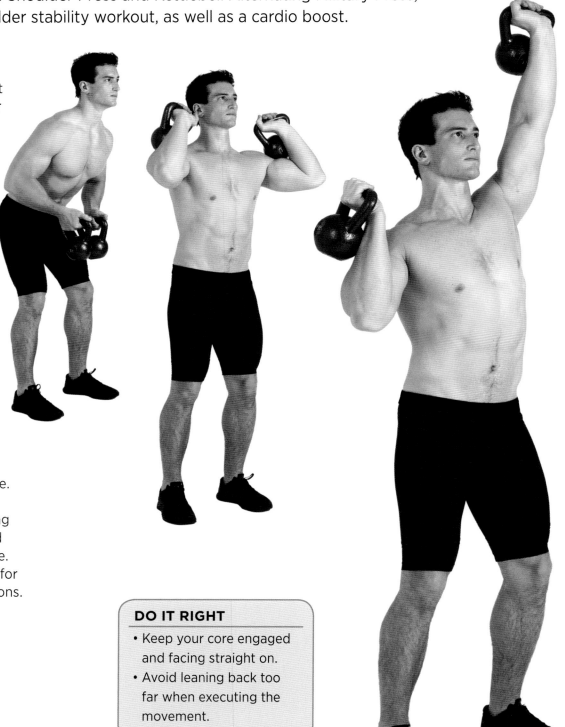

DO IT RIGHT
- Keep your core engaged and facing straight on.
- Avoid leaning back too far when executing the movement.

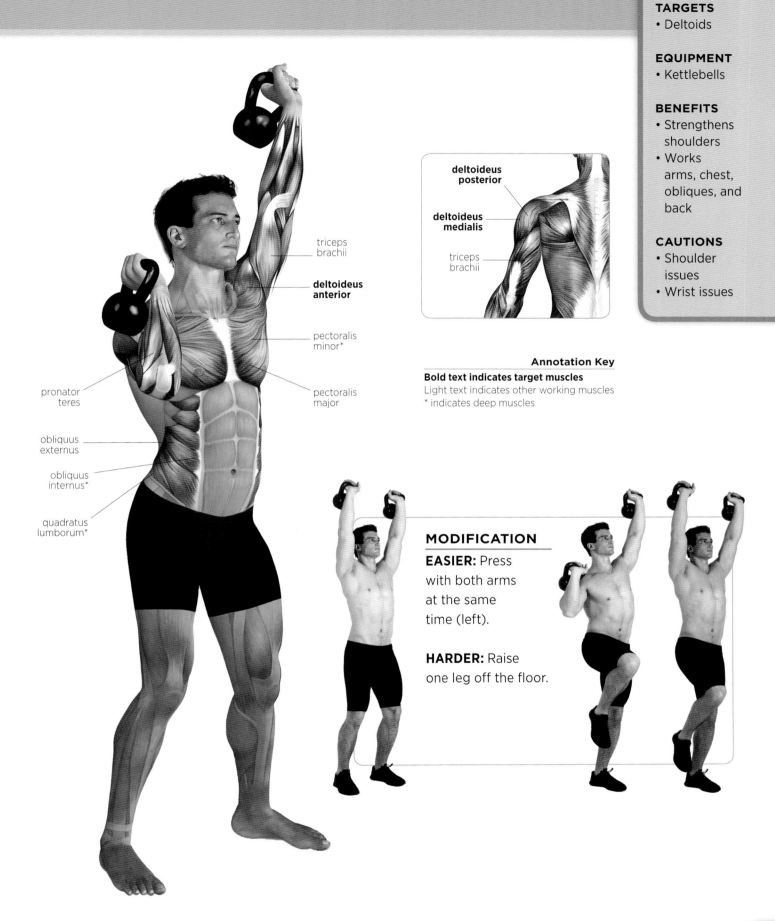

TARGETS
• Deltoids

EQUIPMENT
• Kettlebells

BENEFITS
• Strengthens shoulders
• Works arms, chest, obliques, and back

CAUTIONS
• Shoulder issues
• Wrist issues

triceps brachii

deltoideus anterior

pectoralis minor*

pronator teres

pectoralis major

obliquus externus

obliquus internus*

quadratus lumborum*

deltoideus posterior

deltoideus medialis

triceps brachii

Annotation Key
Bold text indicates target muscles
Light text indicates other working muscles
* indicates deep muscles

MODIFICATION

EASIER: Press with both arms at the same time (left).

HARDER: Raise one leg off the floor.

Bottom-Up Kettlebell Clean

This exercise is one for the forearms. Swinging the kettlebell backward, forward, and upward takes your arm and upper body through a good range of motion. The squeezing action is an excellent forearm-strengthener.

HOW TO DO IT

- Stand with your arms by your sides, holding a kettlebell in your left hand. Your feet should be about shoulder-width apart and your knees slightly bent.

- Swing the kettlebell backward, then bring it forward and above your head forcefully, squeezing the handle as you do so.

- Once your upper arm is parallel to the floor, hold the position, lower your arm, and repeat for the recommended repetitions. Repeat on the opposite side for the recommended repetitions.

DO IT RIGHT

- Keep your back straight throughout.
- Avoid adopting a loose grip.

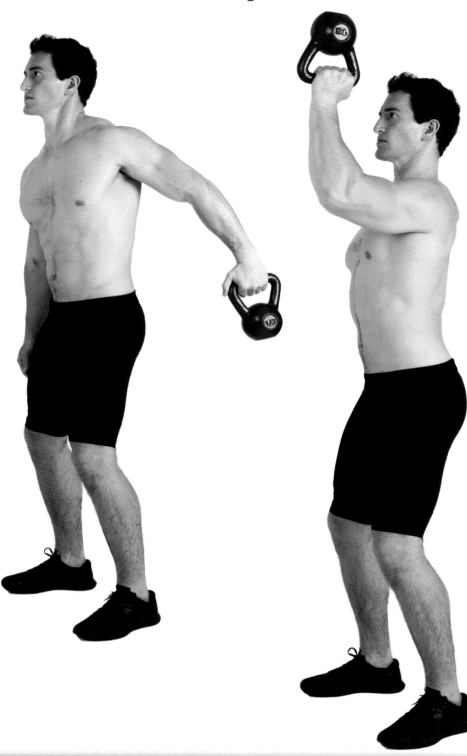

TARGETS
• Forearms

EQUIPMENT
• Kettlebell

BENEFITS
• Strengthens forearms
• Works shoulders, upper arms, and chest

CAUTIONS
• Arm or wrist issues/pain
• Shoulder issues

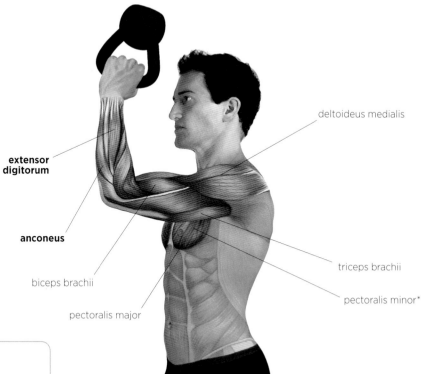

extensor digitorum

anconeus

biceps brachii

pectoralis major

deltoideus medialis

triceps brachii

pectoralis minor*

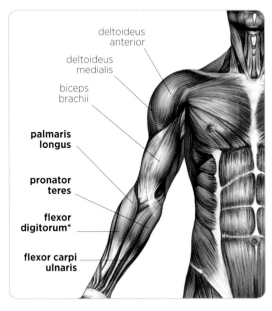

deltoideus anterior

deltoideus medialis

biceps brachii

palmaris longus

pronator teres

flexor digitorum*

flexor carpi ulnaris

MODIFICATION

EASIER: Try the exercise without a kettlebell.

Annotation Key

Bold text indicates target muscles

Light text indicates other working muscles

* indicates deep muscles

Standing Barbell Row

Performing an upright overhand row with a barbell isolates and powers up your shoulders, upper back, and upper arms. It also strengthens two muscles—teres minor and supraspinatus—belonging to the all-important rotator cuff, which stabilizes your shoulders.

HOW TO DO IT

- Stand, holding a barbell down in front of you with both hands, using an overhand grip. Your hands should be shoulder-width apart or slightly narrower, your feet shoulder-width apart, and your pelvis tucked in slightly.

- Rest the barbell against the top of your thighs, arms extended. Your back should be straight. Now bend your knees and arms slightly. This is your starting position.

- Focus on engaging your deltoids to lift the barbell to chest height. Pause at the top of the movement, return to your starting position, and repeat for the recommended repetitions.

DO IT RIGHT

- Make your elbows initiate the movement.
- Raise your elbows higher than your forearms.
- Keep the barbell close to your body as you move it.
- Keep your torso stationary.
- Avoid lifting very heavy weights with this exercise—this can lead to bad form and possible shoulder injury.

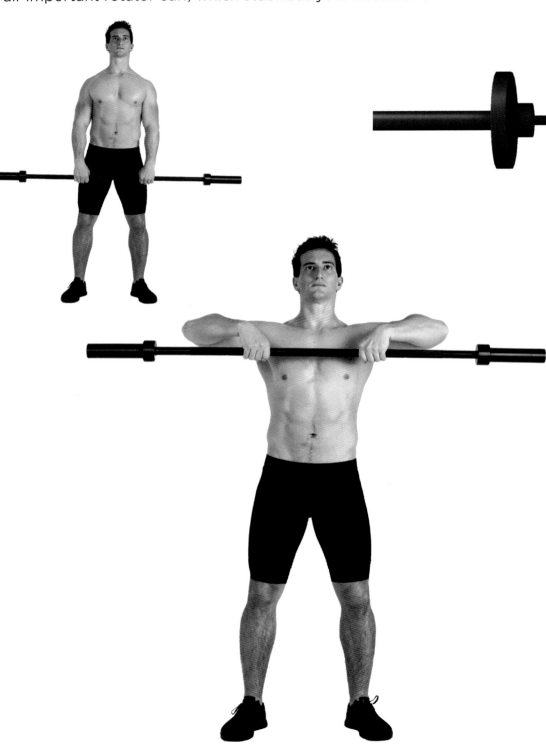

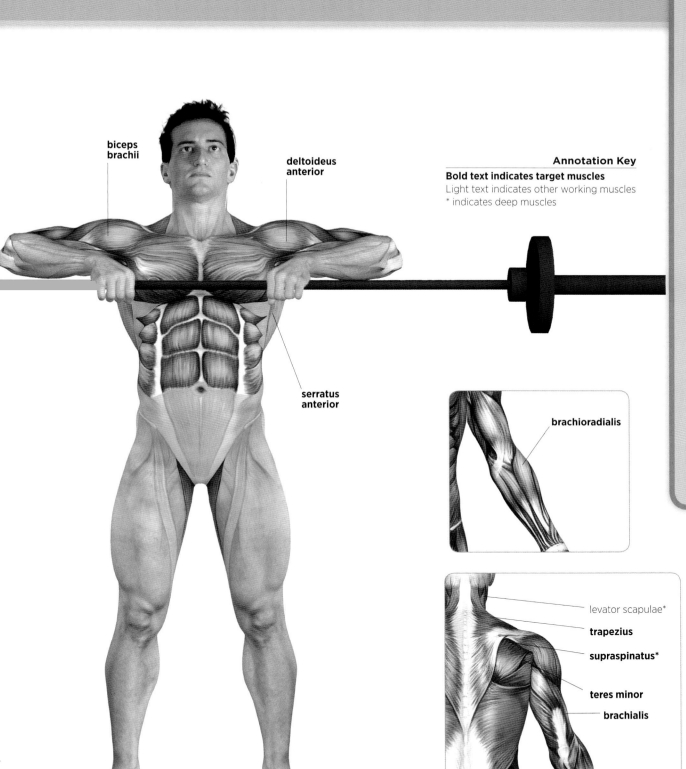

biceps brachii

deltoideus anterior

serratus anterior

brachioradialis

levator scapulae*

trapezius

supraspinatus*

teres minor

brachialis

Annotation Key

Bold text indicates target muscles

Light text indicates other working muscles

* indicates deep muscles

TARGETS

- Deltoids
- Upper trapezius
- Biceps
- Rotator cuff
- Elbow flexors

EQUIPMENT

- Barbell

BENEFITS

- Strengthens and stabilizes shoulders and upper back
- Strengthens biceps and elbow flexors
- Stabilizes the sides of the chest

CAUTIONS

- Shoulder pain/issues
- Wrist issues
- Elbow or upper-back issues

Barbell Curl

You will find the classic Barbell Curl in many arm-building workouts. It effectively targets your biceps, while relying on other arm and shoulder muscles as stabilizers.

HOW TO DO IT

- Stand, holding a barbell down in front of you with both hands, using an underhand grip. Your hands as well as your feet should be shoulder-width apart, your knees slightly bent, and your pelvis tucked in slightly.

- Keep your elbows as close to the sides of your body as possible. With your upper arms stationary, bend your arms at the elbow and curl the barbell up toward your upper chest.

- When the barbell is at the top of the movement, pause and then slowly lower it back down. Repeat for the recommended repetitions.

DO IT RIGHT

- Keep your upper arms stationary throughout.
- If you sway or lean backward, do the exercise leaning against a wall with your feet some way in front.
- Avoid bending at the wrists; keep them aligned with your forearms.
- Avoid raising your shoulders

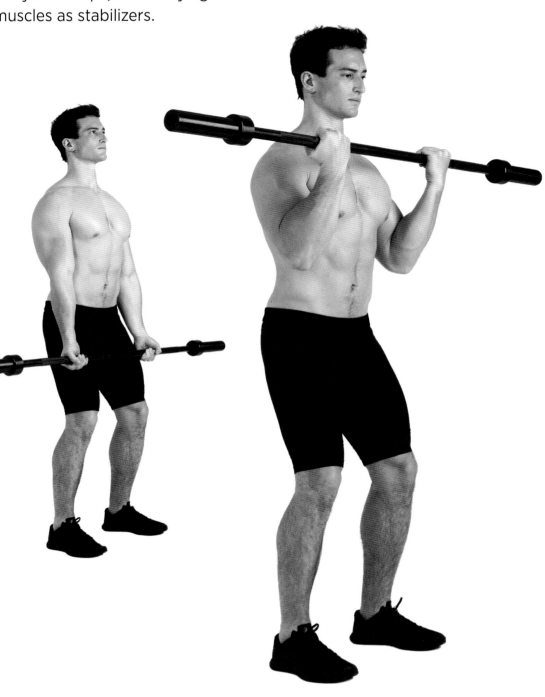

TARGETS
- Biceps
- Elbow flexors

EQUIPMENT
- Barbell

BENEFITS
- Increases biceps strength and mass

CAUTIONS
- Wrist issues

levator scapulae*

trapezius

deltoideus anterior

biceps brachii

brachialis

brachioradialis

flexor carpi ulnaris

flexor carpi radialis

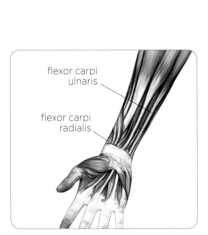

Annotation Key

Bold text indicates target muscles
Light text indicates other working muscles
* indicates deep muscles

MODIFICATION

SIMILAR DIFFICULTY: Perform the exercise using a narrower grip if you want to work the outside of your biceps more. However, this may be harder on your elbows and wrists.

HARDER: Try performing the exercise using a wider grip. This decreases your range of motion.

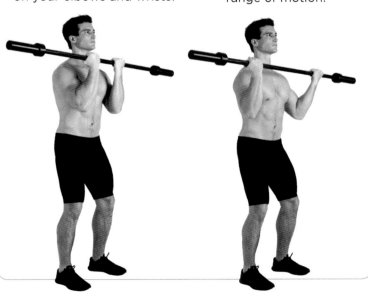

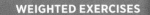

Zipper

Zipper is perfect for building strength in the chest, shoulders, and triceps. It also reinforces the connection between upper-body strength and lower-body stability. The movement imitates someone unzipping a jacket and then pulling it wide open.

HOW TO DO IT

- Stand with your arms by your sides, holding a dumbbell in each hand. Your legs should be together, with your spine and pelvis in a neutral position.

- Bend your elbows and bring your hands together about level with your bottom ribs.

- Move your elbows in close to your sides. This is your starting position.

- Keeping your fists together, "zip" down your body's midline, and then swing your arms out to your sides until level with your shoulders. Your palms should face backward.

- Keeping your shoulder blades pressed down your back, swing your arms down to your sides and back to your starting position. Building speed, repeat for the recommended repetitions.

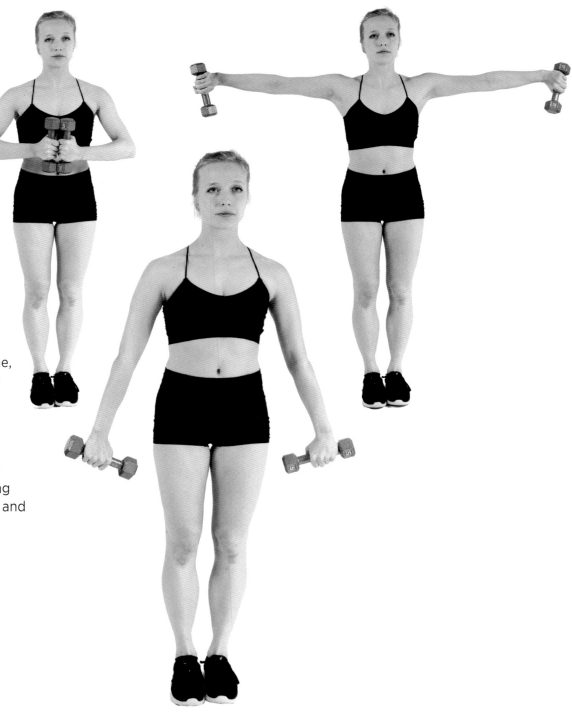

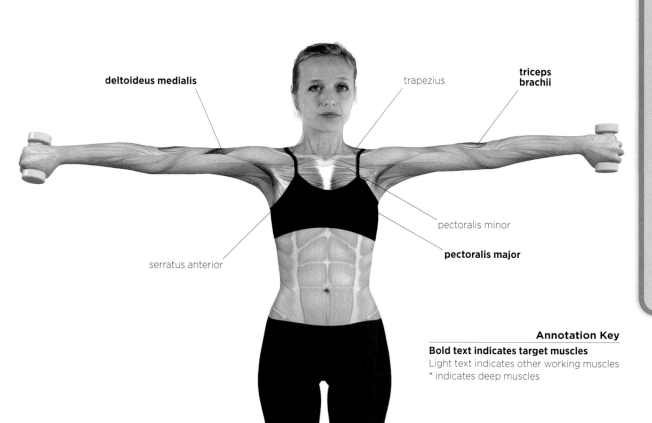

deltoideus medialis

trapezius

triceps brachii

pectoralis minor

serratus anterior

pectoralis major

FACT FILE

TARGETS
- Chest
- Shoulders
- Triceps

EQUIPMENT
- Dumbbells

BENEFITS
- Strengthens and tones chest
- Strengthens and tones upper arms and shoulders
- Promotes good posture

CAUTIONS
- Cervical vertebrae curvature
- Severe neck tension

Annotation Key
Bold text indicates target muscles
Light text indicates other working muscles
* indicates deep muscles

DO IT RIGHT
- Maintain your neutral posture.
- Press your shoulders down your back.
- Make the zipping movement strong.
- Keep your chest open.
- Avoid letting your shoulders roll forward.
- Avoid breaking your rhythm or losing momentum.
- Avoid "forgetting" to keep your lower body in pose.

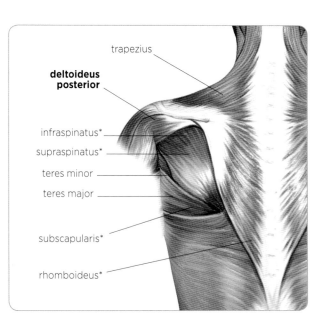

trapezius

deltoideus posterior

infraspinatus*

supraspinatus*

teres minor

teres major

subscapularis*

rhomboideus*

Hammer-Grip Press

This exercise uses the hammer grip—with palms facing—to focus primarily on your chest, especially the upper part. Your shoulders and triceps will benefit from this press, too.

HOW TO DO IT

- Sit on an incline bench, holding a pair of dumbbells on your thighs. This is your starting position.

- Kick up to give some momentum while leaning back on the bench and lift the dumbbells above your chest. Your palms should be facing each other in a hammer-grip position. Keep your elbows bent and your shoulder blades in contact with the bench.

- Raise the dumbbells toward the ceiling until they are directly above your shoulders. Your feet should be on the floor. Hold this top position for the recommended time.

- Slowly lower the dumbbells to your shoulders, and then bring the dumbbells back to your starting position. Repeat for the recommended repetitions.

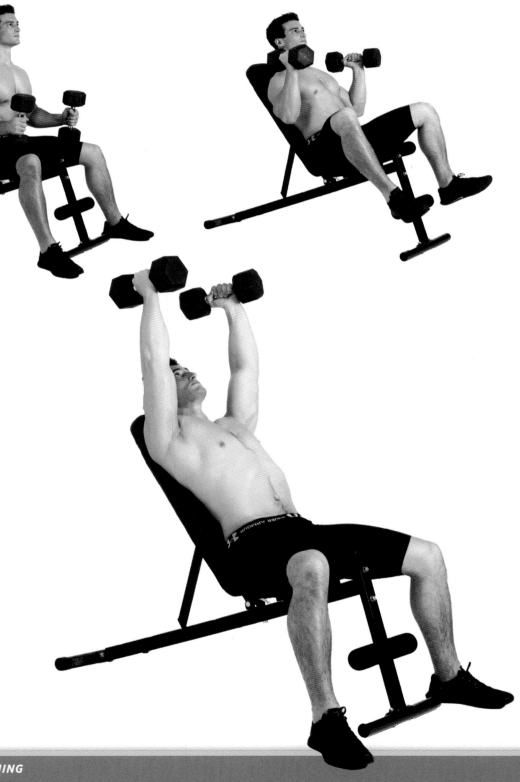

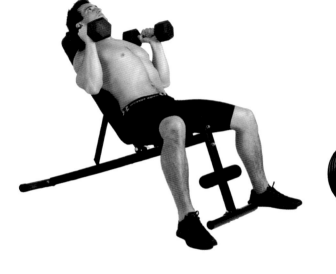

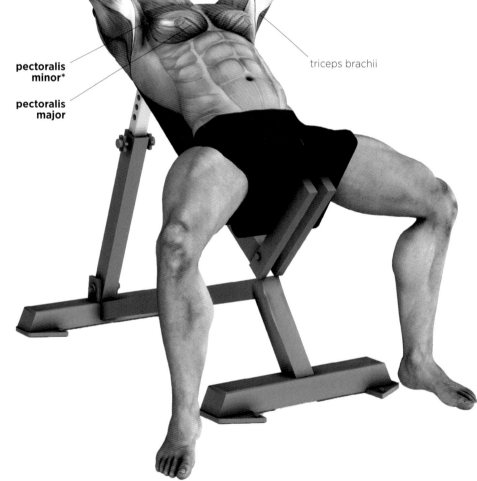

FACT FILE

TARGETS
• Upper chest

EQUIPMENT
• Dumbbells
• Incline bench

BENEFITS
• Strengthens upper chest
• Stabilizes shoulders and upper arms

CAUTIONS
• Shoulder issues
• Wrist issues
• Upper-back issues

Annotation Key

Bold text indicates target muscles

Light text indicates other working muscles

* indicates deep muscles

deltoideus anterior

triceps brachii

pectoralis minor*

pectoralis major

DO IT RIGHT

• Try to isolate your chest muscles as you work.

• Exhale as you lift the dumbbells up, and inhale as you lower them down.

• Keep the dumbbells facing each other as you do the raise.

• Avoid letting your elbows drift out.

• Avoid lifting your feet off the floor for the raise.

• Avoid lifting your glutes and back while doing the exercise.

• Avoid hyperextending your arms at the top of your raise.

Bent-Arm Dumbbell Pullover

The Bent-Arm Dumbbell Pullover chiefly powers your chest, helped by your back muscles. Be sure to keep a slight bend at the elbows or your triceps will be doing the work instead of your chest.

HOW TO DO IT

- Place a dumbbell in a vertical position onto a flat bench, and lower your upper body onto the bench.

- Pick up the dumbbell by the top weight, keeping the dumbbell in a vertical position.

- Lift the dumbbell onto your chest, and slightly lower your body on the bench so that your head, neck, and upper back are supported by it.

- Keeping your palms under the top weight as far as possible, raise the dumbbell above your chest. This is your starting position.

- With your elbows slightly bent, lower the dumbbell over and behind you. Do not lower the dumbbell lower than your head.

- Carefully return to your starting position, and repeat for the recommended repetitions.

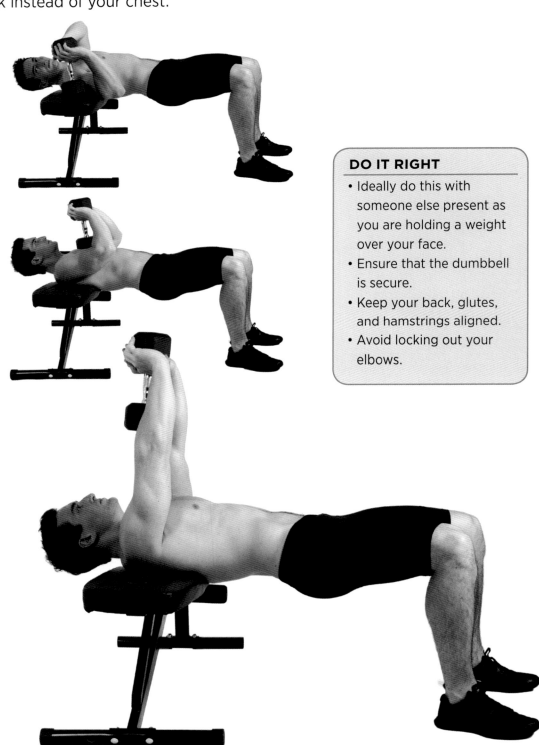

DO IT RIGHT

- Ideally do this with someone else present as you are holding a weight over your face.
- Ensure that the dumbbell is secure.
- Keep your back, glutes, and hamstrings aligned.
- Avoid locking out your elbows.

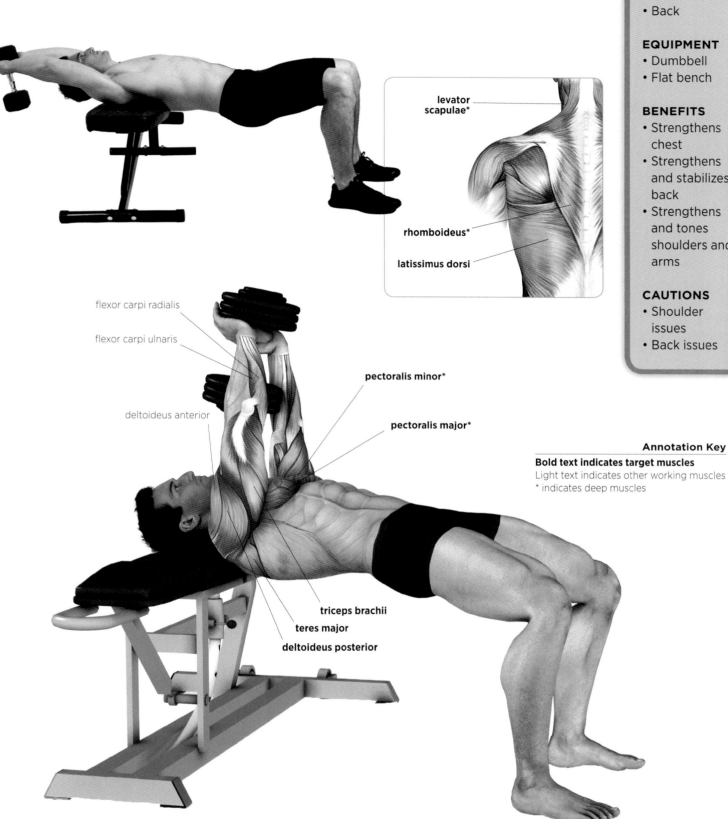

TARGETS
- Upper, middle, and lower chest
- Back

EQUIPMENT
- Dumbbell
- Flat bench

BENEFITS
- Strengthens chest
- Strengthens and stabilizes back
- Strengthens and tones shoulders and arms

CAUTIONS
- Shoulder issues
- Back issues

levator scapulae*

rhomboideus*

latissimus dorsi

flexor carpi radialis

flexor carpi ulnaris

deltoideus anterior

pectoralis minor*

pectoralis major*

Annotation Key

Bold text indicates target muscles
Light text indicates other working muscles
* indicates deep muscles

triceps brachii

teres major

deltoideus posterior

Dumbbell Fly

This is essentially a Hammer-Grip Press (pages 176–177) with an arm-opening movement added. This means that the whole routine not only strengthens your chest, but also your shoulders and biceps.

HOW TO DO IT

- Sit on an incline bench, holding a pair of dumbbells on your thighs. This is your starting position.

- Kick up to give some momentum while leaning back on the bench and lift the dumbbells above your chest. Your palms should be facing each other in a hammer-grip position. Keep your elbows bent and your shoulder blades in contact with the bench.

- Raise the dumbbells toward the ceiling until they are directly above your shoulders. Your feet should be on the floor. Hold this top position for the recommended time.

- Keeping your elbows bent, push your hands apart until your hands drop to just below the height of your chest. Return to your starting position by squeezing your chest and bringing the dumbbells back along the same path as the descent. Repeat for the recommended repetitions.

DO IT RIGHT

- In the final step, inhale as you drop your arms wide, exhale as you return to your starting position.
- Your chest and rib cage should rise as the dumbbells descend.
- Keep your grip strong and your upper arms, both biceps and triceps, contracted.
- Keep your spine and shoulders in the same position as you return to your starting position.
- Avoid moving your head or chin forward or off the bench.
- Avoid elevating your shoulders.
- Avoid bending your elbows excessively as the dumbbells descend, or flattening them as the dumbbells ascend.

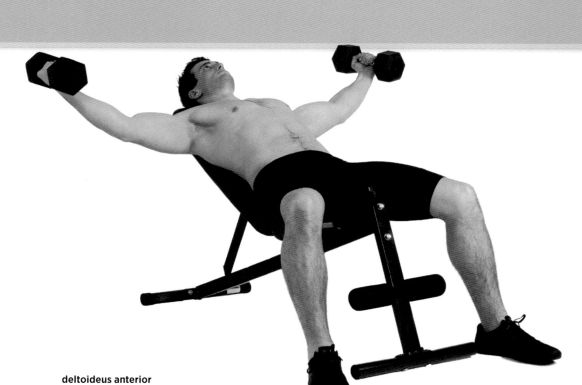

FACT FILE

TARGETS
• Middle chest

EQUIPMENT
• Dumbbells
• Incline bench

BENEFITS
• Strengthens chest
• Stabilizes shoulders, upper arms, and core

CAUTIONS
• Shoulder issues
• Back issues
• Wrist issue

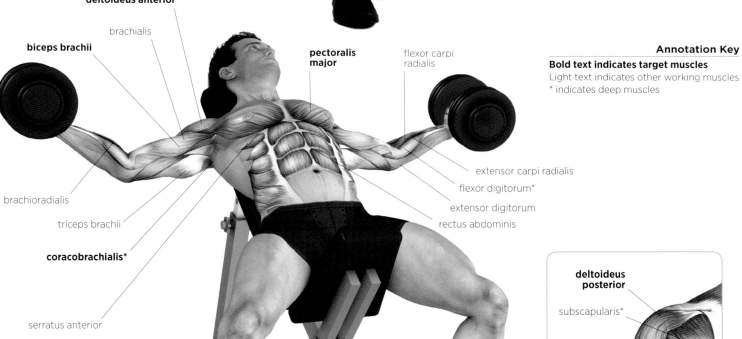

deltoideus anterior

brachialis

biceps brachii

pectoralis major

flexor carpi radialis

brachioradialis

triceps brachii

coracobrachialis*

serratus anterior

extensor carpi radialis

flexor digitorum*

extensor digitorum

rectus abdominis

Annotation Key

Bold text indicates target muscles
Light text indicates other working muscles
* indicates deep muscles

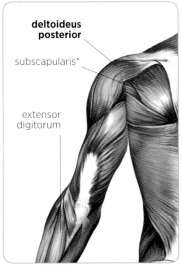

deltoideus posterior

subscapularis*

extensor digitorum

Swiss Ball Fly

This exercise is a great way to isolate your pectorals. Doing this fly—exercises where your arms move through an arc—on a Swiss ball offers you a really good range of movement. It also engages your abdominals.

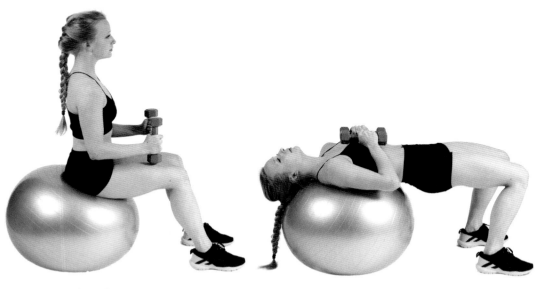

DO IT RIGHT

- When lifting the weights up, keep your arms directly above your shoulders.
- Keep your torso stable and feet planted throughout the exercise.
- Engage your abdominals throughout.
- Keep your buttocks and hips lifted so your upper legs, torso, and neck form a straight line.
- Move your arms smoothly and with control.
- Avoid arching your back.
- Avoid swinging your arms.

HOW TO DO IT

- Sit on a Swiss ball holding a dumbbell in each hand.

- Faceup, roll down slowly and carefully until your head, neck, and upper back are on the ball and properly supported. Your body should be extended with your torso long, knees bent at an angle as close to 90 degrees as possible, and feet planted firmly on the floor, a little wider than shoulder-width apart.

- Extend your arms upward, palms facing, straight above your chest. Keep steady, with your abdominals engaged. This is your starting position.

- Keeping the rest of your body stable, bring your arms out to your sides in a smooth, controlled movement.

- Return your arms to your starting position, and repeat for the recommended repetitions.

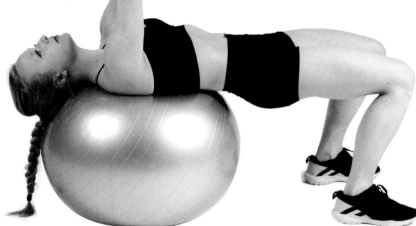

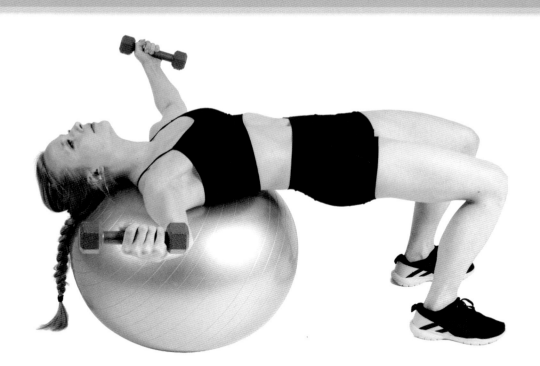

FACT FILE

TARGETS
- Pectorals

EQUIPMENT
- Dumbbells
- Swiss ball

BENEFITS
- Strengthens and tones pectorals
- Works and stabilizes shoulders, core, and triceps

CAUTIONS
- Shoulder issues
- Stability issues

Annotation Key
Bold text indicates target muscles
Light text indicates other working muscles
* indicates deep muscles

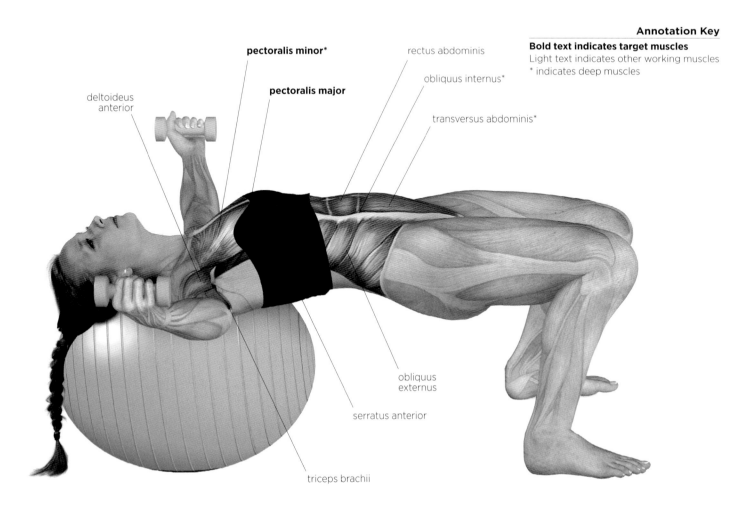

pectoralis minor*

pectoralis major

deltoideus anterior

rectus abdominis

obliquus internus*

transversus abdominis*

obliquus externus

serratus anterior

triceps brachii

Seated Dumbbell Russian Twist

There's nothing like a good torso twist to develop core durability. The Seated Dumbbell Russian Twist engages and strengthens your abdominals as well as your back. Quads and upper arms get worked too.

HOW TO DO IT

- Holding a dumbbell in both hands, sit with your legs extended in front of you, knees bent and feet about hip-width apart. Lean back slightly.

- Engage your core muscles as you bring the dumbbell to your right side, twisting your torso as you go but keeping your head straight ahead.

- Bring the dumbbell back to the middle of your body and then twist with it to your left, again keeping your gaze ahead. Repeat for the recommended repetitions.

DO IT RIGHT

- Engage your core.
- Anchor your heels to the floor.
- Move smoothly.
- Avoid arching or rounding your back.
- Avoid hunching your shoulders.
- Avoid swinging your arms or moving in a jerky manner.
- Avoid allowing your heels to lift off the floor.
- Avoid tensing your neck as you twist.

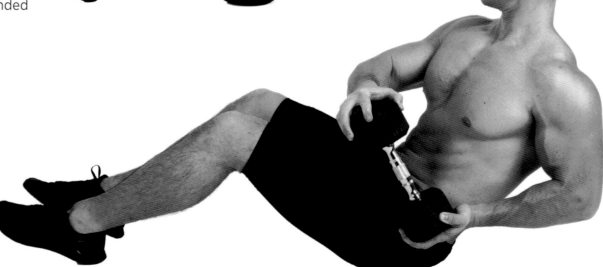

MODIFICATION

SIMILAR DIFFICULTY: Instead of looking straight ahead as you twist, take your head with you. Don't overstrain your neck or swing round too far or too fast. Observe carefully how this shifts the way your muscles are worked.

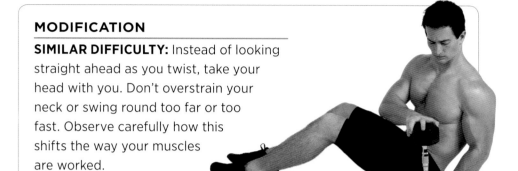

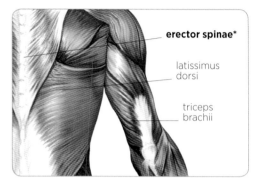

transversus abdominis*

tensor fascie latae

iliopsoas*

vastus intermedius*

rectus femoris

vastus lateralis

erector spinae*

latissimus dorsi

triceps brachii

Annotation Key
Bold text indicates target muscles
Light text indicates other working muscles
* indicates deep muscles

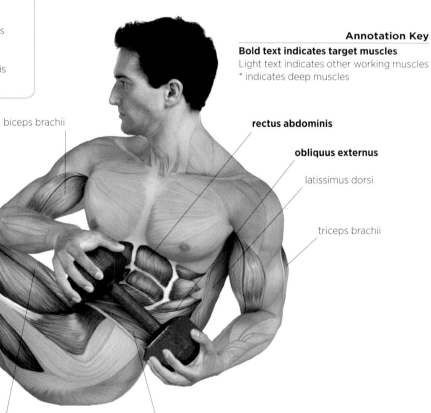

biceps brachii

rectus femoris

vastus lateralis

rectus abdominis

obliquus externus

latissimus dorsi

triceps brachii

soleus

vastus intermedius*

obliquus internus*

C-Curve Arm Cross

This routine is named for the C-curve used in Pilates, which is all about forging a strong connection between your spine and abdominals. Using small dumbbells adds greater upper-body resistance.

HOW TO DO IT

- To get into position on the ball, sit with legs bent up and pressed together and feet flat. Have your Bosu/Swiss ball close by. Extend your arms out in front, straighten your legs, and roll back to about 45 degrees. Place the ball behind you to support your back. Pick up your dumbbells.

- Engage your abdominals and, with your legs pressed together and feet pointed, raise your legs off the floor. Go as far as is comfortable.

- With your palms facing down, cross your right arm over your left and then your left arm over your right in quick, controlled movements.

- Keep alternating arms for the recommended number of times. Pause and repeat for the recommended repetitions.

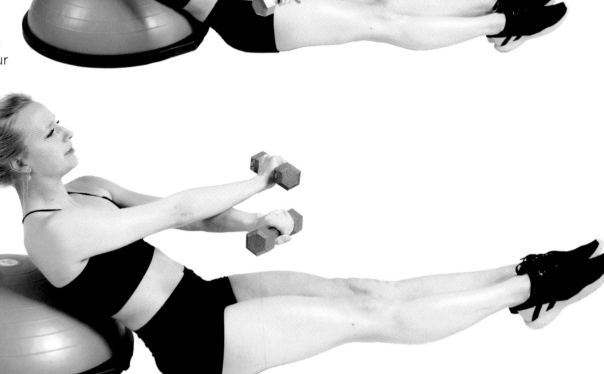

> ### DO IT RIGHT
> - Keep your arm movements steady and controlled.
> - Keep your shoulder blades pressed down your back.
> - Keep your abdominals engaged.
> - Avoid totally locking your elbows or knees.

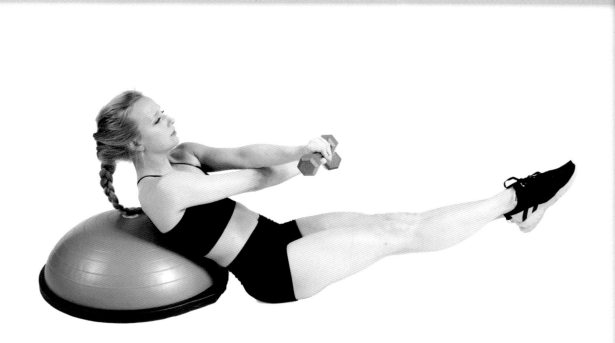

FACT FILE

TARGETS
- Abdominals
- Trapezius

EQUIPMENT
- Half-dome balance ball
- Dumbbells

BENEFITS
- Increases abdominal strength
- Strengthens upper body
- Stabilizes shoulder girdle

CAUTIONS
- Back issues
- Shoulder issues

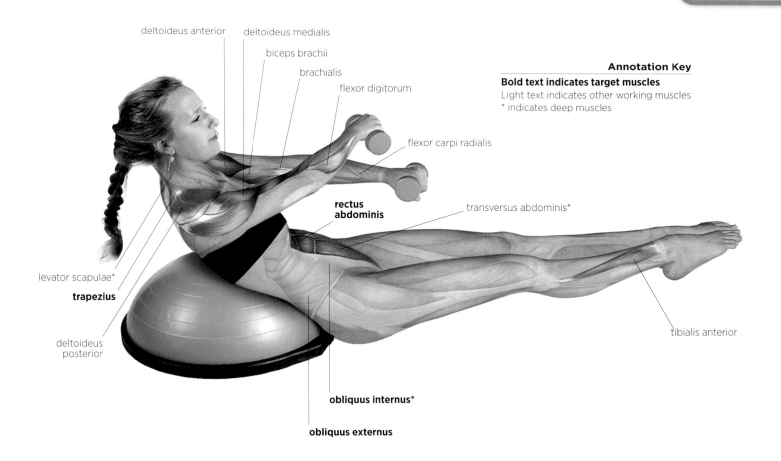

deltoideus anterior

deltoideus medialis

biceps brachii

brachialis

flexor digitorum

flexor carpi radialis

Annotation Key
Bold text indicates target muscles
Light text indicates other working muscles
* indicates deep muscles

rectus abdominis

transversus abdominis*

levator scapulae*

trapezius

deltoideus posterior

tibialis anterior

obliquus internus*

obliquus externus

Single-Arm T-Row

The Single-Arm T-Row is a tough exercise that builds both strength and stability in the core and upper body. Don't use so much weight that you are unable to maintain proper form.

HOW TO DO IT

- Start in a Plank position, holding a dumbbell in each hand.

- Adjust your stance so that there is a reasonable distance between your legs. This is whatever makes you feel stable and firm; it might be quite wide.

- Pull your right-hand dumbbell in to chest level.

- Rotate your torso to the right while raising your right arm toward the ceiling.

- Slowly lower the weight back to the ground to return to the Plank position. Repeat with the opposite arm. Alternate sides for the recommended repetitions.

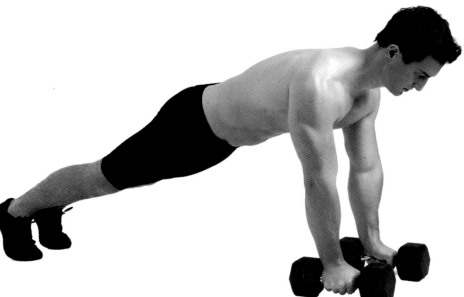

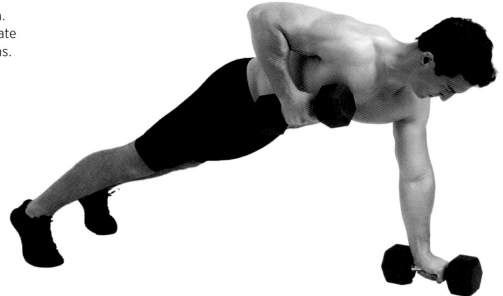

DO IT RIGHT

- Make sure your stance is wide enough for stability.
- Move the weight slowly, so you're not knocked off balance.
- Avoid using a weight heavier than you can comfortably lift over your head.
- Avoid attempting this movement before you can perform the Plank (pages 114–115), Alternating Floor Row (pages 142–143), and Standing Single-Leg Row (pages 140–141) exercises without any pain.

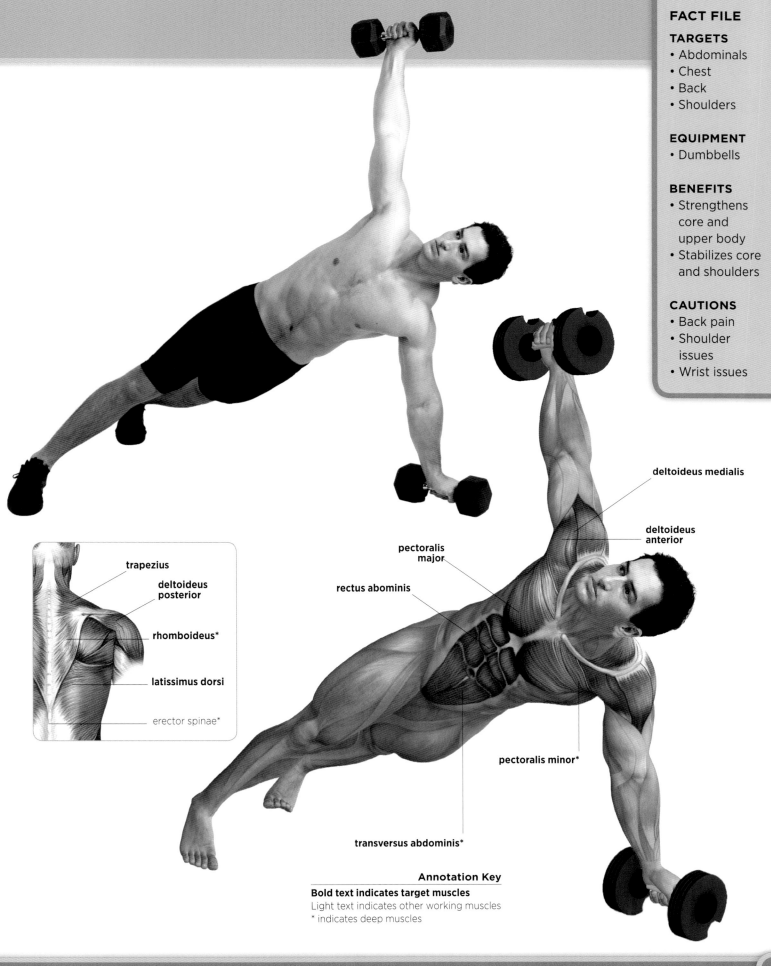

deltoideus medialis

deltoideus anterior

pectoralis major

rectus abominis

deltoideus posterior

trapezius

rhomboideus*

latissimus dorsi

erector spinae*

pectoralis minor*

transversus abdominis*

Annotation Key
Bold text indicates target muscles
Light text indicates other working muscles
* indicates deep muscles

Alternating Renegade Row

Also known as Commando Row, the Renegade Row hits a range of muscles, offering the benefits of a weighted row and a Plank. It is especially good for your core, but also works your arm and back muscles.

HOW TO DO IT

- With a kettlebell in each hand, plant yourself on the floor in a Plank position.

- While staying up on your toes and keeping your core stable, pull the kettlebell in your right hand up toward your chest while straightening your left arm and pushing that kettlebell into the floor.

- Lower your right arm, and repeat with the opposite arm. Continue alternating arms for the recommended repetitions.

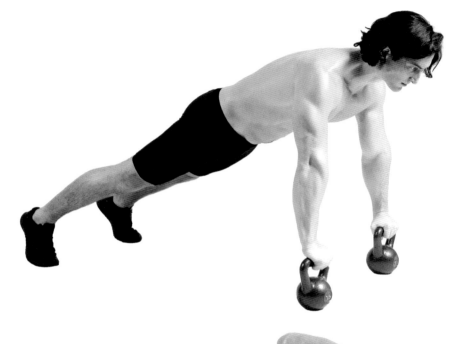

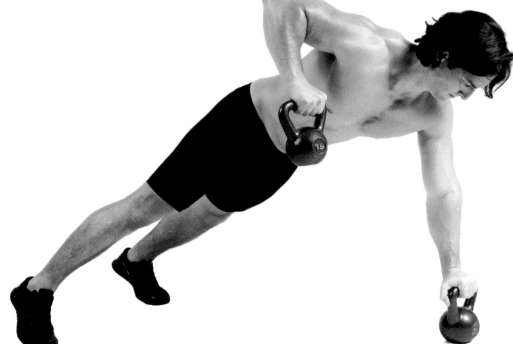

DO IT RIGHT

- Make sure the kettlebells have a flat surface on the bottom for stability.
- Keep your core stable and straight on.
- Avoid allowing your hips to sag.
- Avoid dropping or slamming the weight into the floor.

FACT FILE

TARGETS
- Lats
- Abdominals
- Arms
- Trapezius

EQUIPMENT
- Kettlebells/ Dumbbells for modification

BENEFITS
- Builds strength in the core and back

CAUTIONS
- Back issues
- Shoulder issues

MODIFICATION

EASIER: Row with just one kettlebell—or dumbbell—while keeping the other hand empty and planted flat on the floor. Switch hands after a few repetitions.

HARDER: As you lift one arm, also lift the opposite leg. Again, you can use dumbbells instead of kettlebells.

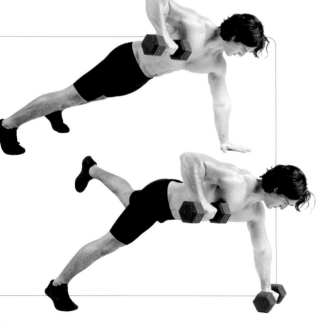

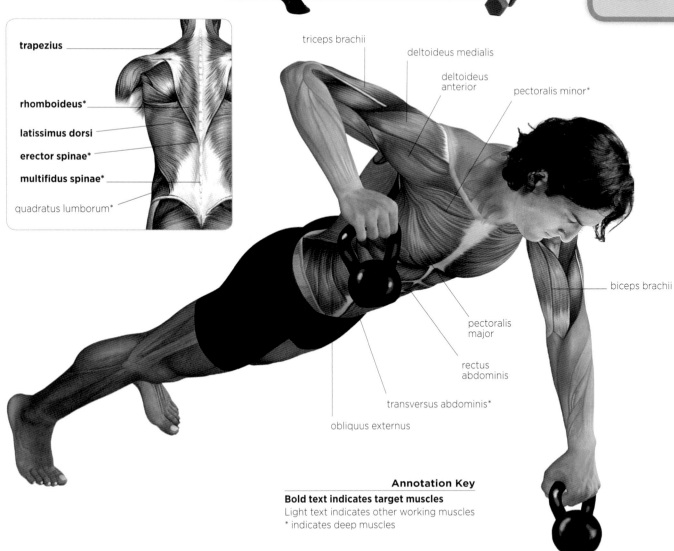

trapezius

rhomboideus*

latissimus dorsi

erector spinae*

multifidus spinae*

quadratus lumborum*

triceps brachii

deltoideus medialis

deltoideus anterior

pectoralis minor*

biceps brachii

pectoralis major

rectus abdominis

transversus abdominis*

obliquus externus

Annotation Key

Bold text indicates target muscles
Light text indicates other working muscles
* indicates deep muscles

Dumbbell Shin Raise

The Dumbbell Shin Raise strengthens the tibialis anterior—the main muscle of your shin that plays a huge role in ankle flexion. When you point your feet in this exercise, you are stretching this muscle.

HOW TO DO IT

- Sit on the front edge of a flat bench with a dumbbell on the floor in front of you. Clasp the dumbbell with your feet.

- Shimmy back onto the bench so that only your feet hang off the bench. Keeping your legs straight and torso sitting up straight, point your feet slowly.

- Still keeping your legs straight and torso sitting up straight, flex your feet slowly. Repeat for the recommended repetitions.

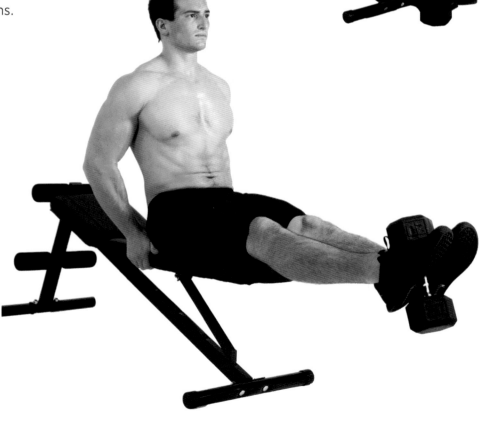

DO IT RIGHT

- Try to go through as full a range of movement as possible (without straining) while pointing and flexing your feet.
- Keep your neck and jaw relaxed throughout.
- Avoid bending your knees while performing this exercise.

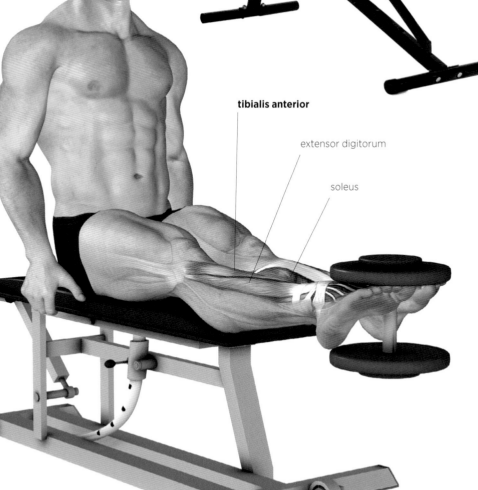

FACT FILE

TARGETS
- Main shin muscle

EQUIPMENT
- Dumbbell
- Flat bench/ seat

BENEFITS
- Strengthens shins

CAUTIONS
- Ankle issues

tibialis anterior

extensor digitorum

soleus

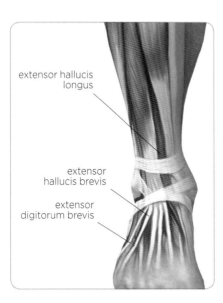

extensor hallucis longus

extensor hallucis brevis

extensor digitorum brevis

Annotation Key

Bold text indicates target muscles
Light text indicates other working muscles
* indicates deep muscles

Dumbbell Calf Raise

This very simple classic does great things for strengthening your gastrocnemius and soleus—your important calf muscles. Using dumbbells just adds a little valuable resistance.

HOW TO DO IT

- Stand holding a pair of dumbbells at your sides with your toes placed on the edge of a raised platform.

- Rise up on your toes, contracting your calf muscles at the top, and then lower your heels back down past the edge of the platform for a full stretch. Repeat for the recommended repetitions.

DO IT RIGHT

- Maintain a full range of up-down motion.
- Keep your toes pointed straight forward throughout.
- Strongly contract your calf muscles with each repetition.
- Avoid bouncy repetitions.

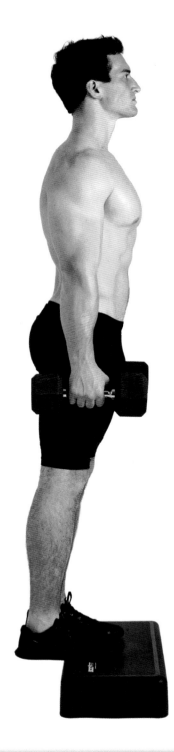
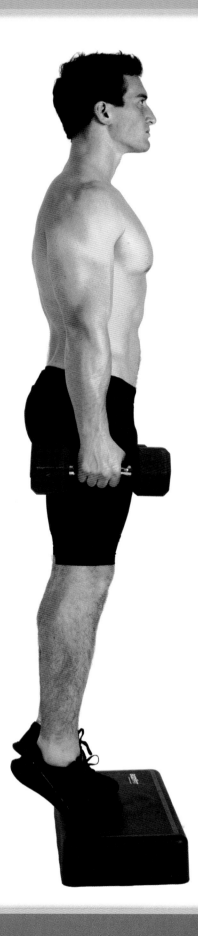

FACT FILE

TARGETS
• Calves

EQUIPMENT
• Dumbbells
• Platform, step, or sturdy, fixed block

BENEFITS
• Strengthens calf muscles

CAUTIONS
• Ankle issues

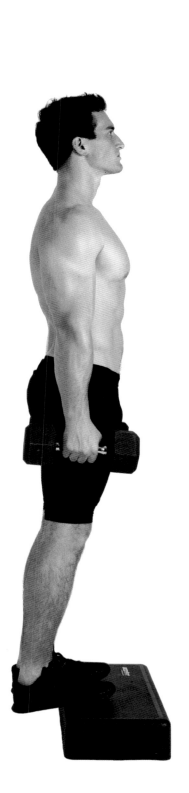

gastrocnemius

tibialis anterior

soleus

extensor hallucis

MODIFICATION

SIMILAR DIFFICULTY:
Point your toes inward throughout the exercise.

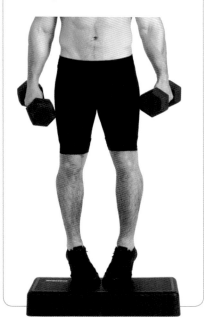

Annotation Key

Bold text indicates target muscles
Light text indicates other working muscles
* indicates deep muscles

Dumbbell Lying Hip Abduction

Hip mobility is so vital, and a complex web of muscles moves your legs away from the midline of your body (abduction), as well as flexing and rotating your hip-joint area. These include the tensor fasciae latae muscle and certain glutes.

HOW TO DO IT

- Lie on your left side, with your right leg stacked on top of the left and your left arm supporting you, forearm on the floor and palm down. Extend your right arm along the side of your body, a dumbbell in your hand.

- Maintaining the position of the rest of your body, smoothly raise your top leg. Try allowing your top arm to rise slightly, too. If desired, hold briefly.

- Lower to your starting position, and repeat for the recommended repetitions. Repeat on the opposite side for the recommended repetitions.

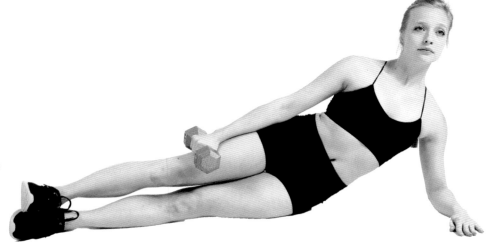

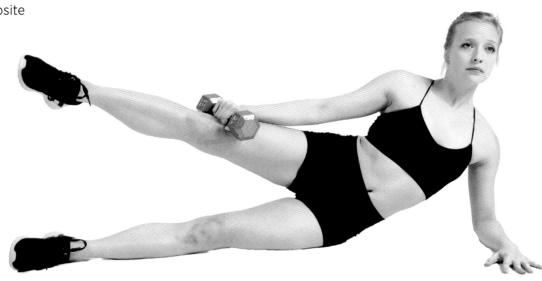

DO IT RIGHT

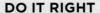

- Keep your torso facing forward.
- Keep your legs extended.
- Anchor your bottom arm and leg to the floor.
- Gaze forward.
- Avoid tilting or twisting your hips as you raise your leg.
- Avoid tensing or twisting your neck.
- Avoid hunching your shoulders.

FACT FILE

TARGETS
• Upper leg/
  hip-joint
  mobilizers

EQUIPMENT
• Dumbbell

BENEFITS
• Strengthens
  and tones
  outer thighs
• Improves hip
  mobility
• Boosts
  performance
  in tennis and
  all field sports

CAUTIONS
• Hip issues
• Shoulder
  issues

MODIFICATION

HARDER: Try moving into a Side Plank position. Focus on keeping your body in a straight line as you hold.

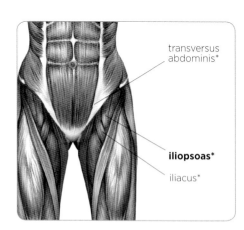

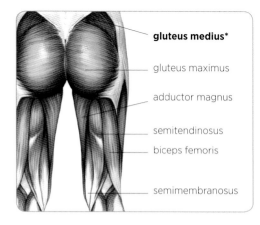

gluteus medius*

gluteus maximus

adductor magnus

semitendinosus

biceps femoris

semimembranosus

transversus abdominis*

iliopsoas*

iliacus*

Annotation Key
Bold text indicates target muscles
Light text indicates other working muscles
* indicates deep muscles

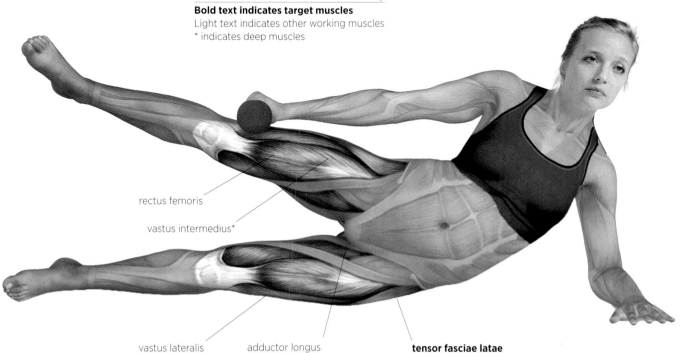

rectus femoris

vastus intermedius*

vastus lateralis

adductor longus

tensor fasciae latae

Dumbbell Lunge

This exercise is another simple classic—with dumbbell resistance added—that your stronger, toned glutes and quads will really thank you for doing. Make sure you move in a smooth flow.

HOW TO DO IT

- Stand with your arms at your sides, holding dumbbells. Your legs are together or a little apart.

- Keeping your head up and spine neutral, take a big step forward with your left leg.

- In one movement as you step forward, bend your front knee to a 90-degree angle and drop your front thigh until it is parallel to the floor. Your right, back, knee will drop behind you so that you are balancing on the toes of your back foot, creating a straight line from your spine to the back of your knee.

- Push through your front heel to stand upright, and return to your starting position. Repeat on the opposite leg. Alternate sides for the recommended repetitions.

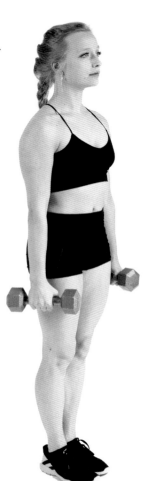

DO IT RIGHT

- Keep your body facing forward as you step one leg in front of you.
- Stand upright.
- Gaze forward.
- Ease into the lunge.
- Make sure that your front knee is facing forward.
- Avoid turning your body to one side.
- Avoid allowing your knee to extend past your foot.
- Avoid arching your back.

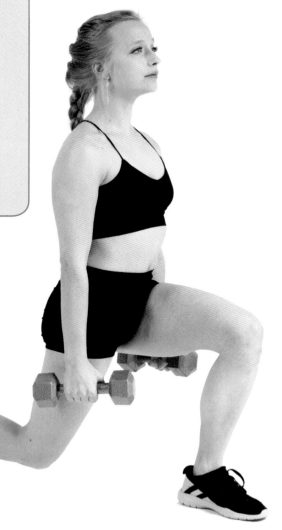

TARGETS
• Glutes
• Quads

EQUIPMENT
• Dumbbells

BENEFITS
• Strengthens
  and tones
  quads and
  glutes
• Stabilizes
  core,
  hamstrings,
  inner thighs,
  and lower legs

CAUTIONS
• Knee issues

Annotation Key

Bold text indicates target muscles

Light text indicates other working muscles

* indicates deep muscles

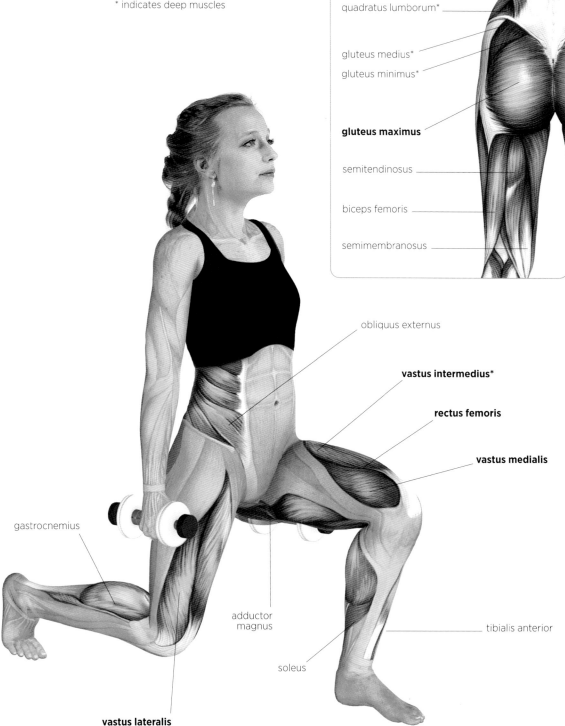

erector spinae*

quadratus lumborum*

gluteus medius*

gluteus minimus*

gluteus maximus

semitendinosus

biceps femoris

semimembranosus

obliquus externus

vastus intermedius*

rectus femoris

vastus medialis

gastrocnemius

adductor
magnus

tibialis anterior

soleus

vastus lateralis

Dumbbell Walking Lunge

This routine could hardly be more straightforward, yet regular practice builds considerable durability and strength into your lower body. It also helps to stabilize and balance muscles in your core.

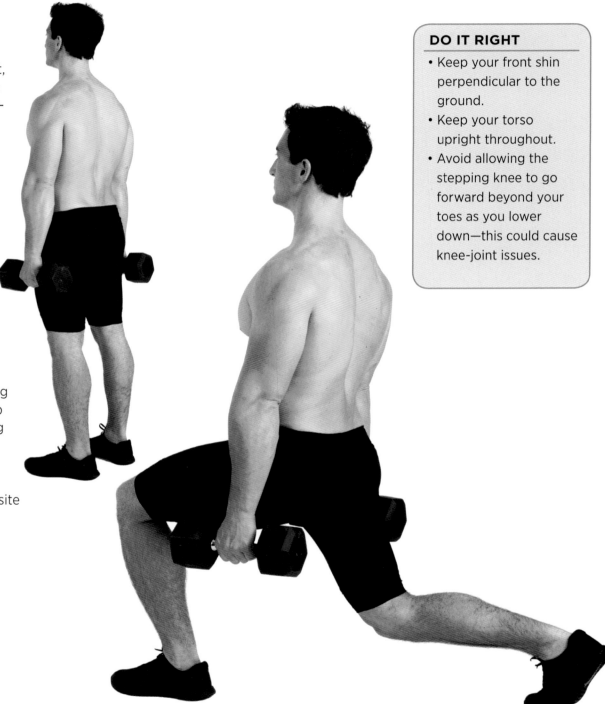

HOW TO DO IT

- Stand with your feet about hip-width apart, holding a dumbbell in each hand in hammer-grip position, palms facing. Keep your arms close to the sides of your body.

- Step forward with your left leg until your left foot is approximately two feet from your right foot, keeping your torso upright as you lower your upper body.

- Concentrating on using your left heel, push up and forward, returning to your starting standing position.

- Repeat with the opposite leg. Alternating legs, keep lunge-walking forward for the recommended repetitions.

DO IT RIGHT

- Keep your front shin perpendicular to the ground.
- Keep your torso upright throughout.
- Avoid allowing the stepping knee to go forward beyond your toes as you lower down—this could cause knee-joint issues.

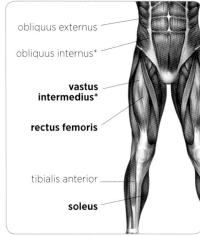

FACT FILE

TARGETS
- Quads
- Glutes
- Inner thighs and calves

EQUIPMENT
- Dumbbells

BENEFITS
- Strengthens and builds durability into legs and glutes

CAUTIONS
- Back issues
- Knee issues

MODIFICATION

EASIER: For a version using body-weight resistance rather than dumbbells, place your hands on your hips instead of holding weights.

Annotation Key

Bold text indicates target muscles
Light text indicates other working muscles
* indicates deep muscles

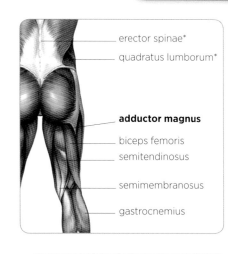

erector spinae*

quadratus lumborum*

adductor magnus

biceps femoris

semitendinosus

semimembranosus

gastrocnemius

vastus lateralis

gluteus medius*

gluteus minimus*

obliquus externus

obliquus internus*

semimembranosus

vastus intermedius*

rectus femoris

gluteus maximus

tibialis anterior

soleus

adductor magnus

Side Lunge and Press

Although Side Lunge and Press is a combo exercise that works out both your upper and lower body, the lunge to the side is a fantastic leg strengthener. It targets your quads as well as mobilizing your hip and gluteal areas.

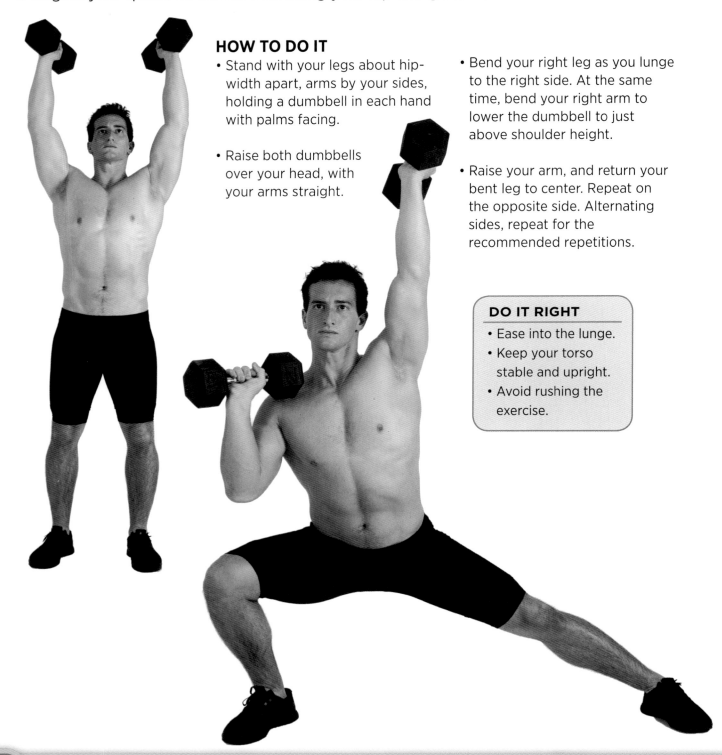

HOW TO DO IT

- Stand with your legs about hip-width apart, arms by your sides, holding a dumbbell in each hand with palms facing.

- Raise both dumbbells over your head, with your arms straight.

- Bend your right leg as you lunge to the right side. At the same time, bend your right arm to lower the dumbbell to just above shoulder height.

- Raise your arm, and return your bent leg to center. Repeat on the opposite side. Alternating sides, repeat for the recommended repetitions.

DO IT RIGHT

- Ease into the lunge.
- Keep your torso stable and upright.
- Avoid rushing the exercise.

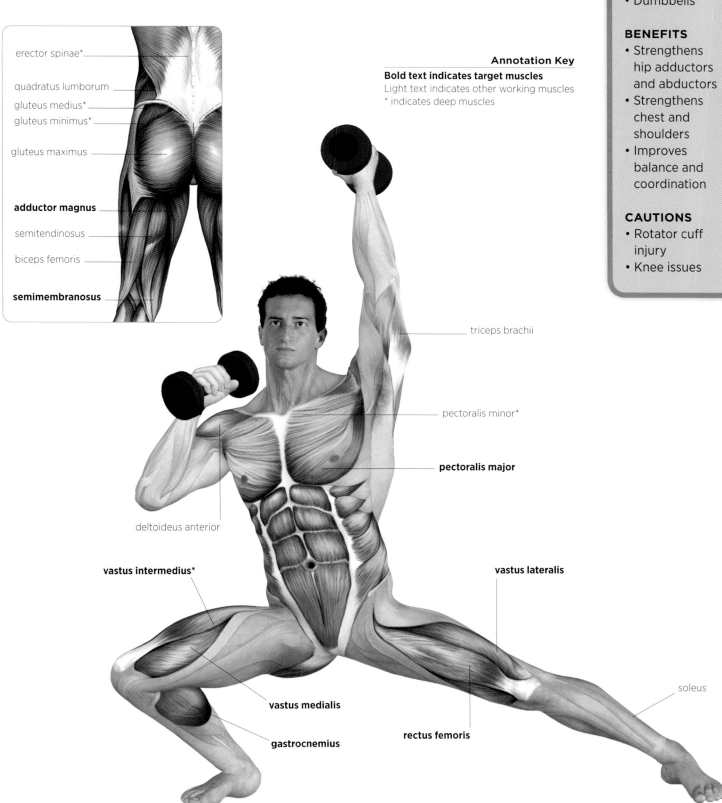

FACT FILE

TARGETS
- Thighs/hips
- Chest

EQUIPMENT
- Dumbbells

BENEFITS
- Strengthens hip adductors and abductors
- Strengthens chest and shoulders
- Improves balance and coordination

CAUTIONS
- Rotator cuff injury
- Knee issues

erector spinae*

quadratus lumborum

gluteus medius*

gluteus minimus*

gluteus maximus

adductor magnus

semitendinosus

biceps femoris

semimembranosus

Annotation Key

Bold text indicates target muscles
Light text indicates other working muscles
* indicates deep muscles

triceps brachii

pectoralis minor*

pectoralis major

deltoideus anterior

vastus intermedius*

vastus lateralis

vastus medialis

gastrocnemius

rectus femoris

soleus

Sumo Squat

This version of the squat is a great way to give your buttocks a deep workout while strengthening your thighs. It also pays attention to your inner-thigh adductors, which move your legs in toward your body.

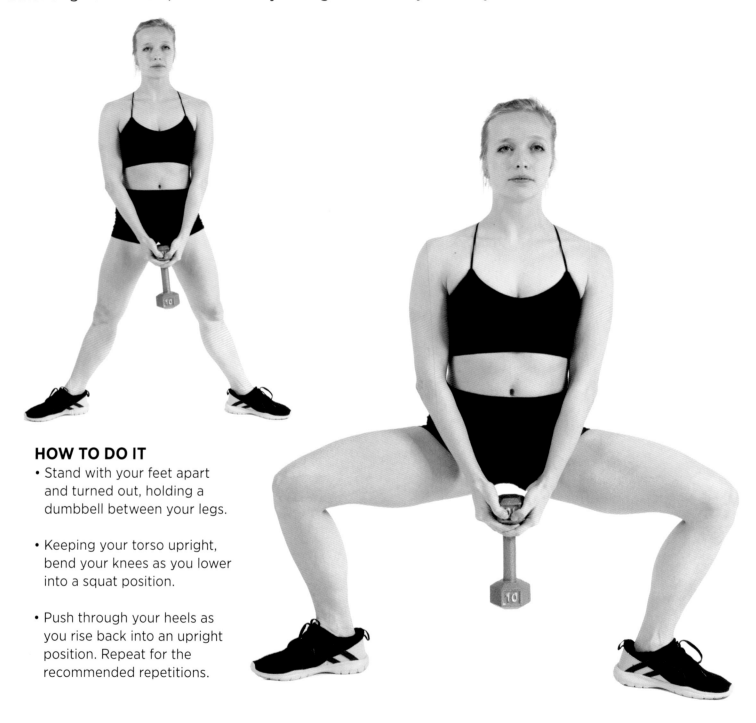

HOW TO DO IT

- Stand with your feet apart and turned out, holding a dumbbell between your legs.

- Keeping your torso upright, bend your knees as you lower into a squat position.

- Push through your heels as you rise back into an upright position. Repeat for the recommended repetitions.

TARGETS
• Glutes
• Quads

EQUIPMENT
• Dumbbell

BENEFITS
• Strengthens
  and tones
  buttocks and
  thighs

CAUTIONS
• Lower-back
  issues

DO IT RIGHT

• Gaze forward.
• Keep your chest lifted and
  your shoulders down.
• Engage your core.
• Avoid letting your knees
  extend past your feet.
• Avoid arching your back
  or slumping forward.
• Avoid hunching your
  shoulders.
• Avoid twisting your torso.

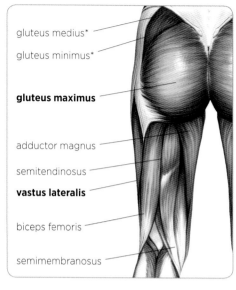

gluteus medius*
gluteus minimus*
gluteus maximus
adductor magnus
semitendinosus
vastus lateralis
biceps femoris
semimembranosus

Annotation Key
Bold text indicates target muscles
Light text indicates other working muscles
* indicates deep muscles

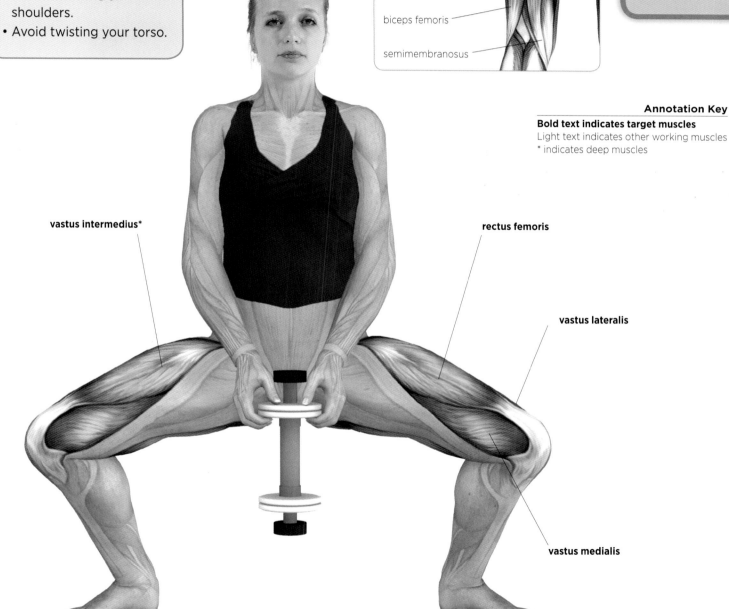

vastus intermedius*

rectus femoris

vastus lateralis

vastus medialis

Goblet Squat

Squatting in combination with holding weight at chest level forces your glutes to take the strain while stabilizing your deltoids and upper arms.

HOW TO DO IT

- While in a standing position, hold a kettlebell with both hands fairly close to your chest. Your legs should be a little more than shoulder-width apart, with your toes pointing slightly outward.

- Squat down until your thighs are parallel to the floor, bringing your elbows toward your thighs.

- Keep your back flat as you push through your heels back to the standing position. Repeat for the recommended repetitions.

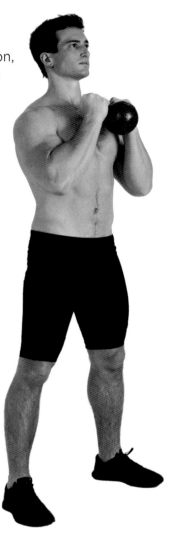

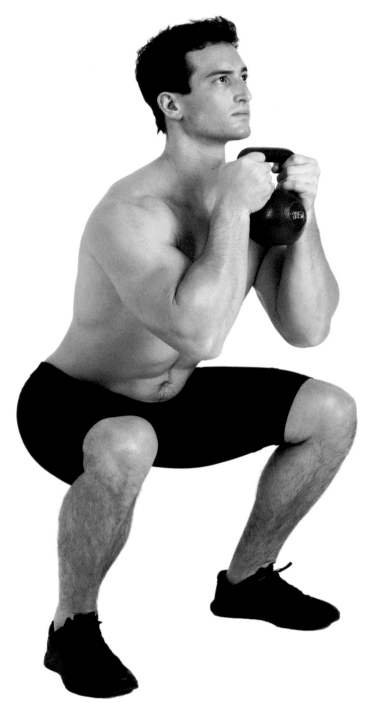

DO IT RIGHT

- Always employ a full range of motion.
- Avoid hyperextending your knees past your toes.

TARGETS
• Quads

EQUIPMENT
• Kettlebell

BENEFITS
• Builds strength in the quads

CAUTIONS
• Back issues
• Hip issues

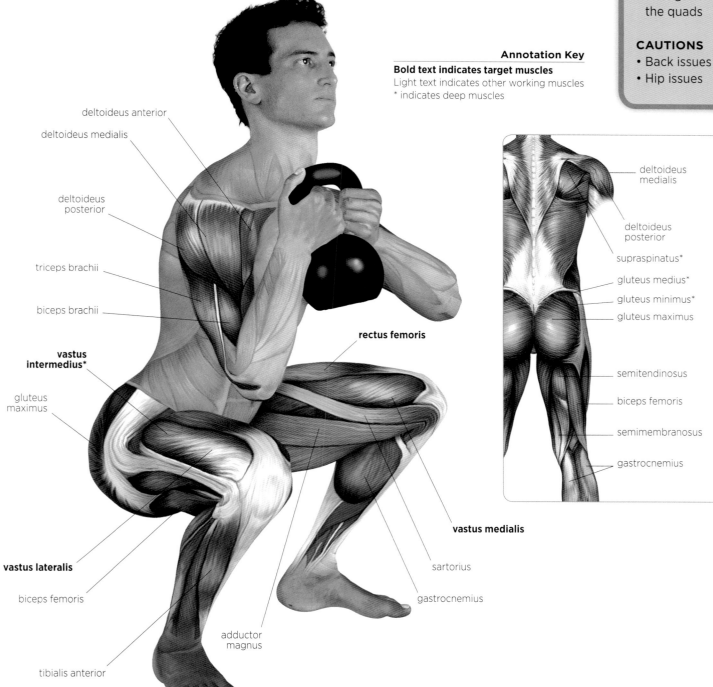

Annotation Key

Bold text indicates target muscles
Light text indicates other working muscles
* indicates deep muscles

deltoideus anterior

deltoideus medialis

deltoideus posterior

triceps brachii

biceps brachii

vastus intermedius*

gluteus maximus

vastus lateralis

biceps femoris

tibialis anterior

adductor magnus

rectus femoris

vastus medialis

sartorius

gastrocnemius

deltoideus medialis

deltoideus posterior

supraspinatus*

gluteus medius*

gluteus minimus*

gluteus maximus

semitendinosus

biceps femoris

semimembranosus

gastrocnemius

Barbell Squat

Just squatting down using no equipment at all is a great workout. Add a barbell into the equation and you have a dynamite strengthener for the lower body. Keep your back straight at all times.

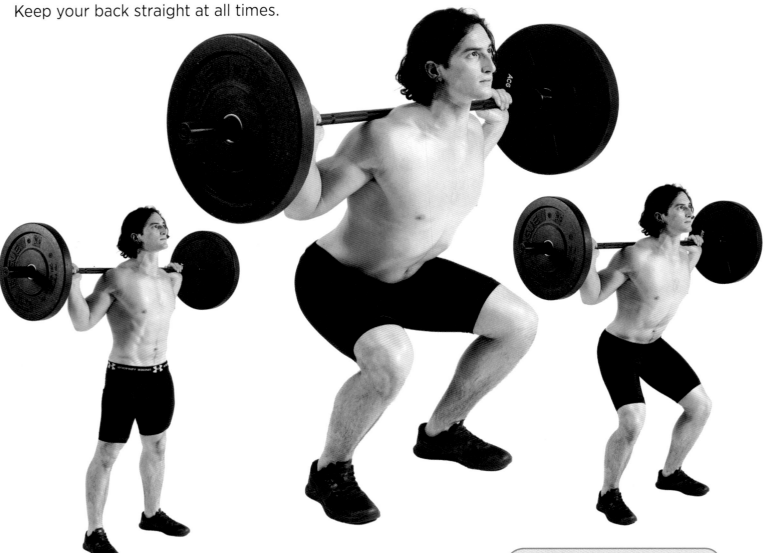

HOW TO DO IT

- Begin standing in front of a barbell situated at eye level in a power rack. With your feet shoulder-width apart, duck beneath the barbell, so that it comes to rest across the back of your shoulders. Walk the barbell out of the rack.

- Bend your knees, and lower yourself until your thighs are parallel to the ground. Be sure to keep your back flat as you do this.

- Push through your heels to stand erect. Repeat for the recommended repetitions.

DO IT RIGHT

- Inhale as you bend your knees and lower yourself; exhale as you stand up again.
- Squat deep while keeping your thighs parallel to the ground.
- Avoid hyperextending your knees past your toes.

TARGETS
- Quads
- Glutes
- Hamstrings

EQUIPMENT
- Barbell
- Power rack

BENEFITS
- Increases strength, power, and mass in your thighs
- Stabilizes core

CAUTIONS
- Seek advice from a medical/ fitness practitioner if you haven't done this before
- Back issues
- Shoulder issues

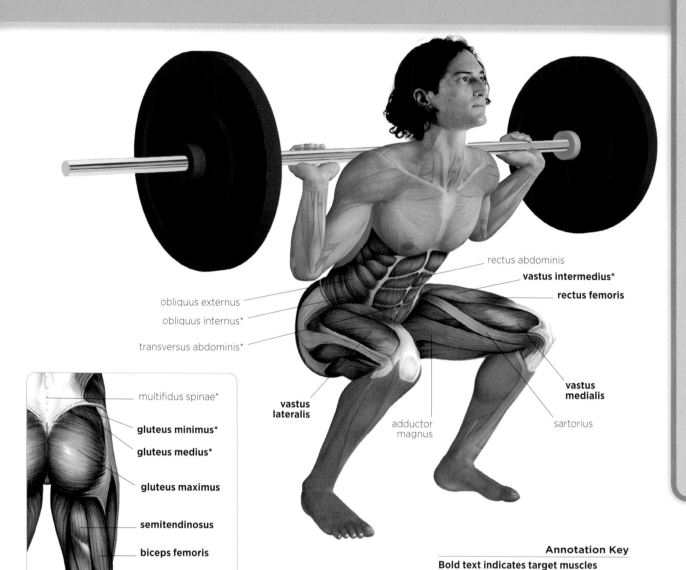

multifidus spinae*

gluteus minimus*

gluteus medius*

gluteus maximus

semitendinosus

biceps femoris

semimembranosus

obliquus externus

obliquus internus*

transversus abdominis*

vastus
lateralis

rectus abdominis

vastus intermedius*

rectus femoris

vastus
medialis

adductor
magnus

sartorius

Annotation Key
Bold text indicates target muscles
Light text indicates other working muscles
* indicates deep muscles

MODIFICATION

EASIER: Simply squat down and stand up as explained here but without a barbell, which uses your own body weight instead.

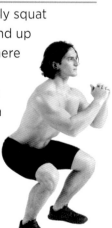

MODIFICATION

HARDER: Bring your feet closer together to increase the range of motion required, making the exercise more difficult.

Clean-and-Press

The Clean-and-Press works with a body bar to target your upper body and arms while also strengthening and stabilizing your quads and hamstrings.

HOW TO DO IT

- Begin in a high squatting position so that your upper legs are parallel with the floor. Hold the body bar in front of you, arms straight.

- Using the muscles in our legs as well as your abdominals, rise to stand as you bend your arms to bring the bar to shoulder height. If you choose, extend one foot in front of the other.

- Move your feet to parallel position, hip-width or wider apart, and bring the body bar above your head. Hold for the recommended time.

- Keep your alignment as you bring the bar down to shoulder height in a controlled manner.

- Repeat the lift overhead and the controlled lowering for the recommended repetitions.

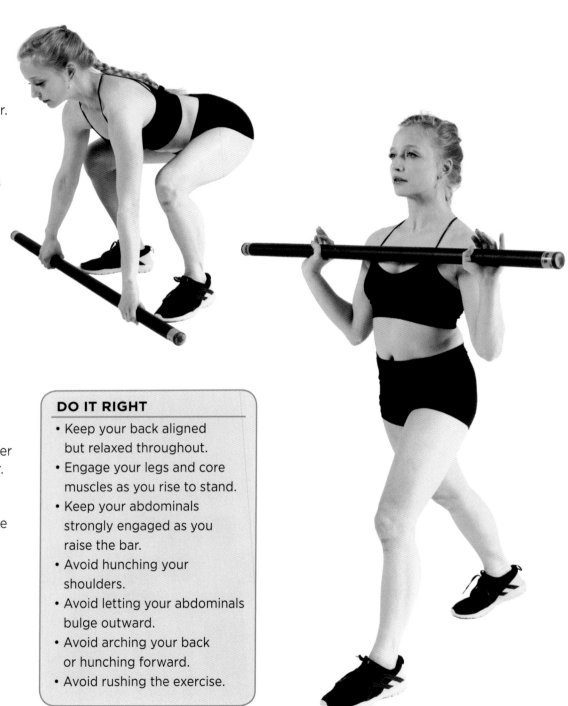

DO IT RIGHT

- Keep your back aligned but relaxed throughout.
- Engage your legs and core muscles as you rise to stand.
- Keep your abdominals strongly engaged as you raise the bar.
- Avoid hunching your shoulders.
- Avoid letting your abdominals bulge outward.
- Avoid arching your back or hunching forward.
- Avoid rushing the exercise.

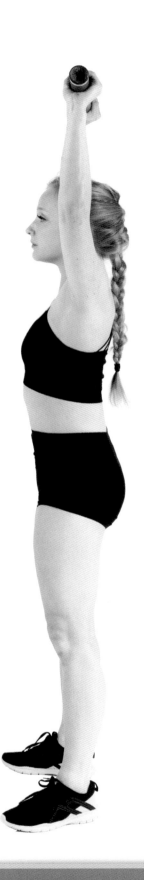

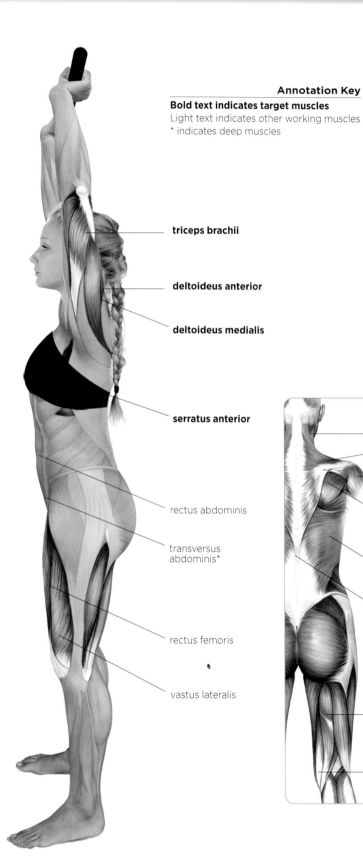

FACT FILE

TARGETS
- Back
- Shoulders
- Ribs/torso
- Triceps

EQUIPMENT
- Body bar

BENEFITS
- Strengthens and tones much of the body
- Boosts performance in tennis, volleyball, and all sports

CAUTIONS
- Back issues

Annotation Key

Bold text indicates target muscles
Light text indicates other working muscles
* indicates deep muscles

triceps brachii

deltoideus anterior

deltoideus medialis

serratus anterior

rectus abdominis

transversus abdominis*

rectus femoris

vastus lateralis

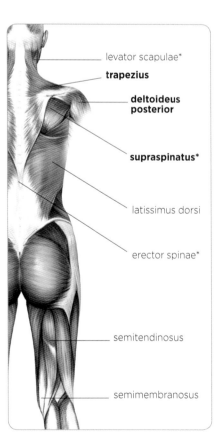

levator scapulae*

trapezius

deltoideus posterior

supraspinatus*

latissimus dorsi

erector spinae*

semitendinosus

semimembranosus

Curling Step-and Raise

The Curling Step-and-Raise is a great strengthener for your upper body and lower body, too. As well as working your core and biceps, it will power your inner thighs and stabilize your pelvis.

HOW TO DO IT

- Stand with your arms at your sides, holding a dumbbell in each hand, palms facing forward. Position a stable step/platform beside your left foot.

- Place your left foot on the step/platform.

- Shift your weight onto your left foot. Bend your elbows, curling the dumbbells toward your chest. At the same time, raise your right knee as the foot comes off the floor. Continue raising and curling until your right leg forms a 90-degree angle and your dumbbells are around shoulder height.

- Lowering the dumbbells, cross your right leg over your left leg, which should bend as you lower your right leg to the floor, left of the platform.

- Step your left leg onto the floor so that you are in starting position on the other side of the step.

- Repeat on the opposite side, and continue alternating sides for the recommended repetitions.

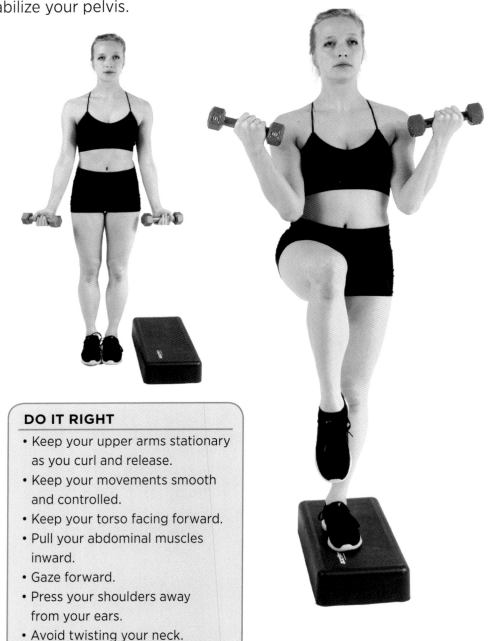

DO IT RIGHT

- Keep your upper arms stationary as you curl and release.
- Keep your movements smooth and controlled.
- Keep your torso facing forward.
- Pull your abdominal muscles inward.
- Gaze forward.
- Press your shoulders away from your ears.
- Avoid twisting your neck.
- Avoid hunching your shoulders.
- Avoid arching your back or hunching forward.
- Avoid rushing the exercise.

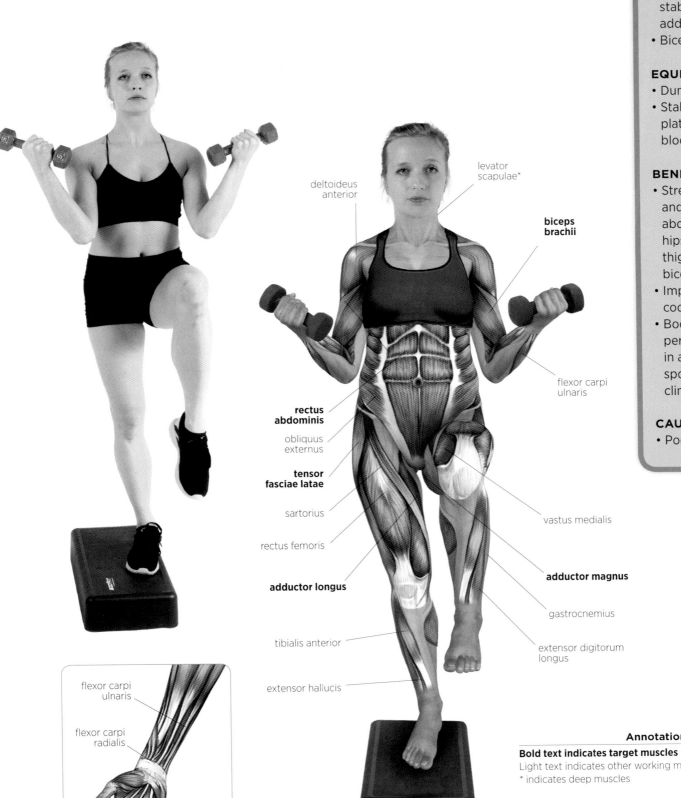

TARGETS
- Abdominals
- Thigh stabilizers and adductors
- Biceps

EQUIPMENT
- Dumbbells
- Stable step, platform, or block

BENEFITS
- Strengthens and tones abdominals, hips, inner thighs, and biceps
- Improves coordination
- Boosts performance in all field sports and climbing stairs

CAUTIONS
- Poor balance

deltoideus anterior

levator scapulae*

biceps brachii

flexor carpi ulnaris

rectus abdominis

obliquus externus

tensor fasciae latae

sartorius

rectus femoris

adductor longus

vastus medialis

adductor magnus

gastrocnemius

tibialis anterior

extensor digitorum longus

extensor hallucis

flexor carpi ulnaris

flexor carpi radialis

Annotation Key
Bold text indicates target muscles
Light text indicates other working muscles
* indicates deep muscles

Knee Raise with Lateral Extension

Performing a straightforward flexed and straight leg raise such as this builds power in your core and shoulders while also developing strength in both your upper and lower legs.

HOW TO DO IT

- Stand with your feet hip-width apart and your arms at the front of your body, holding a dumbbell in each hand. This is your starting position.

- Shifting weight onto your left leg, bend your right knee and raise the leg. At the same time, raise your arms until the weights are around shoulder height, palms facing down. Take a moment or two to find your balance.

- Keeping your arms and upper body stationary, extend your right leg out to the side. Try holding briefly.

- Moving with control, lower your arms and return your right leg to your starting position.

- Repeat for the recommended repetitions on this side and then for the same number on the opposite side. Keep alternating sides for the recommended repetitions.

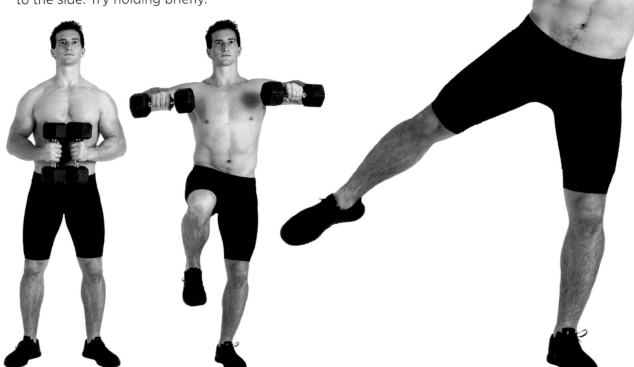

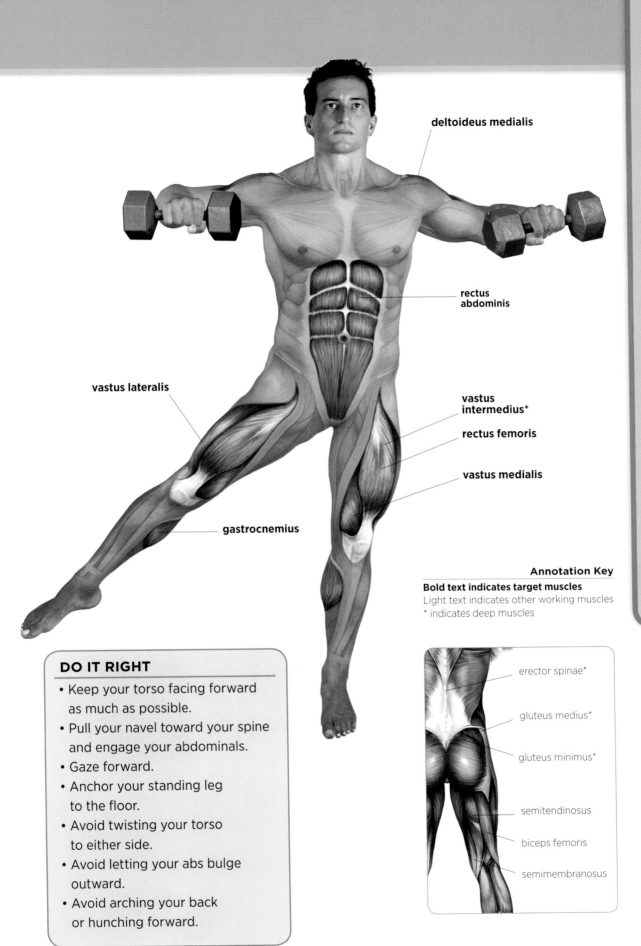

deltoideus medialis

rectus abdominis

vastus lateralis

vastus intermedius*

rectus femoris

vastus medialis

gastrocnemius

erector spinae*

gluteus medius*

gluteus minimus*

semitendinosus

biceps femoris

semimembranosus

FACT FILE

TARGETS
- Abdominals
- Deltoids
- Quads
- Calves

EQUIPMENT
- Dumbbells

BENEFITS
- Improves balance, coordination, and range of motion
- Strengthens and tones core, shoulder, leg, and arm muscles
- Stabilizes core
- Boosts performance in football, tennis, squash, baseball, rollerblading, skating, and skiing

CAUTIONS
- Knee issues
- Balance issues

Annotation Key

Bold text indicates target muscles
Light text indicates other working muscles
* indicates deep muscles

DO IT RIGHT

- Keep your torso facing forward as much as possible.
- Pull your navel toward your spine and engage your abdominals.
- Gaze forward.
- Anchor your standing leg to the floor.
- Avoid twisting your torso to either side.
- Avoid letting your abs bulge outward.
- Avoid arching your back or hunching forward.

Barbell Power Clean and Jerk

While targeting your upper arms, shoulders, and back, this exercise will work a huge number of other muscles at the same time. It is especially effective for stabilizing your core and thighs.

HOW TO DO IT

- Begin standing behind a barbell, with your feet shoulder-width apart. Squat down and grab the barbell with a wide overhand grip.

- As you return to a standing position, flip the barbell towards you so your palms face upward until the barbell is nearly touching your upper chest.

- Push the barbell up and overhead, holding it at arms' length.

- Lower the barbell back to your upper chest, palms still up. Reverse your flip so your palms face down, and return the barbell to the floor. Repeat for the recommended repetitions.

DO IT RIGHT

- Use your legs to help with the start of the movement.
- Avoid overarching your back.

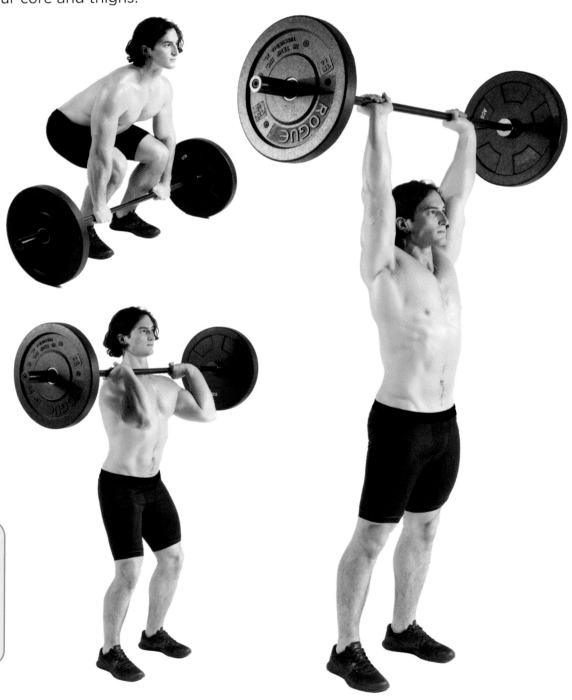

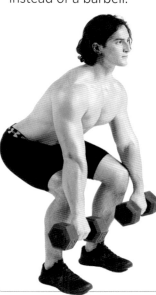

FACT FILE

TARGETS
- Shoulder girdle
- Back
- Triceps

EQUIPMENT
- Barbell/ dumbbells for modification

BENEFITS
- Increases power, strength, and mass in the shoulders and upper back
- Works torso, upper legs, and upper arms

CAUTIONS
- Back issues
- Shoulder issues
- Seek medical/ fitness professional advice if you have not done this before

MODIFICATION

EASIER: Use a very light bar or just your own body weight.

HARDER: Use dumbbells (below) instead of a barbell.

brachialis

biceps brachii

teres major

serratus anterior

latissimus dorsi

obliquus externus

tractus iliotibialis

tensor fasciae latae

vastus lateralis

rectus femoris

triceps brachii

deltoideus medialis

deltoideus anterior

rectus abdominis

transversus abdominis*

adductor longus

vastus intermedius*

sartorius

vastus medialis

gracilis*

adductor magnus

Annotation Key

Bold text indicates target muscles
Light text indicates other working muscles
* indicates deep muscles

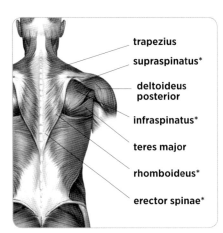

trapezius

supraspinatus*

deltoideus posterior

infraspinatus*

teres major

rhomboideus*

erector spinae*

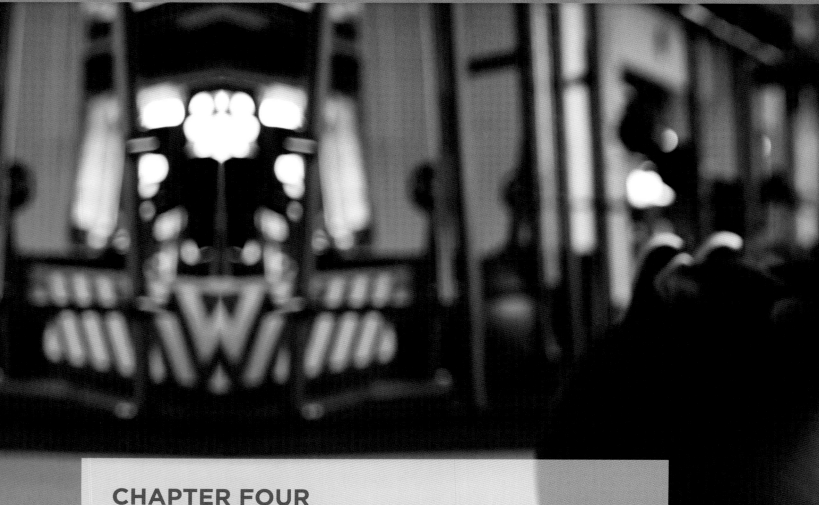

CHAPTER FOUR
EQUIPMENT EXERCISES

From foam rollers and cables, to resistance bands and Swiss balls, you'll find that equipment can really enhance your strength training. Either singly or in combination, some simple pieces of equipment act to lend your body a vital helping hand. They may offer your body support, get it into prime position to work muscles in a specific way, or provide resistance for it to work against.

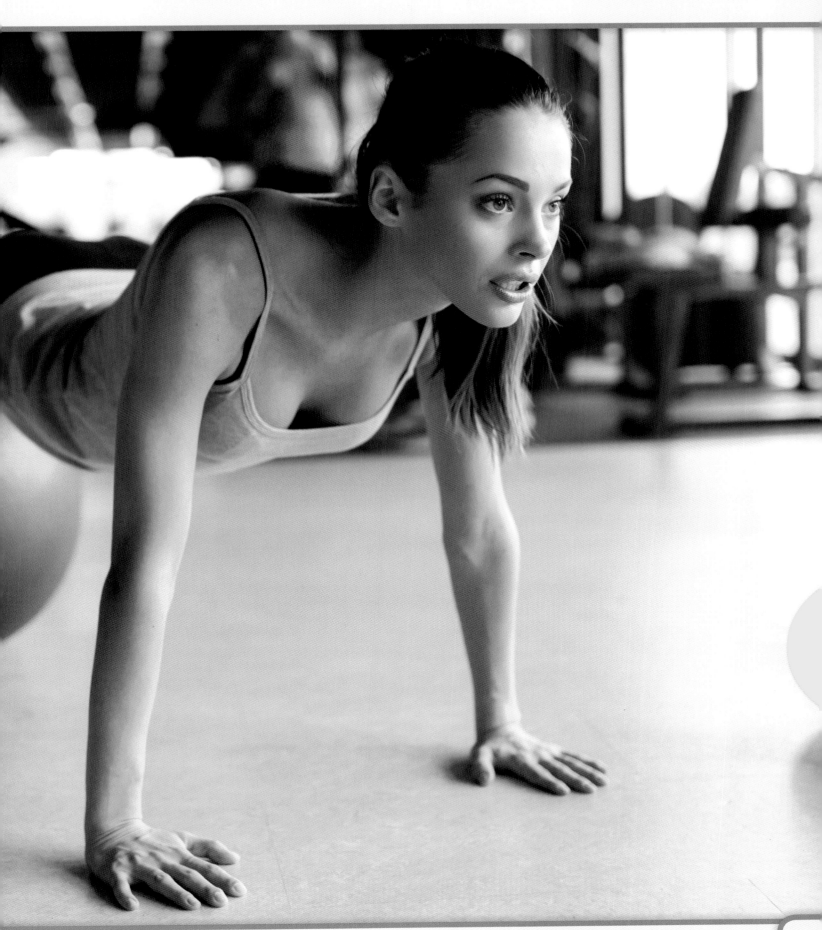

Swiss Ball Crossover

This exercise offers a wonderful releaser and strengthener for your lower back. It also powers your abdominals, including your obliques, and works your thigh muscles.

HOW TO DO IT

- Lie on your back, with your arms extended out to your sides. Place your legs on a Swiss ball, with your buttocks close to the ball.

- Brace your abs, and lower your legs to your right, as close to the floor as you can go without raising your shoulders off the floor.

- Return to your starting position, and repeat on the opposite side. Alternate sides for the recommended repetitions.

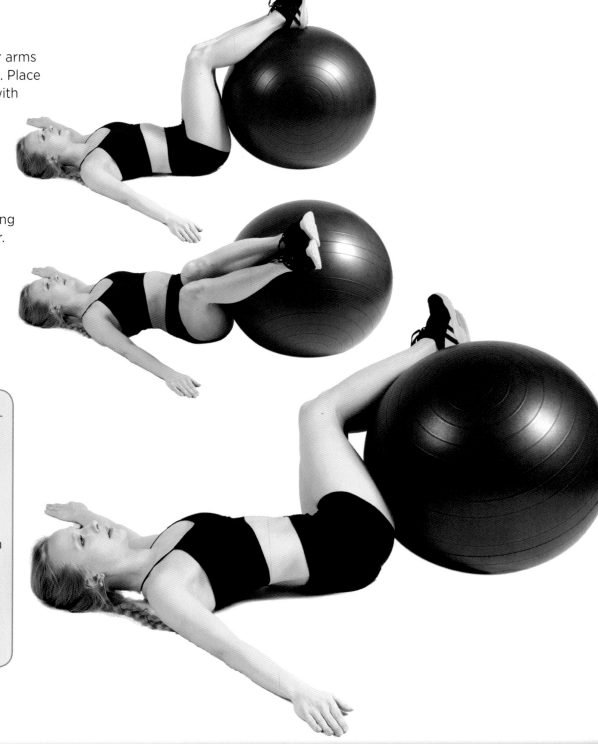

DO IT RIGHT

- Keep your core engaged and as stable as possible throughout.
- Keep your arms anchored to the floor.
- Keep your legs firmly over the ball to maintain your body's positioning.
- Avoid swinging your legs too quickly; keep the movement smooth and controlled.

FACT FILE

TARGETS
- Lower back
- Abdominals

EQUIPMENT
- Swiss ball

BENEFITS
- Helps to strengthen and tone abdominals
- Stabilizes core

CAUTIONS
- Lower-back issues

MODIFICATION

EASIER: Try performing the exercise without a Swiss ball. Start with your legs lifted and bent at an angle of 90 degrees or a little more. Try to keep your upper body as stable as possible as you perform the crossover, alternating sides.

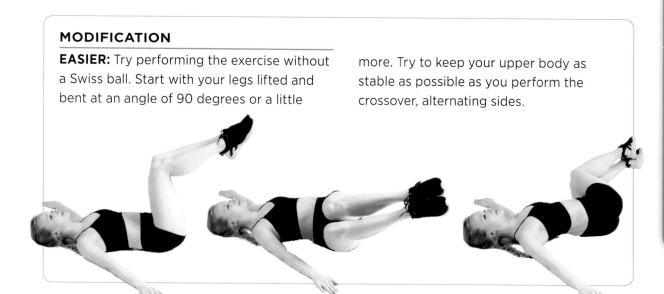

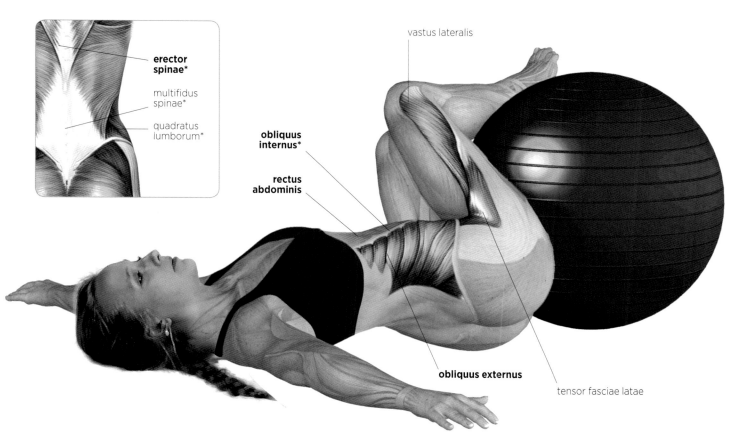

erector spinae*

multifidus spinae*

quadratus lumborum*

vastus lateralis

obliquus internus*

rectus abdominis

obliquus externus

tensor fasciae latae

Annotation Key

Bold text indicates target muscles
Light text indicates other working muscles
* indicates deep muscles

Neutral-Grip Pull-Up

A classic strength exercise, this Pull-Up is "neutral" because it uses a shoulder-width grip rather than a wide or narrow one. The basic routine is a fundamental upper-body movement that is especially effective at targeting your back's latissimus dorsi.

HOW TO DO IT

- Standing in front of a pull-up bar, either reach up or you may need to step on a stool. Place your hands shoulder-width apart on the bar using an overgrip (palms facing away from you), and hang with your arms straight.

- Pull yourself up until your chest touches the bar. Hold for just a moment, and then lower yourself slowly to your hanging position. Repeat for the recommended repetitions.

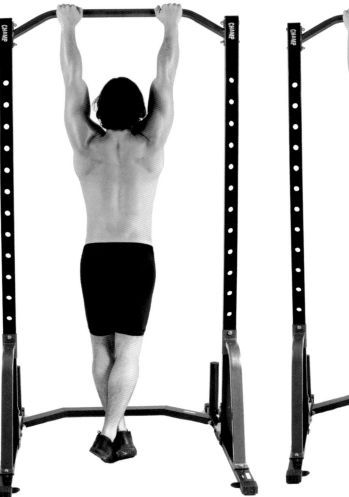
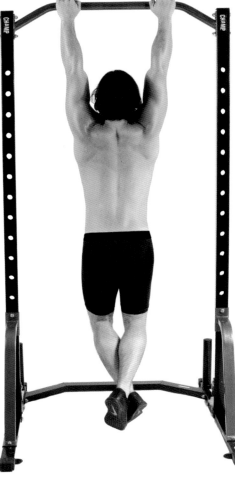

DO IT RIGHT

- Be sure your arms are straight in the hanging position—or it doesn't count!
- To strengthen your grip while performing pull-ups, grip your thumb over the top of the bar rather than wrapping it around the bar.
- Avoid kipping (swinging) your body—this can injure your rotator cuffs.

MODIFICATION

SIMILAR DIFFICULTY: Try moving your hands much closer together on the bar to perform a close-grip version of this Pull-Up. Feel the differences in how your muscles are working. You may feel more activity lower down your back.

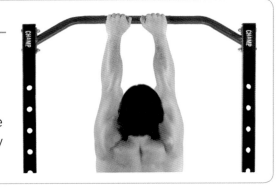

FACT FILE

TARGETS
• Back, including lats
• Shoulders
• Upper arms
• Chest

EQUIPMENT
• Pull-up bar

BENEFITS
• Strengthens upper body

CAUTIONS
• Shoulder issues
• Wrist issues

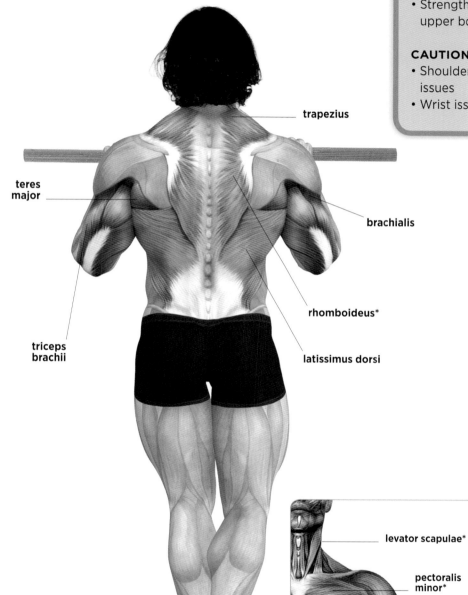

trapezius

teres major

brachialis

triceps brachii

rhomboideus*

latissimus dorsi

levator scapulae*

pectoralis minor*

pectoralis major

biceps brachii

Annotation Key
Bold text indicates target muscles
Light text indicates other working muscles
* indicates deep muscles

Wide-Grip Pull-Up

Varying your grip width when doing Pull-Ups makes a real difference. Hands close together brings certain shoulder muscles into play a bit more. A wide grip—as here—increases the effort needed by your lats and is a challenging but great back-strengthener.

HOW TO DO IT

- Standing in front of a pull-up bar, either reach up or you may need to step on a stool. Place your hands as wide apart as possible on the bar using an overgrip (palms facing away from you), and hang with your arms straight.

- Pull yourself up until your chest touches the bar. Hold for just a moment, and then lower yourself slowly to your hanging position. Repeat for the recommended repetitions.

DO IT RIGHT

- Start and end the movement from the dead hang position.
- Pull your body as high onto the bar as possible—your chin over the bar is the minimum height.
- Avoid kipping (swinging) your body—this can injure your rotator cuffs.

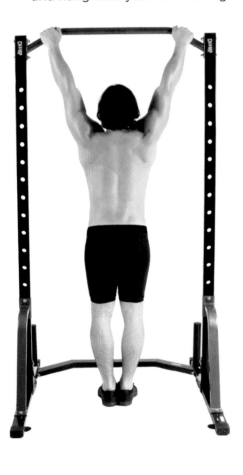

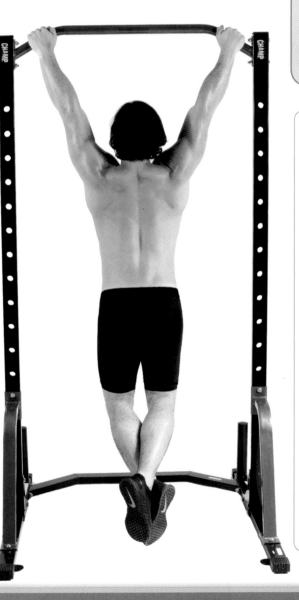

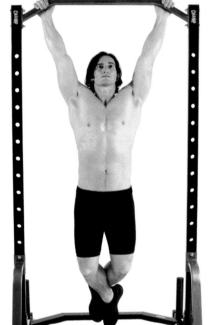

FRONT VIEW

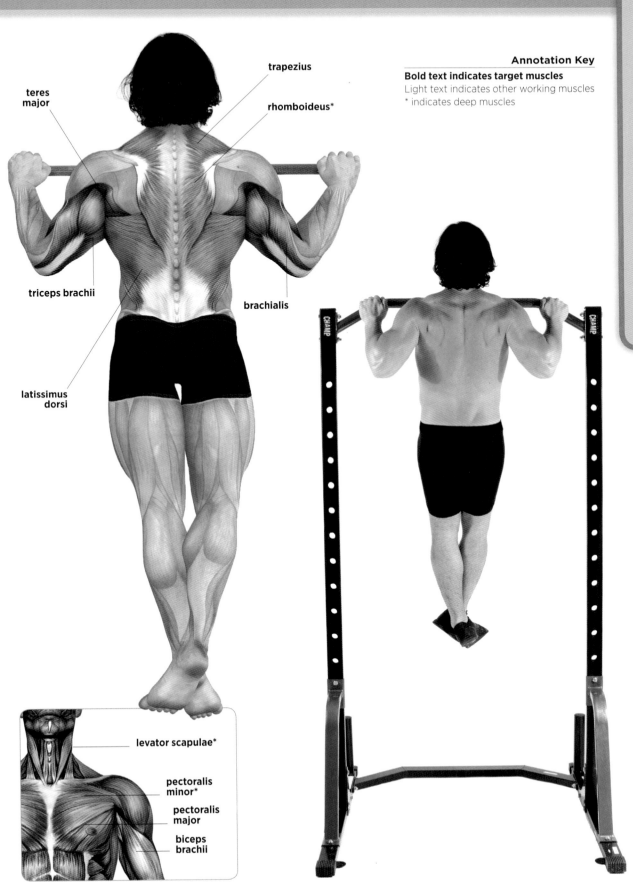

trapezius

teres
major

rhomboideus*

triceps brachii

brachialis

latissimus
dorsi

levator scapulae*

pectoralis
minor*

pectoralis
major

biceps
brachii

FACT FILE

TARGETS
- Back, especially lats
- Shoulders
- Upper arms
- Chest

EQUIPMENT
- Pull-up bar

BENEFITS
- Strengthens latissimus dorsi
- Strengthens upper body

CAUTIONS
- Shoulder issues
- Wrist issues

Reverse-Grip Pull-Up

Also called a Chin-Up, Reverse Grip Pull-Up has you grasp the bar with your palms facing you. Doing this places more focus on your biceps. The reverse variation is well worth adding to any routine for strengthening your upper body.

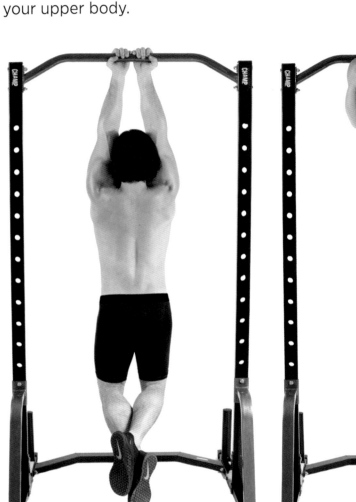
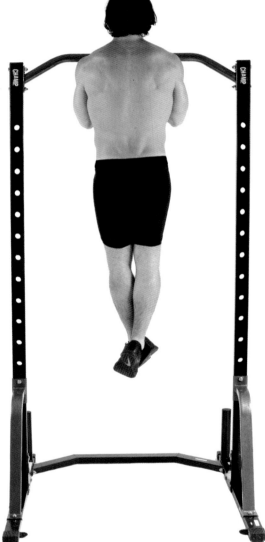

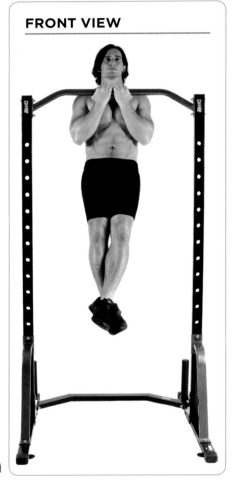

FRONT VIEW

HOW TO DO IT

- Standing in front of a pull-up bar, either reach up or you may need to step on a stool. Place your hands in either a neutral, closer, or wider position on the bar using an undergrip (palms facing toward you), and hang with your arms straight.

- Pull yourself up until your chin is over the bar. Hold for just a moment, and then lower yourself slowly to your hanging position, stopping just before your arms are completely straight. Repeat for the recommended repetitions.

DO IT RIGHT

- Pull your body as high onto the bar as possible—your chin over the bar is the minimum height.
- Avoid kipping (swinging) your body— this can injure your rotator cuffs.

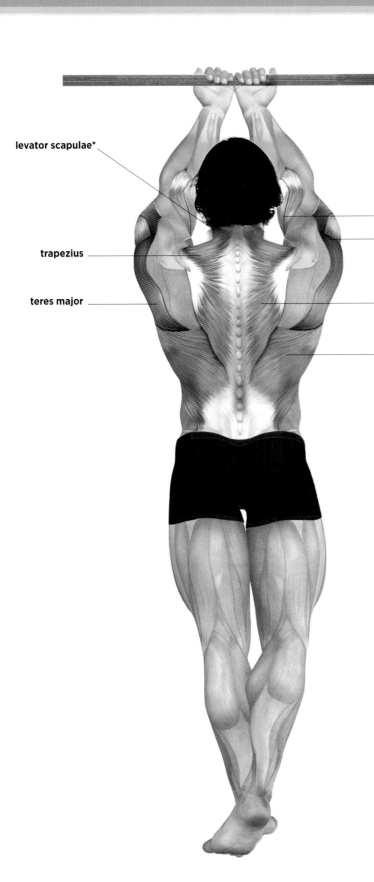

TARGETS
• Back
• Shoulders
• Upper arms
• Chest

EQUIPMENT
• Pull-up bar

BENEFITS
• Strengthens upper body
• Strengthens biceps

CAUTIONS
• Shoulder issues
• Wrist issues

levator scapulae*

triceps brachii

brachialis

trapezius

teres major

rhomboideus*

latissimus dorsi

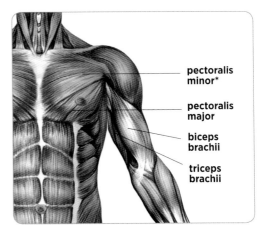

pectoralis minor*

pectoralis major

biceps brachii

triceps brachii

Annotation Key

Bold text indicates target muscles
Light text indicates other working muscles
* indicates deep muscles

Swiss Ball Prone Row with External Rotation

This is a challenging exercise, but one that really comes through for your upper back and also rotator cuffs, while working your core too. Before performing it, try to run through a thorough warm-up to loosen your shoulder girdle.

HOW TO DO IT

• Begin facedown on top of a Swiss ball, with your torso supported. Balance on your toes, with your legs separated for stability.

• Bend your arms so that they form 90-degree angles, pulled up so your upper arms are parallel to the floor and lined up roughly with your shoulders. This is your starting position.

• Swing your forearms and pointed hands up to point ahead of you. Your arms are still at a 90-degree angle, but this time with your forearms parallel to the floor.

• Drop your forearms back down again. Now drop your arms down, straightening them, so that your fingers nearly touch the floor.

• Bring your arms back up to your starting position, and repeat for the recommended repetitions.

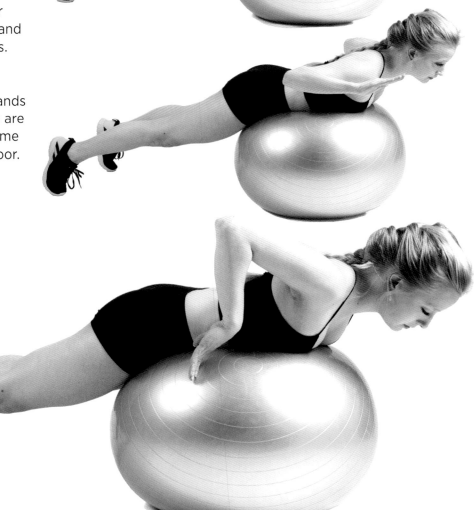

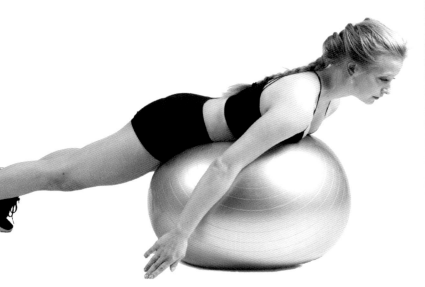

DO IT RIGHT

- Remain as stable as possible on top of the ball.
- Keep your fingers active and outstretched.
- Avoid straining your neck by trying to look up.

FACT FILE

TARGETS
- Lats
- Rhomboids

EQUIPMENT
- Swiss ball

BENEFITS
- Strengthens upper back and shoulders
- Improves balance and posture

CAUTIONS
- Lower-back issues
- Rotator cuff injury

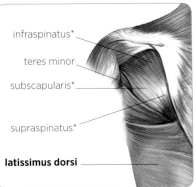

- infraspinatus*
- teres minor
- subscapularis*
- supraspinatus*
- **latissimus dorsi**

Annotation Key

Bold text indicates target muscles
Light text indicates other working muscles
* indicates deep muscles

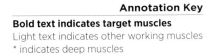

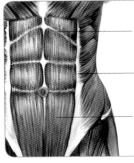

- **rectus abdominis**
- obliquus internus*
- transversus abdominis

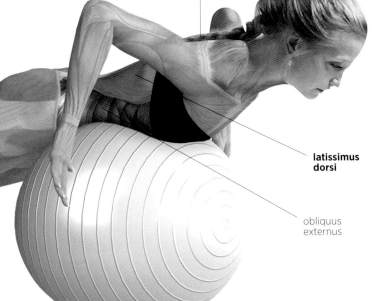

- rhomboideus*
- **latissimus dorsi**
- obliquus externus

Swiss Ball Back Extension

This is a wonderful exercise for strengthening your middle and lower back through using the weight of your body over a ball. And because your glutes do plenty of work here, they also get strengthened—along with quite a few other areas.

HOW TO DO IT

- Lie prone over a Swiss ball, with your upper chest and head hanging off the edge of the ball.

- Firmly plant your feet to stabilize yourself over the ball, and place your hands on either side of your head. This is your starting position.

- With arms bent and elbows out, raise your upper body off the ball.

- Slowly and carefully lower your body to your starting position, and repeat for the recommended number of repetitions.

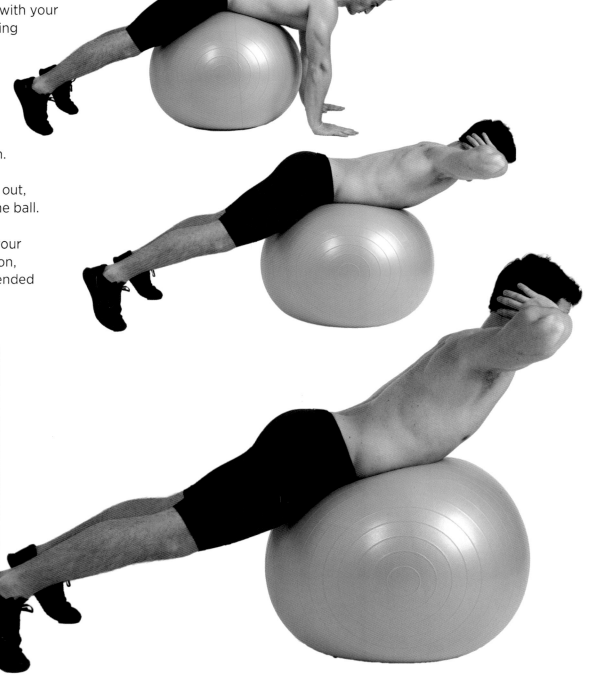

DO IT RIGHT

- Engage your glutes and thighs throughout.
- Keep your lower-body muscles taut.
- Keep your head in a neutral (natural and not up or down) position.
- Maintain a wide base for extra balance.
- Avoid lifting your shoulders.
- Avoid lifting your hips off the ball.

FACT FILE

TARGETS
- Middle back
- Lower back
- Glutes
- Shoulders and chest
- Arms and legs

EQUIPMENT
- Swiss ball

BENEFITS
- Strengthens back extensor muscles
- Stabilizes core
- Strengthens abdominals

CAUTIONS
- Neck issues
- Lower-back pain

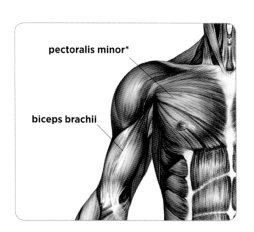

pectoralis minor*

biceps brachii

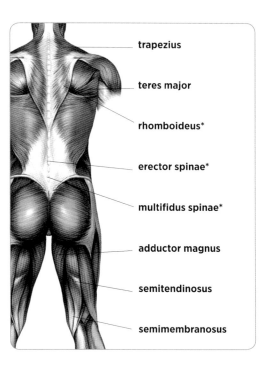

trapezius

teres major

rhomboideus*

erector spinae*

multifidus spinae*

adductor magnus

semitendinosus

semimembranosus

Annotation Key

Bold text indicates target muscles
Light text indicates other working muscles
* indicates deep muscles

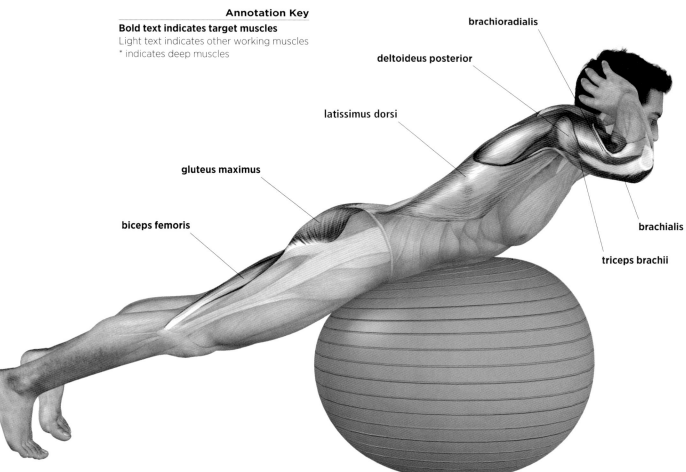

brachioradialis

deltoideus posterior

latissimus dorsi

gluteus maximus

biceps femoris

brachialis

triceps brachii

Single-Arm Band Pull

The Single-Arm Band Pull makes use of pulling a resistance band to target your back, particularly the latissimus dorsi, as well as the front of your core.

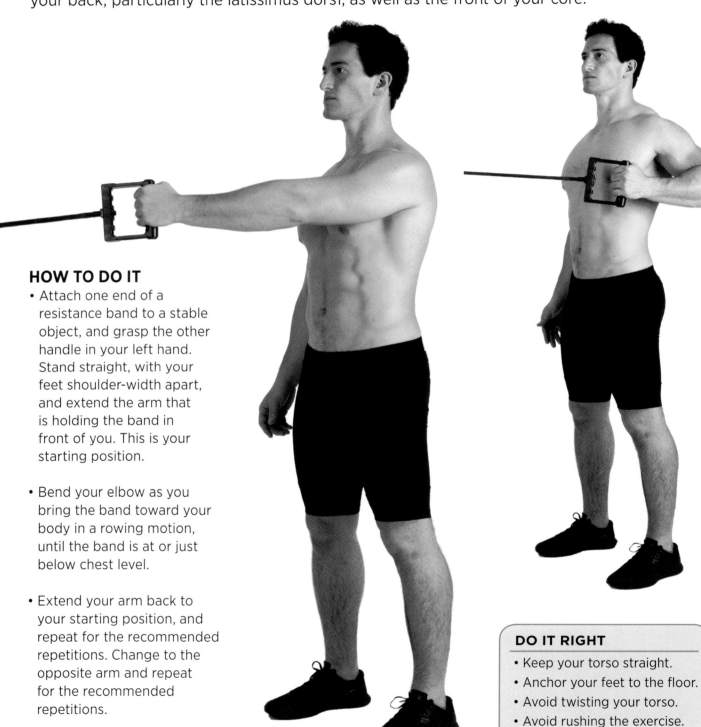

HOW TO DO IT

• Attach one end of a resistance band to a stable object, and grasp the other handle in your left hand. Stand straight, with your feet shoulder-width apart, and extend the arm that is holding the band in front of you. This is your starting position.

• Bend your elbow as you bring the band toward your body in a rowing motion, until the band is at or just below chest level.

• Extend your arm back to your starting position, and repeat for the recommended repetitions. Change to the opposite arm and repeat for the recommended repetitions.

DO IT RIGHT
• Keep your torso straight.
• Anchor your feet to the floor.
• Avoid twisting your torso.
• Avoid rushing the exercise.

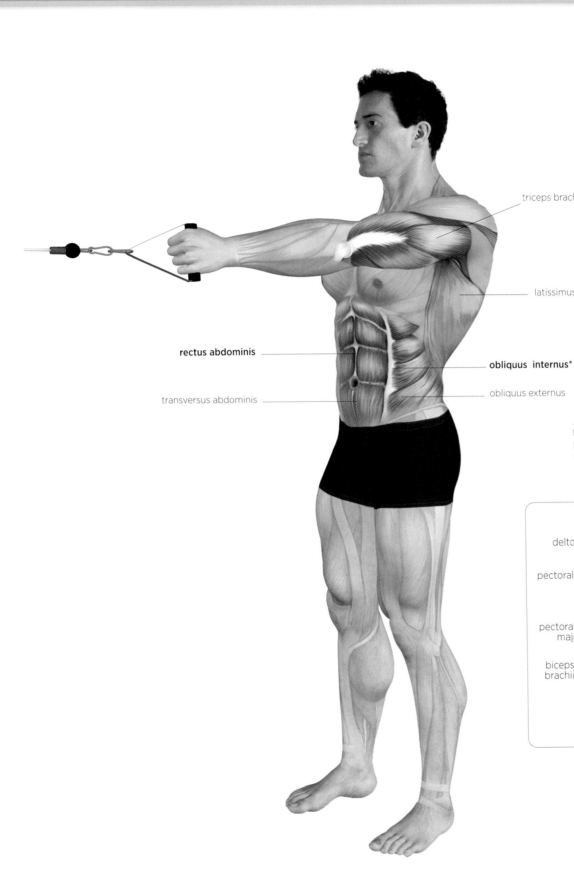

TARGETS
- Latissimus dorsi
- Abdominals
- Upper arms

EQUIPMENT
- Resistance band

BENEFITS
- Strengthens back
- Tones and defines abdominals and upper arms

CAUTIONS
- Lower-back issues

triceps brachii

latissimus dorsi

rectus abdominis

obliquus internus*

transversus abdominis

obliquus externus

Annotation Key
Bold text indicates target muscles
Light text indicates other working muscles
* indicates deep muscles

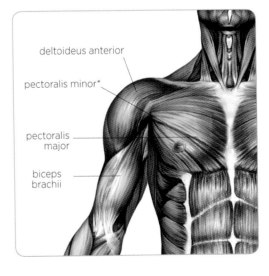

deltoideus anterior

pectoralis minor*

pectoralis major

biceps brachii

Pyramid Cable Press

This is the perfect routine to strengthen an assembly of muscles that rotate the whole shoulder and upper–arm area. Proceed slowly and with control to get the most from it—and don't be tempted to work with too much weight.

HOW TO DO IT

• Set both sides of a cable machine to the lowest settings. Attach a single-handle grip to each side.

• Center yourself between the cable uprights, with your feet shoulder-width apart and your pelvis tucked in. Pick up the handle grips one at a time.

• Starting with your palms facing up, curl the weight in. Rotate your palms to face forward, with your arms in a 90-degree bend.

• Press the cable weight upward in a pyramid motion to a near touch at the top range of the movement.

• Slowly and deliberately lower the weight to the starting position, and repeat for the recommended repetitions.

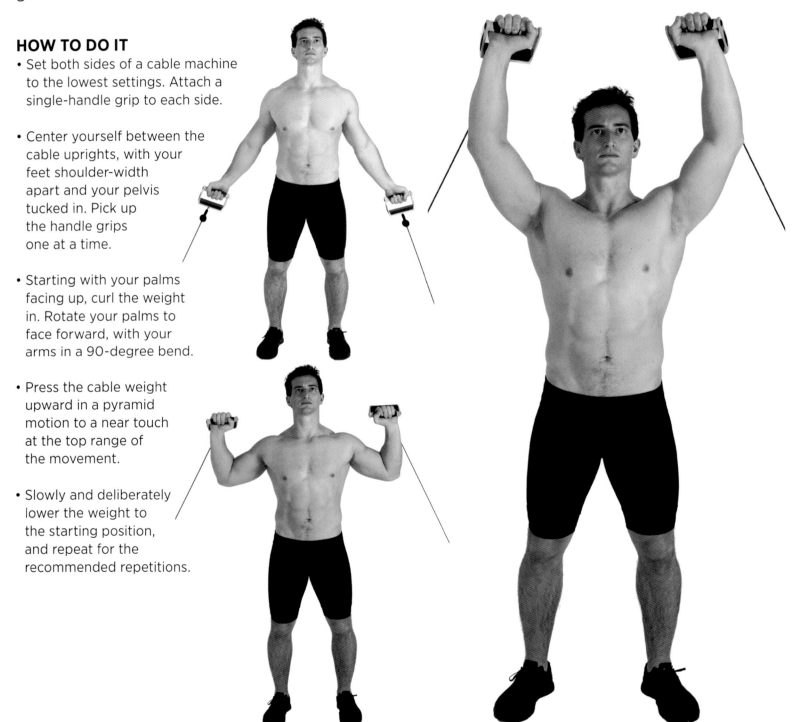

FACT FILE

TARGETS
- Deltoids
- Shoulder blade muscles
- Supraspinatus rotator cuff
- Biceps and triceps
- Trapezius

EQUIPMENT
- Cable machine

BENEFITS
- Strengthens shoulders, upper back, and upper arms
- Stabilizes neck muscles that lift the shoulder blades

CAUTIONS
- Shoulder issues
- Wrist issues

biceps brachii

deltoideus medialis

triceps brachii

deltoideus anterior

serratus anterior

DO IT RIGHT

- Maintain a consistent speed of movement throughout.
- Exhale as you press the cable weight up; inhale as you lower it back down.
- Avoid lifting overly heavy weights—this could strain your biceps as you get into your starting position and even cause injury.
- Avoid bending your knees to give assistance and momentum.

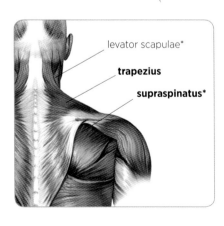

levator scapulae*

trapezius

supraspinatus*

Annotation Key
Bold text indicates target muscles
Light text indicates other working muscles
* indicates deep muscles

Bent-Over Cable Raise

Doing the Bent-Over Cable Raise will benefit your deltoids in general, but especially the deltoids encasing the back, side, and top of your shoulders. Your upper arms get a good workout, too.

HOW TO DO IT

- Set a cable machine with a single-handle grip to its lowest setting.

- Stand with your right shoulder parallel to the cable machine.

- With your left hand, grasp the handle with your palm facing inward, hammer-grip style. This is your starting position.

- With your feet parallel and shoulder-width apart, slightly bend your knees as you lean over, flattening your back.

- Extend your left arm out to the left side.

- Carefully bring the cable weight back to your starting position, and repeat for the recommended repetitions. Repeat, with your opposite hand holding the handle grip, for the recommended repetitions.

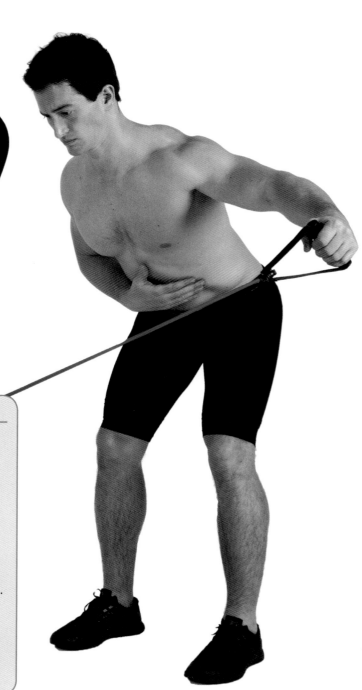

DO IT RIGHT

- Try to get a stretch in your rear deltoid at the starting-position stage.
- Engage your glutes and thighs.
- Keep your shoulders down and back.
- Avoid using momentum to execute the movement.
- Avoid dropping your head.
- Avoid letting your chest or shoulders roll inward.

TARGETS
- Rear and side deltoids

EQUIPMENT
- Cable machine

BENEFITS
- Focuses on strengthening the backs and sides of your shoulders
- Stabilizes and works upper arms

CAUTIONS
- Back issues
- Wrist issues

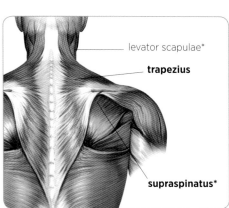

levator scapulae*

trapezius

supraspinatus*

Annotation Key

Bold text indicates target muscles
Light text indicates other working muscles
* indicates deep muscles

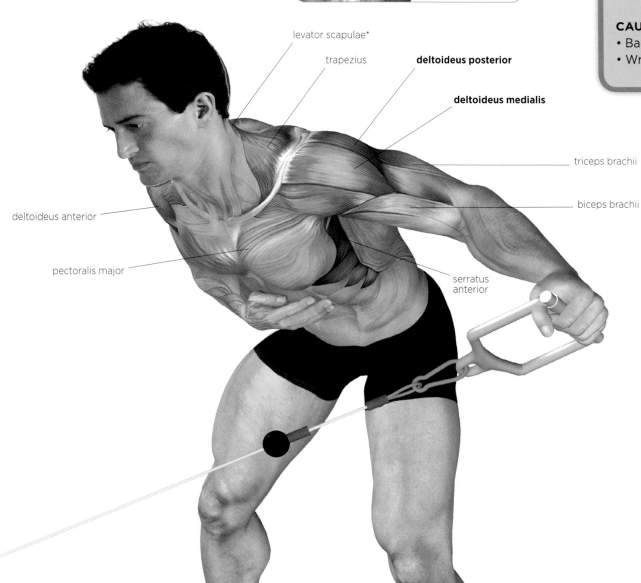

levator scapulae*

trapezius

deltoideus posterior

deltoideus medialis

triceps brachii

biceps brachii

deltoideus anterior

pectoralis major

serratus anterior

Resistance Band Overhead Press

This closely focused routine concentrates on strengthening your anterior—front—deltoids. These let you bend you arms at the shoulder and rotate your arms and shoulders inward. It also stabilizes other muscles around the area, including your upper arms.

HOW TO DO IT

• Stand with your left leg extended about a foot behind you. Position the resistance band beneath the foot of your front, right, leg. Hold the handles in both hands, with arms bent, so that the resistance band is taut. Your palms should face forward.

• Straighten both arms so that they are fully extended above your head a few inches in front of your shoulders.

• Lower your arms to your starting position and then repeat for the recommended repetitions.

DO IT RIGHT
• Keep the rest of your body stable as you extend your arms.
• Gaze forward throughout.
• Keep your abs engaged and pulled in.
• Extend both arms at the same time.
• Avoid twisting your torso.

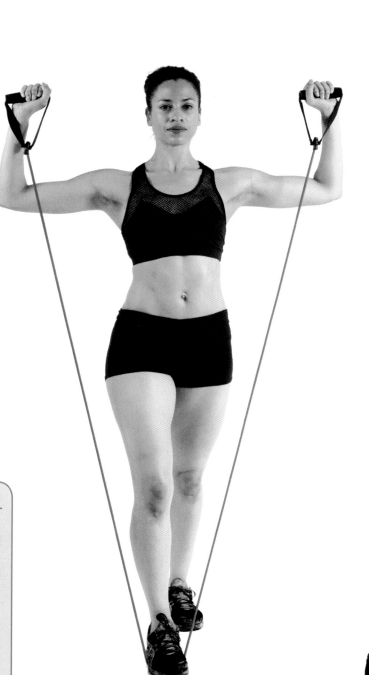
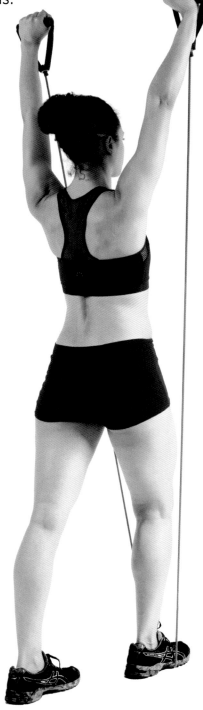

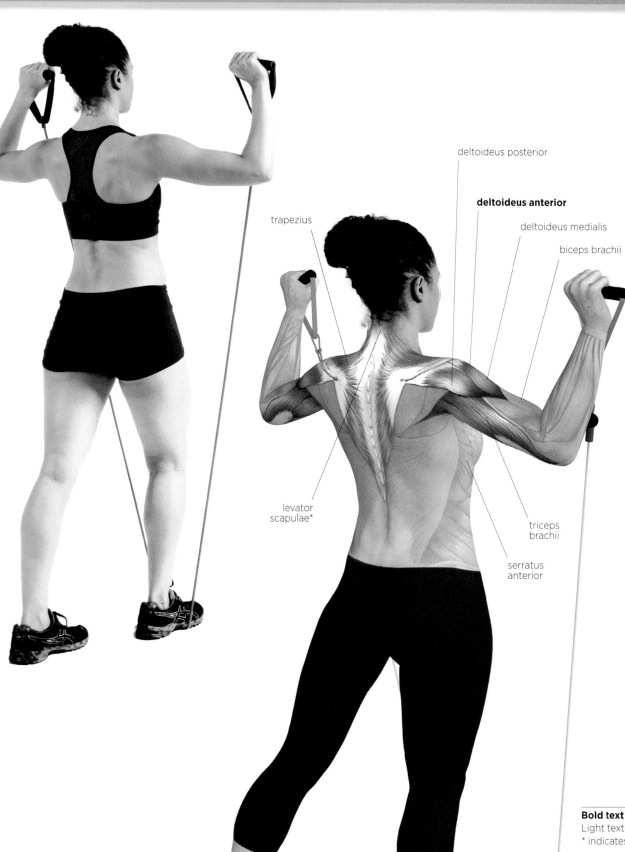

FACT FILE

TARGETS
- Anterior (front) deltoids

EQUIPMENT
- Resistance band

BENEFITS
- Strengthens and tones shoulders
- Works and stabilizes upper arms

CAUTIONS
- Shoulder issues

deltoideus posterior

deltoideus anterior

deltoideus medialis

trapezius

biceps brachii

levator scapulae*

triceps brachii

serratus anterior

Annotation Key

Bold text indicates target muscles
Light text indicates other working muscles
* indicates deep muscles

Resistance Band Lateral Raise

This is one for your deltoideus medialis shoulder muscles—otherwise variously known as the lateral, side, or middle deltoids. These are your shoulder abductors, letting you move your shoulders out and away from your body.

HOW TO DO IT

- Stand with your arms at your sides and feet about hip-width apart on top of your resistance band. Hold one handle in each hand, palms facing inward.

- Keeping your palms down, raise your arms out to your sides so that they are parallel to the floor. Raise them to around shoulder height, but not much above that.

- Lower, and repeat for the recommended repetitions.

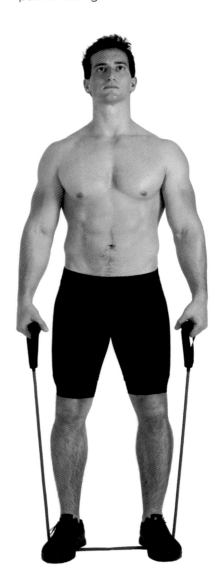

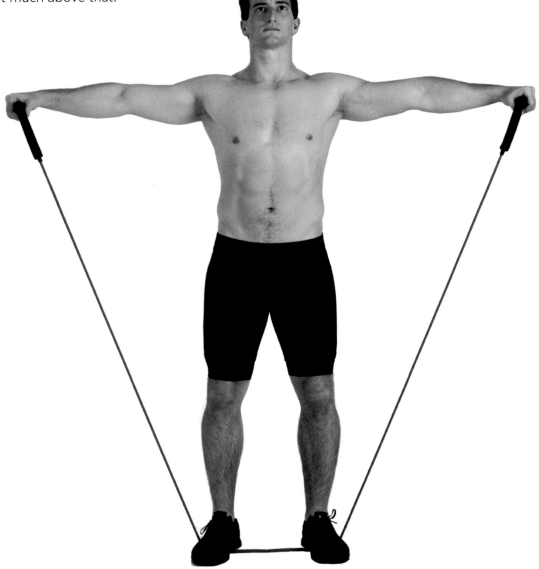

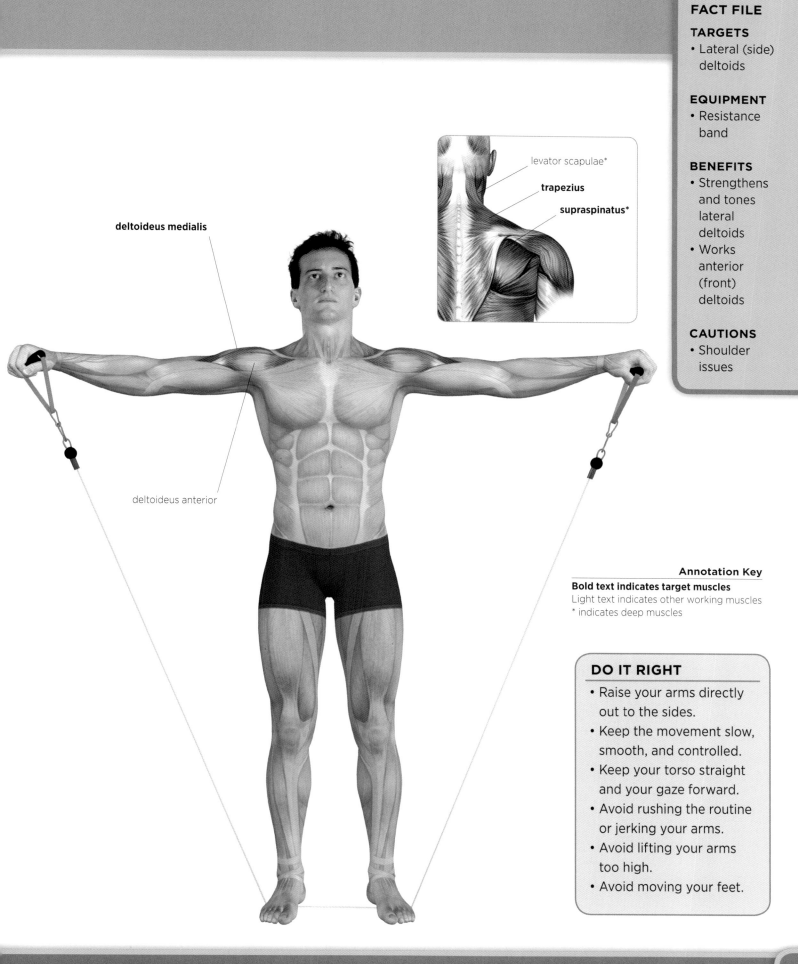

TARGETS
• Lateral (side) deltoids

EQUIPMENT
• Resistance band

BENEFITS
• Strengthens and tones lateral deltoids
• Works anterior (front) deltoids

CAUTIONS
• Shoulder issues

levator scapulae*

trapezius

supraspinatus*

deltoideus medialis

deltoideus anterior

Annotation Key
Bold text indicates target muscles
Light text indicates other working muscles
* indicates deep muscles

DO IT RIGHT
• Raise your arms directly out to the sides.
• Keep the movement slow, smooth, and controlled.
• Keep your torso straight and your gaze forward.
• Avoid rushing the routine or jerking your arms.
• Avoid lifting your arms too high.
• Avoid moving your feet.

Resistance Band Biceps Curl

Bring some power and strength to your all-important biceps, at the front of your upper arms, with this simple classic exercise. Curls make you work other arm muscles, too.

HOW TO DO IT

• Stand with your feet a little way apart on top of your resistance band. Grasp both handles of the band in your hands, palms facing forward.

• Move your elbows and upper arms to your sides and bend your elbows slightly.

• Curl the resistance band upward, quite tightly.

• Lower, and repeat for the recommended repetitions.

DO IT RIGHT
• Keep your elbows at your sides, not splayed out.
• Avoid rushing the routine.

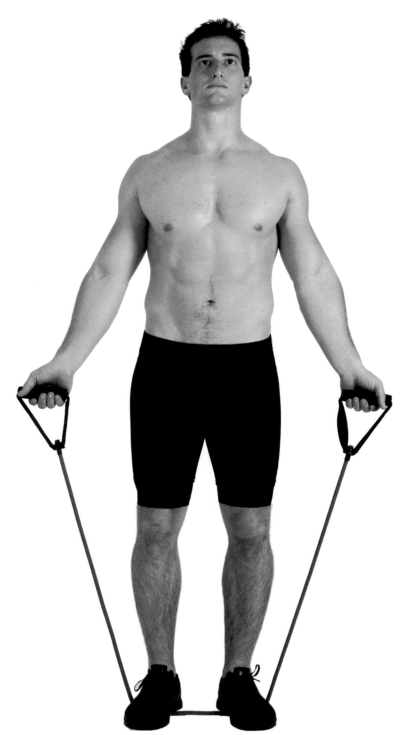

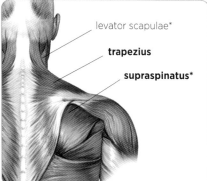

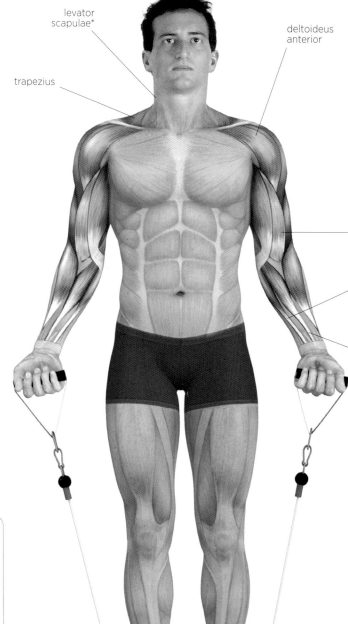

FACT FILE

TARGETS
• Biceps

EQUIPMENT
• Resistance band

BENEFITS
• Strengthens and tones biceps

CAUTIONS
• Wrist or elbow pain

levator scapulae*

trapezius

deltoideus anterior

biceps brachii

flexor carpi ulnaris

flexor carpi radialis

levator scapulae*

trapezius

supraspinatus*

Annotation Key

Bold text indicates target muscles
Light text indicates other working muscles
* indicates deep muscles

Resistance Band Single-Arm Row

All you need is a basic resistance band to enjoy this highly effective strengthener and toner for your biceps—as well as for the latissimus dorsi muscle of your back. Stablized deltoids are another bonus of this routine.

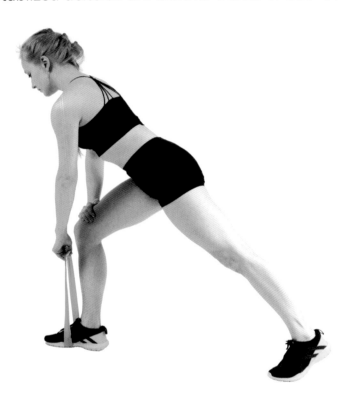

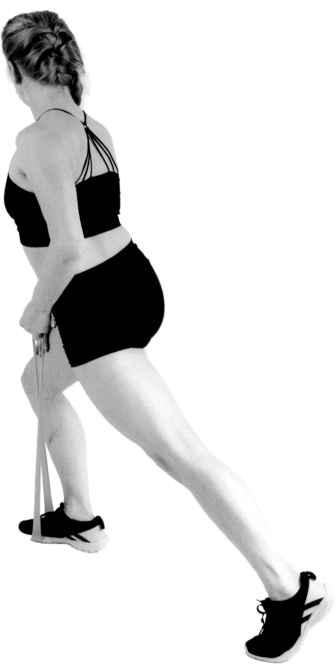

HOW TO DO IT

- Stand with your right leg extended a long way in front of your left, with your front, right, leg bent and the heel of your back, left, foot off the floor. Either trap one end of a resistance band under your right foot and grasp the other end with your left hand, or use a looped band around your right foot, held with your left hand.

- Rest your free right hand above your right knee, and lean forward.

- Bend your left arm as you pull the resistance band up toward your chest.

- Lower, and repeat for the recommended repetitions. Repeat on the opposite side for the recommended repetitions.

FACT FILE

TARGETS
- Biceps
- Latissimus dorsi

EQUIPMENT
- Resistance band

BENEFITS
- Strengthens and tones biceps
- Improves back stabilization

CAUTIONS
- Lower-back issues

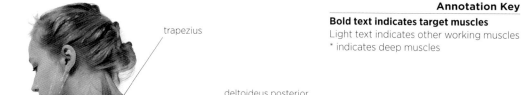

Annotation Key
Bold text indicates target muscles
Light text indicates other working muscles
* indicates deep muscles

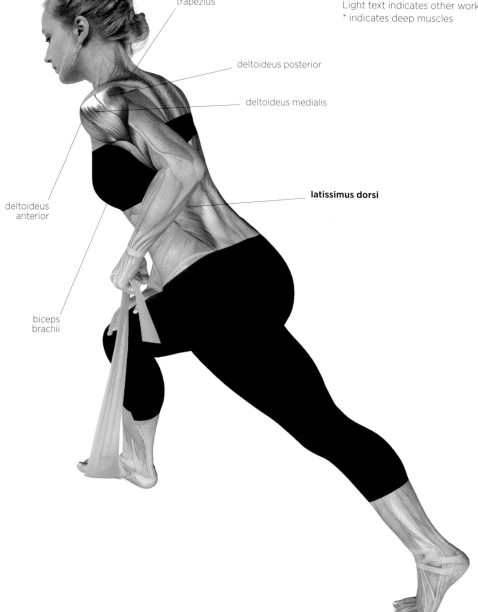

trapezius

deltoideus posterior

deltoideus medialis

latissimus dorsi

deltoideus anterior

biceps brachii

DO IT RIGHT
- Keep your back flat throughout.
- Lean forward so your back leg and torso form a straight line.
- Move smoothly and with control, engaging your arm muscles.
- Avoid allowing the resistance band to come loose from beneath your front foot.
- Avoid arching your back or neck.
- Avoid curving your back forward.
- Avoid hunching your shoulders.
- Avoid rushing through the movement, or jerking your arm.

Swiss Ball W

Named for the W shape that your bent arms and shoulders form at the top of this movement, the Swiss Ball W targets your rear deltoids. These muscles let you rotate your arms and shoulders outward and behind you.

HOW TO DO IT

- Lie facedown on a Swiss ball with your back flat, your chest off the ball, and your legs elongated. Bend your elbows, keeping them fairly close to your sides and not splayed out.

- Keeping your elbows bent, squeeze your shoulder blades together as you raise your upper arms. Your arms should form a W at the top of the movement.

- Hold for a few moments, slowly lower to your starting position, and repeat for the recommended repetitions.

DO IT RIGHT

- Keep your arms bent throughout.
- Use a reverse "hugging" motion when you raise your arms.
- Avoid excessive speed or momentum.

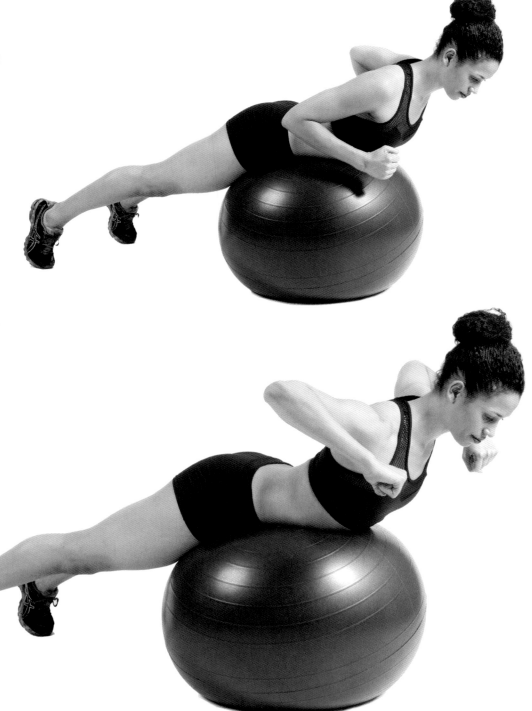

TARGETS
- Posterior (rear) deltoids
- Core

EQUIPMENT
- Swiss ball/ dumbbells for modifications

BENEFITS
- Strengthens back of shoulders
- Stabilizes core
- Helps improve posture

CAUTIONS
- Shoulder issues
- Severe lower-back pain

MODIFICATION

HARDER: Hold a dumbbell in each hand.

HARDER: Holding dumbbells, stretch your arms straight out to the sides, as a variant or added into the W routine. This will work your arm and shoulder muscles slightly differently.

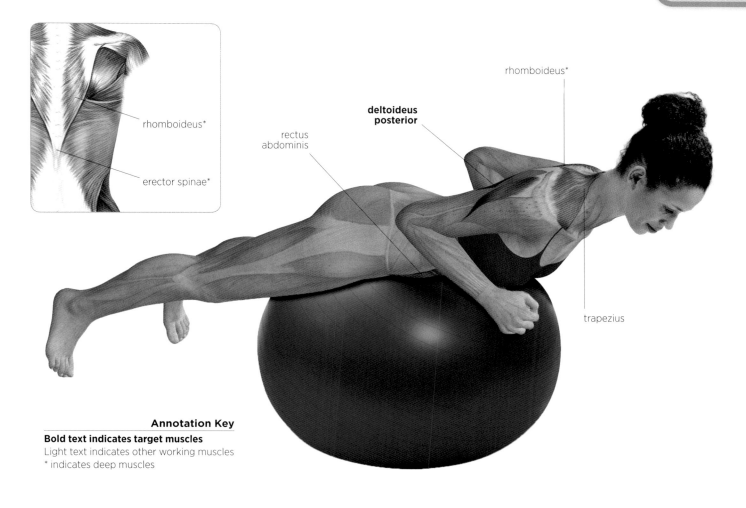

rhomboideus*

rhomboideus*

erector spinae*

deltoideus posterior

rectus abdominis

trapezius

Annotation Key
Bold text indicates target muscles
Light text indicates other working muscles
* indicates deep muscles

Foam Roller Triceps Dip

The serratus anterior muscles play a vital role in mobilizing and stabilizing your shoulder blades. Often under-worked, they take center stage in this routine, along with your deltoids and triceps—and aided by your abdominals.

HOW TO DO IT

- Sit on the floor with your legs outstretched, the foam roller behind you. Place both hands on the foam roller, with your fingers facing toward your buttocks and your elbows bent.

- Press through your legs and straighten your arms to lift your hips and shoulders. Raise your body up, keeping your legs straight.

- Keeping your shoulders pressed down away from your ears, bend your elbows and dip your trunk up and then down. The foam roller should not move. Repeat for the recommended repetitions.

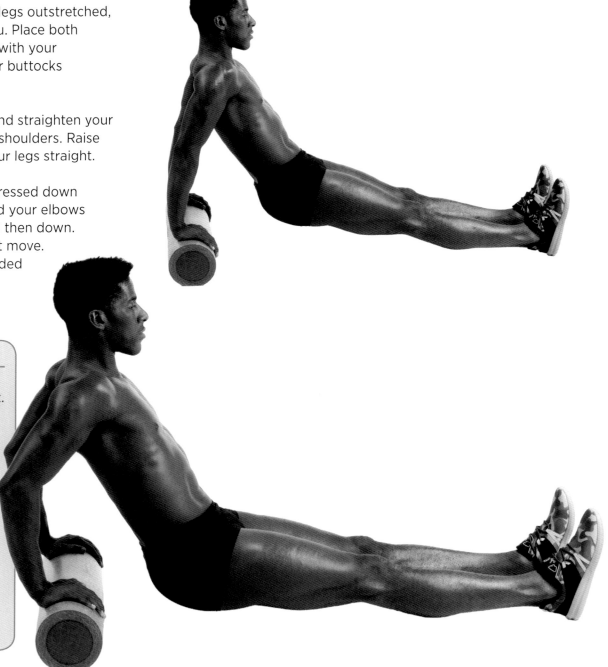

DO IT RIGHT

- Keep your legs firm, with your knees straight.
- Keep your neck and shoulders relaxed throughout.
- Keep your hands pressed firmly to the roller.
- Avoid allowing your shoulders to lift toward your ears.
- Avoid shifting the roller as you move up and down.

TARGETS
- Shoulder stabilizers
- Triceps
- Deltoids
- Abdominals

EQUIPMENT
- Foam roller

BENEFITS
- Improves shoulder and upper-arm strength and stability
- Works and stabilizes core

CAUTIONS
- Wrist pain
- Shoulder pain
- Discomfort in the back of the knee or knee swelling

Annotation Key

Bold text indicates target muscles
Light text indicates other working muscles
* indicates deep muscles

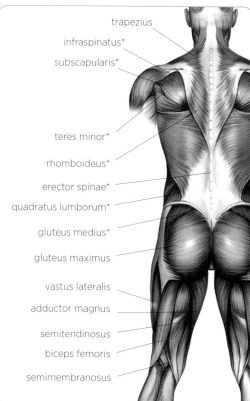

- trapezius
- infraspinatus*
- subscapularis*
- teres minor*
- rhomboideus*
- erector spinae*
- quadratus lumborum*
- gluteus medius*
- gluteus maximus
- vastus lateralis
- adductor magnus
- semitendinosus
- biceps femoris
- semimembranosus

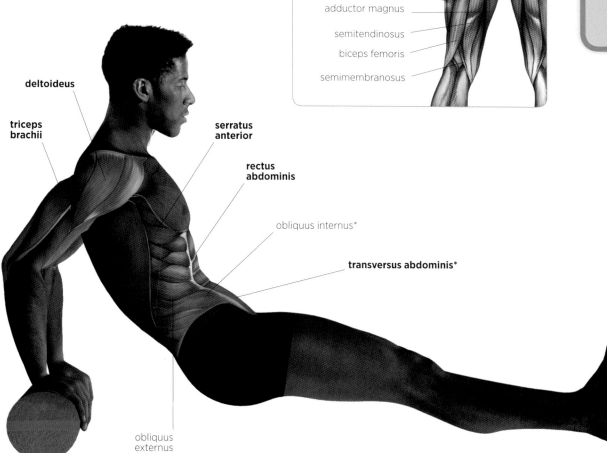

- **deltoideus**
- **triceps brachii**
- **serratus anterior**
- **rectus abdominis**
- obliquus internus*
- **transversus abdominis***
- obliquus externus

Cable Fly

This Cable Fly routine provides excellent strength development for your chest. It also gives a thorough workout to much of the top half of your body.

HOW TO DO IT

- Stand between two high cable machine uprights. Grasp the overhead handle grips in each hand, one at a time.

- Center yourself between the uprights.

- Take a full step back, bringing your hands toward your thighs.

- Step forward with your right leg, lunging slightly with this front leg, as you start the exercise by bringing your arms to just below chest level, palms facing each other. Your weight should be on your front, right, foot.

- Keeping the gentle lunge, extend your arms backward and out to the side until you feel a slight stretch in your chest.

- Bring the weight back to your starting position, and repeat for the recommended repetitions. Alternate lunging legs if you wish.

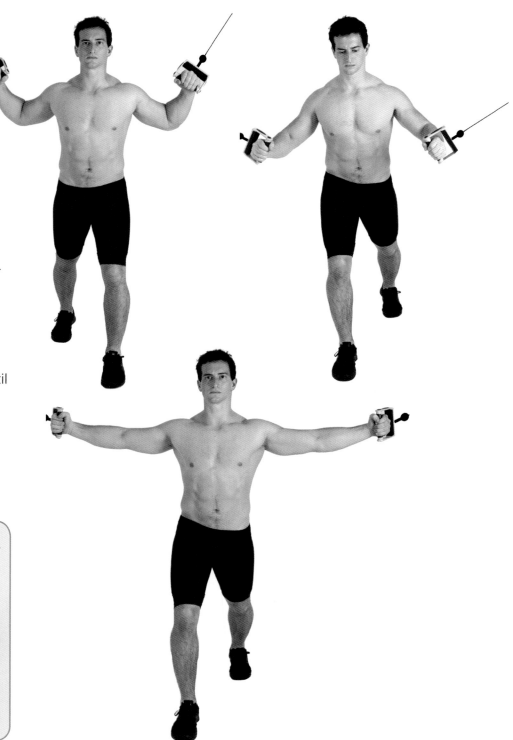

DO IT RIGHT

- Keep your hands facing each other in the hammer.
- Make sure your arms are well stretched out on your pulls.
- Start off with a light weight until you have mastered the movement and feel confident that you are strong enough to increase the weight used.
- Avoid extending your arms too far.

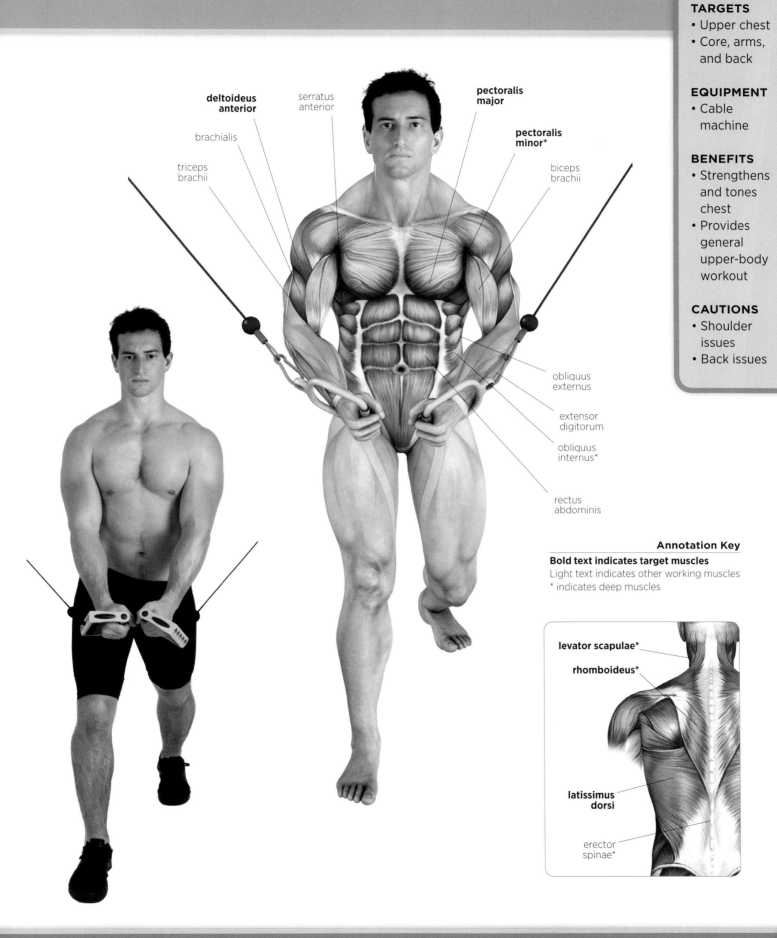

TARGETS
• Upper chest
• Core, arms, and back

EQUIPMENT
• Cable machine

BENEFITS
• Strengthens and tones chest
• Provides general upper-body workout

CAUTIONS
• Shoulder issues
• Back issues

deltoideus anterior

serratus anterior

brachialis

triceps brachii

pectoralis major

pectoralis minor*

biceps brachii

obliquus externus

extensor digitorum

obliquus internus*

rectus abdominis

Annotation Key

Bold text indicates target muscles
Light text indicates other working muscles
* indicates deep muscles

levator scapulae*

rhomboideus*

latissimus dorsi

erector spinae*

Cable Decline Fly

Try working on your chest, as well as your arms, with this Cable Decline Fly. Plus it will strengthen and stabilize your shoulders—as long as you keep them down and firmly in a stable position.

HOW TO DO IT

- Adjust two cables on a cable machine so they are set on the highest setting. Stand between the machine uprights. Grasp the handle grips in each hand, one at a time.

- Center yourself between the uprights. Stand with your feet placed at least around shoulder-width apart.

- With your elbows slightly bent and your palms facing downward, pull your arms down at an angle to meet in front of your body.

- Lower the weights to your starting position, and repeat for the recommended repetitions.

DO IT RIGHT

- Your shoulders to remain down and away from your ears, allowing your chest to elevate.
- Avoid leaning too far forward.
- Avoid swaying your lower back.

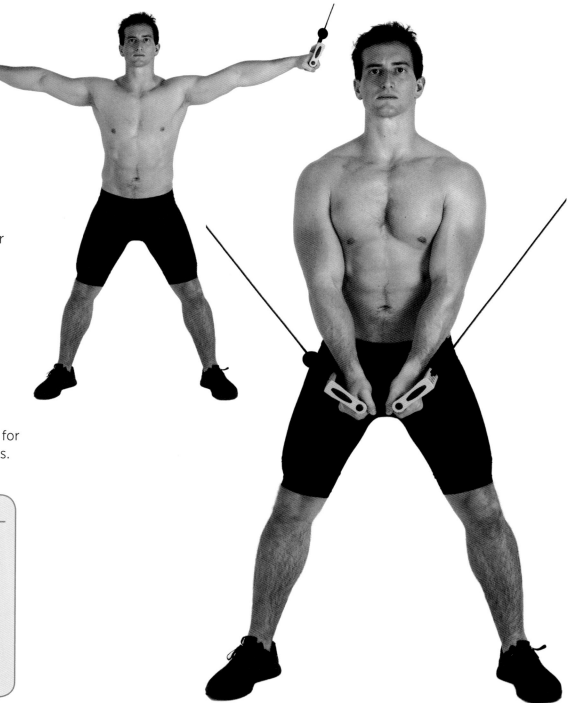

FACT FILE

TARGETS
• Lower chest
• Arms

EQUIPMENT
• Cable machine

BENEFITS
• Strengthens lower chest
• Tones arms
• Stabilizes shoulders

CAUTIONS
• Shoulder issues
• Wrist issues

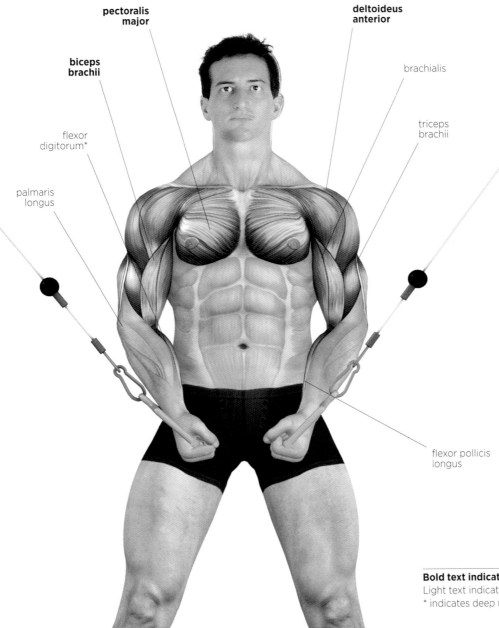

pectoralis major

deltoideus anterior

brachialis

biceps brachii

triceps brachii

flexor digitorum*

palmaris longus

flexor pollicis longus

Annotation Key

Bold text indicates target muscles
Light text indicates other working muscles
* indicates deep muscles

Cable Crossover Fly

The Cable Crossover Fly gives you another variant for working your lower chest. This is great, too, for your shoulders and biceps.

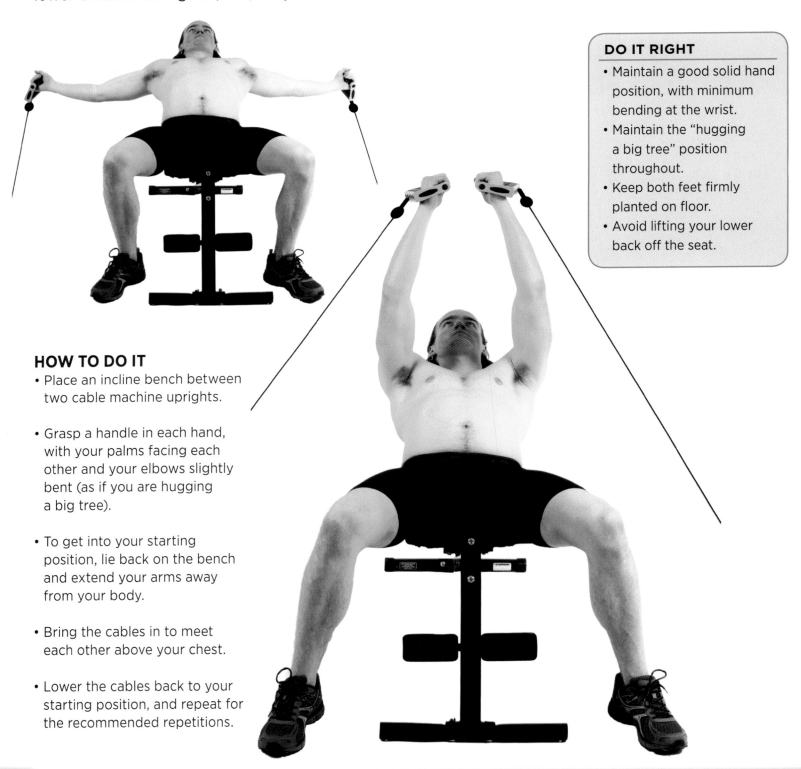

HOW TO DO IT

- Place an incline bench between two cable machine uprights.

- Grasp a handle in each hand, with your palms facing each other and your elbows slightly bent (as if you are hugging a big tree).

- To get into your starting position, lie back on the bench and extend your arms away from your body.

- Bring the cables in to meet each other above your chest.

- Lower the cables back to your starting position, and repeat for the recommended repetitions.

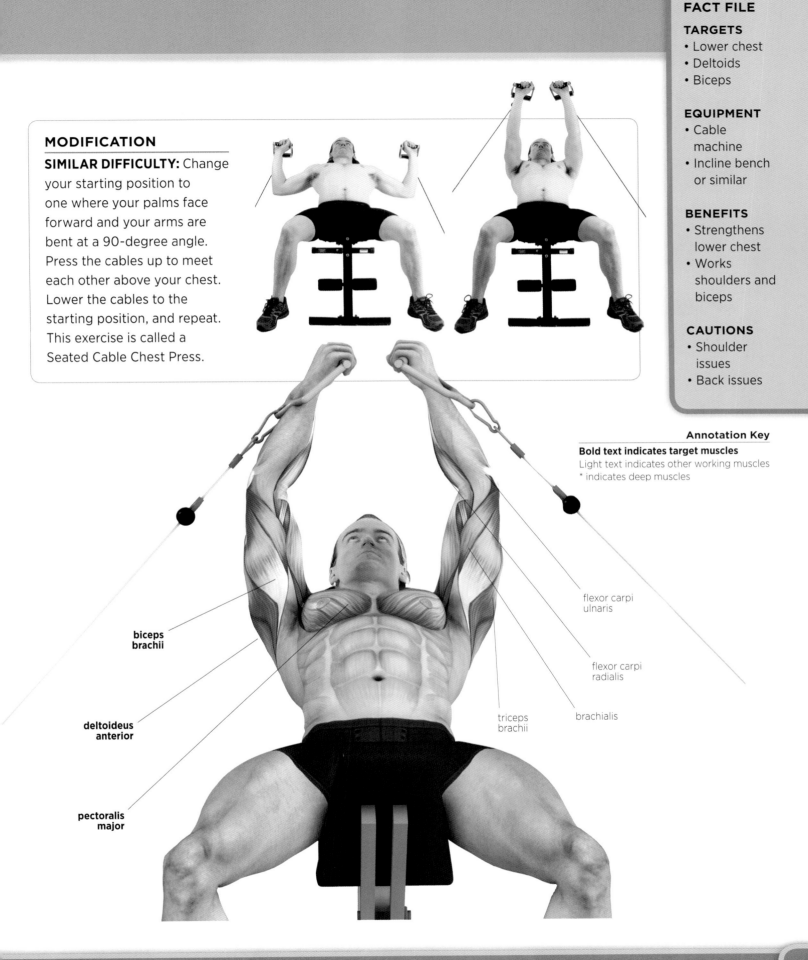

TARGETS
- Lower chest
- Deltoids
- Biceps

EQUIPMENT
- Cable machine
- Incline bench or similar

BENEFITS
- Strengthens lower chest
- Works shoulders and biceps

CAUTIONS
- Shoulder issues
- Back issues

MODIFICATION

SIMILAR DIFFICULTY: Change your starting position to one where your palms face forward and your arms are bent at a 90-degree angle. Press the cables up to meet each other above your chest. Lower the cables to the starting position, and repeat. This exercise is called a Seated Cable Chest Press.

Annotation Key

Bold text indicates target muscles
Light text indicates other working muscles
* indicates deep muscles

flexor carpi ulnaris

flexor carpi radialis

biceps brachii

brachialis

triceps brachii

deltoideus anterior

pectoralis major

Alternating Chest Press

Perform the Alternating Chest Press if you want to concentrate on strengthening the large pectoralis major muscle of your chest. The key to success here is to work smoothly and with control.

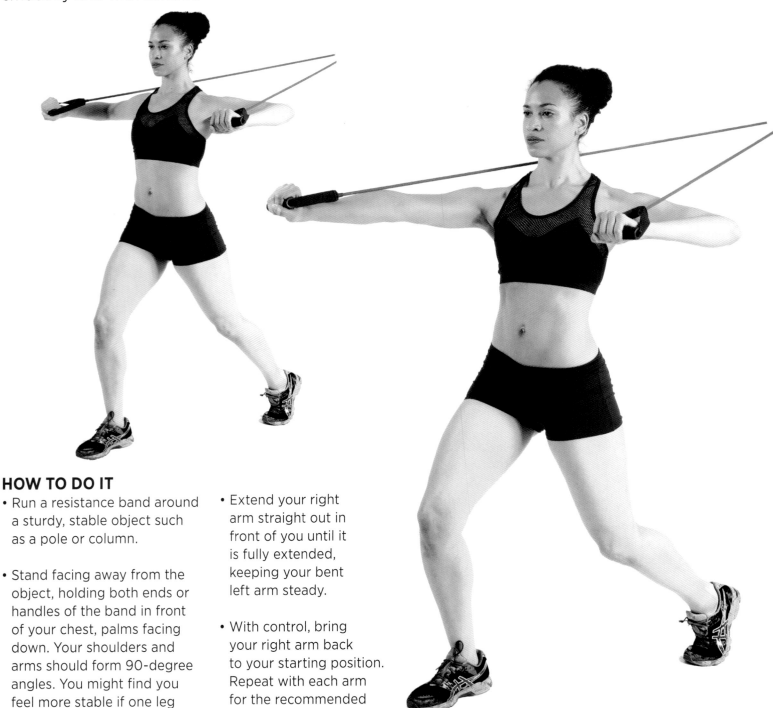

HOW TO DO IT

- Run a resistance band around a sturdy, stable object such as a pole or column.

- Stand facing away from the object, holding both ends or handles of the band in front of your chest, palms facing down. Your shoulders and arms should form 90-degree angles. You might find you feel more stable if one leg is in front of the other.

- Extend your right arm straight out in front of you until it is fully extended, keeping your bent left arm steady.

- With control, bring your right arm back to your starting position. Repeat with each arm for the recommended repetitions.

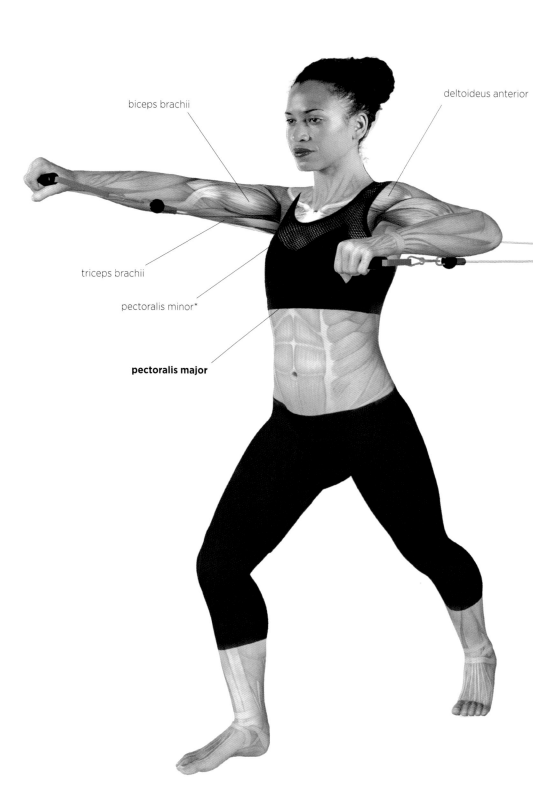

FACT FILE

TARGETS
• Pectorals

EQUIPMENT
• Resistance band

BENEFITS
• Strengthens and tones pectorals
• Stabilizes upper arms and shoulders

CAUTIONS
• Shoulder issues

biceps brachii

deltoideus anterior

triceps brachii

pectoralis minor*

pectoralis major

Annotation Key
Bold text indicates target muscles
Light text indicates other working muscles
* indicates deep muscles

DO IT RIGHT
• Keep one arm motionless as you extend the other fully.
• Maintain a stable torso.
• Keep your feet in place as you extend your arm.
• Engage your abdominal muscles throughout.
• Keep your arms level with your shoulders.
• Avoid twisting your torso.
• Avoid hunching your shoulders.

Resistance Band Standing Fly

This exercise is both easy and very simple—ideal for adding in to any exercise regimen. It is often promoted for its effectiveness in working the back, but in fact is an excellent way to strengthen your pecs.

HOW TO DO IT

- Run a resistance band around a sturdy, stable object such as a pole or column. Stand upright, with your feet planted shoulder-width apart.

- Grasp both ends or handles of the resistance band, and extend your arms in front of you to almost shoulder height, holding the band taut.

- Slowly and with control, bring both arms out to the sides, palms facing forward.

- Return to your starting position, and repeat for the recommended repetitions.

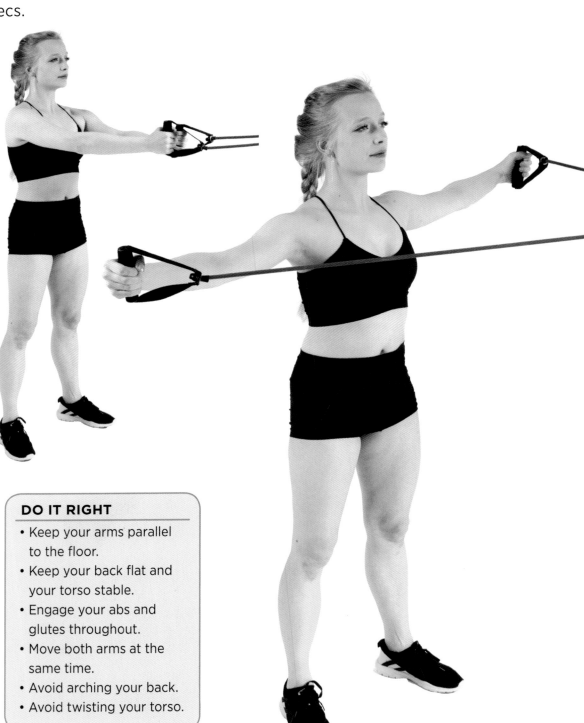

DO IT RIGHT

- Keep your arms parallel to the floor.
- Keep your back flat and your torso stable.
- Engage your abs and glutes throughout.
- Move both arms at the same time.
- Avoid arching your back.
- Avoid twisting your torso.

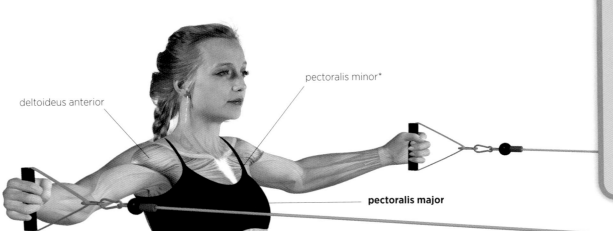

FACT FILE

TARGETS
• Pectorals

EQUIPMENT
• Resistance band

BENEFITS
• Strengthens chest
• Stabilizes shoulders and upper back

CAUTIONS
• Lower-back issues
• Shoulder pain

deltoideus anterior

pectoralis minor*

pectoralis major

latissimus dorsi

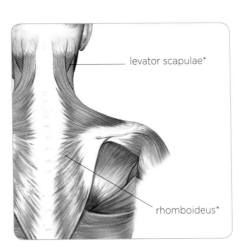

levator scapulae*

rhomboideus*

Annotation Key

Bold text indicates target muscles
Light text indicates other working muscles
* indicates deep muscles

Swiss Ball Push-Up

Here, using a Swiss ball adds helpful resistance to the classic push-up and provides a great chest exercise. It also adds an element of balance that really gets you engaging your abdominals.

HOW TO DO IT

- Place your toes on top of a Swiss ball, and walk your arms out until your legs are fully extended and your body forms a straight line from shoulders to feet, your hands shoulder-width apart.

- Bend your arms to lower your torso until your chest almost touches the floor.

- Press your upper body back up to your starting position and squeeze your chest. Pause at the contracted position, and repeat the up-and-down motion of your body for the recommended repetitions.

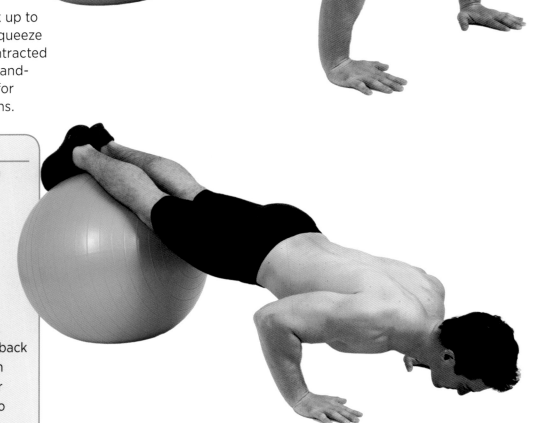

DO IT RIGHT

- Form a straight plane from neck to ankles.
- Inhale as you lower your torso, exhale as you press back up.
- Avoid arching your back during the exercise.
- Avoid rotating your hips.
- Avoid locking your elbows.
- Avoid allowing your lower back and hips to droop—this can put pressure on the lumbar vertebrae and could lead to a back injury.

FACT FILE

TARGETS
- Pectorals
- Deltoids
- Abdominals
- Triceps

EQUIPMENT
- Swiss ball

BENEFITS
- Strengthens chest
- Strengthens shoulders and upper arms
- Stabilizes core

CAUTIONS
- Wrist pain
- Lower-back pain
- Shoulder instability

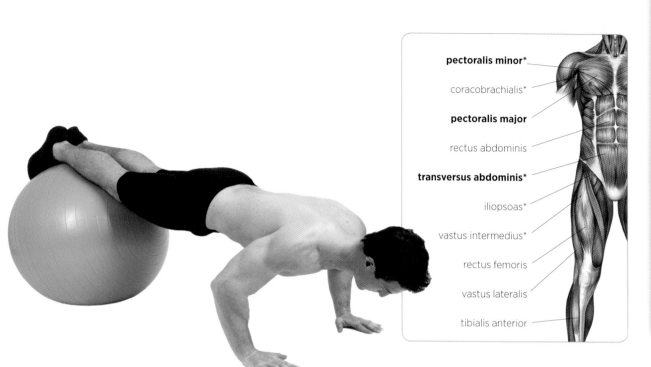

pectoralis minor*

coracobrachialis*

pectoralis major

rectus abdominis

transversus abdominis*

iliopsoas*

vastus intermedius*

rectus femoris

vastus lateralis

tibialis anterior

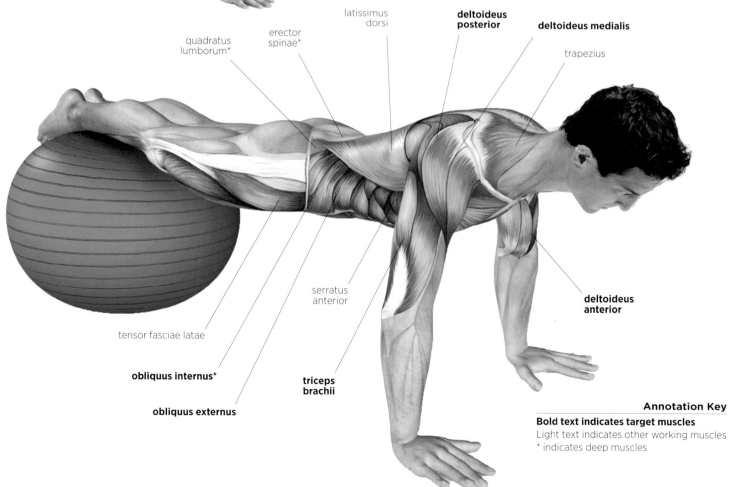

quadratus lumborum*

erector spinae*

latissimus dorsi

deltoideus posterior

deltoideus medialis

trapezius

serratus anterior

tensor fasciae latae

deltoideus anterior

obliquus internus*

triceps brachii

obliquus externus

Annotation Key

Bold text indicates target muscles
Light text indicates other working muscles
* indicates deep muscles

Balance Ball Crunch

There is persuasive evidence to suggest that crunches performed on a balance device of some kind work the abdominals much better than those done without one. And this applies to your lower and upper abs as well as your obliques.

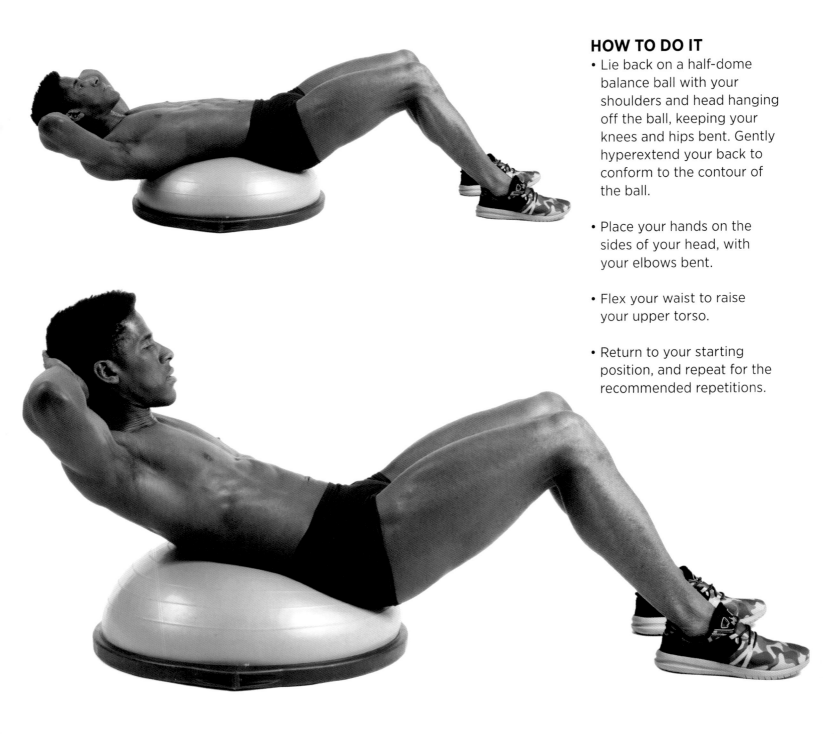

HOW TO DO IT

- Lie back on a half-dome balance ball with your shoulders and head hanging off the ball, keeping your knees and hips bent. Gently hyperextend your back to conform to the contour of the ball.

- Place your hands on the sides of your head, with your elbows bent.

- Flex your waist to raise your upper torso.

- Return to your starting position, and repeat for the recommended repetitions.

TARGETS
• Abdominals

EQUIPMENT
• Half-dome
  balance ball

BENEFITS
• Challenges
  and
  strengthens
  core
• Tones abs
• Increases
  back flexibility

CAUTIONS
• Neck issues

DO IT RIGHT

• Keep your feet planted firmly
  on the floor.
• Engage your abdominal muscles
  to initiate the movement.
• Keep your pelvis in a neutral
  position during
  the crunching motion.
• Keep your neck elongated
  and relaxed.
• Avoid rocking back and forth;
  keep your back stable on
  the ball.
• Avoid holding your breath—
  empty your lungs and take
  catch breaths when necessary.

Annotation Key

Bold text indicates target muscles
Light text indicates other working muscles
* indicates deep muscles

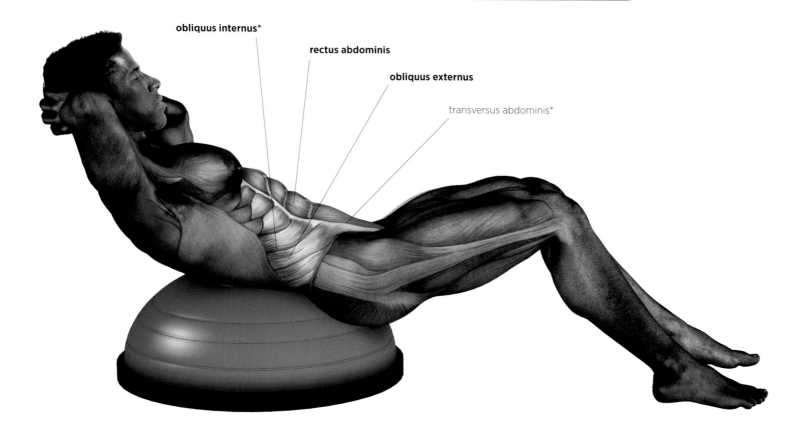

obliquus internus*

rectus abdominis

obliquus externus

transversus abdominis*

Diagonal Crunch with Medicine Ball

Diagonal Crunch with Medicine Ball strengthens your abdominal—including oblique—and intercostal muscles. You will notice the sides of your core getting tighter and stronger through regularly practicing this challenging move.

HOW TO DO IT

- Holding a medicine ball in both hands, lie on your back with your arms and legs extended behind and in front of you so that your body forms one straight line. Your legs should be around shoulder-width apart.

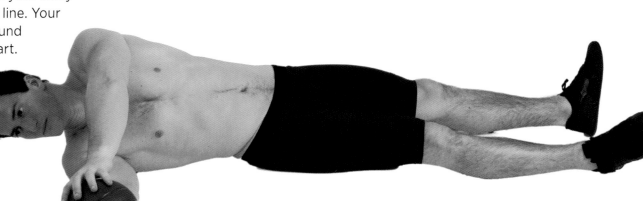

- Using your abdominals to drive the movement, move your arms and torso to your right side.

- Bring your torso to an upright position with the ball planted in between your legs.

- Lower back to your starting position, with the medicine ball held flat on the floor over your head. Repeat on the opposite side, and complete the recommended repetitions per side.

DO IT RIGHT

- Keep your legs and feet stable.
- Move smoothly and with control.
- Use your abdominal muscles to drive the movement.
- Avoid lifting your legs or feet off the floor.
- Avoid jerking your upper body.

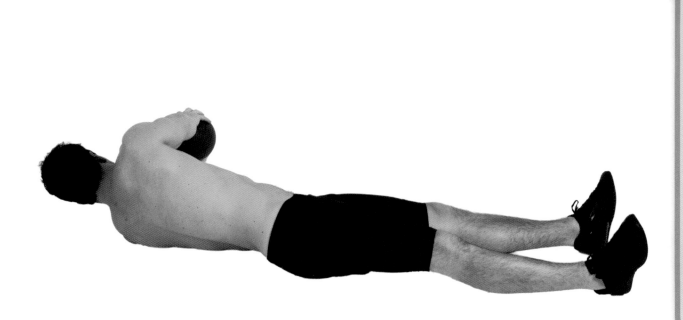

Annotation Key

Bold text indicates target muscles
Light text indicates other working muscles
* indicates deep muscles

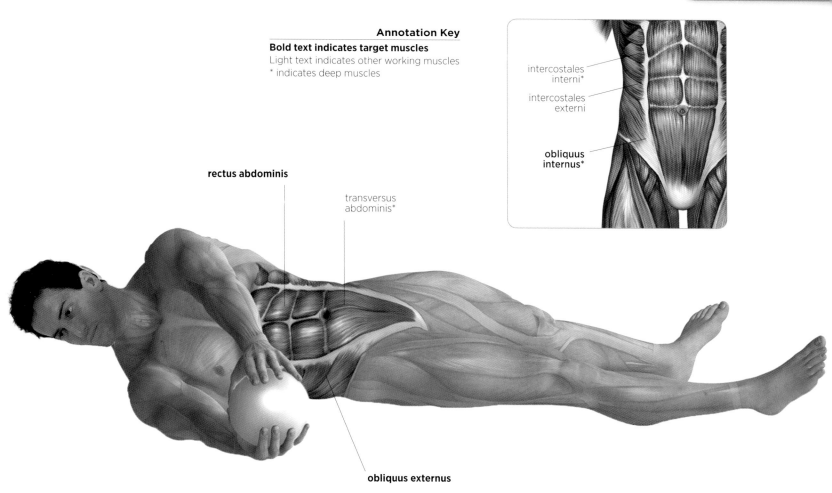

intercostales interni*

intercostales externi

obliquus internus*

rectus abdominis

transversus abdominis*

obliquus externus

Medicine Ball Standing Russian Twist

Medicine Ball Standing Russian Twist is extremely effective for strengthening your major core muscles. Make sure you maintain alignment and stability in the rest of your body as you keep your core as engaged as possible.

HOW TO DO IT

- Stand with your legs slightly wider than shoulder-distance apart. Hold a medicine ball in front of you with your arms extended, firm and straight.

- Rotate your arms and torso to the right, back to center, and then to the left.

- Return to center and repeat, alternating sides for the recommended repetitions.

DO IT RIGHT

- Twist in a smooth, controlled motion.
- Keep your arms extended.
- Keep both feet anchored to the floor.
- Move your head round with your torso.
- Avoid letting go of the ball.
- Avoid totally locking your arms or legs.
- Avoid hunching your shoulders or slumping forward.

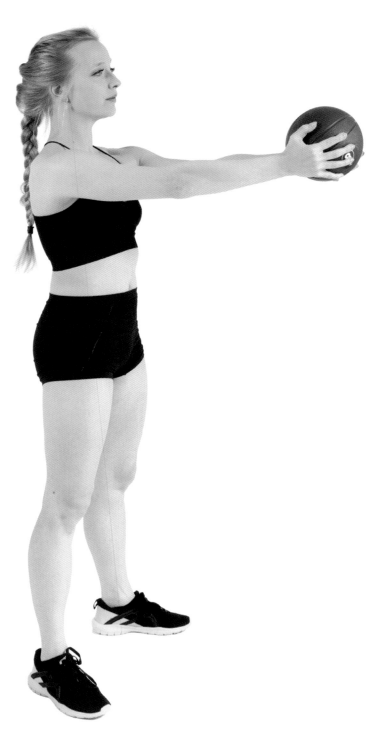

TARGETS
• Transverse abdominals
• Obliques

EQUIPMENT
• Medicine ball

BENEFITS
• Strengthens core
• Tightens abdominals, especially obliques
• Stabilizes back

CAUTIONS
• Lower-back issues

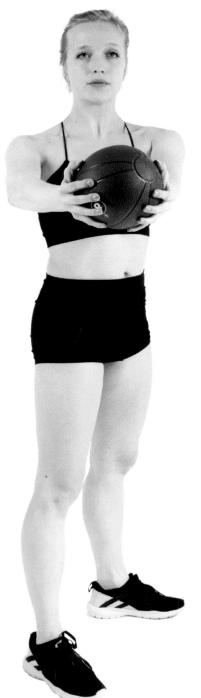

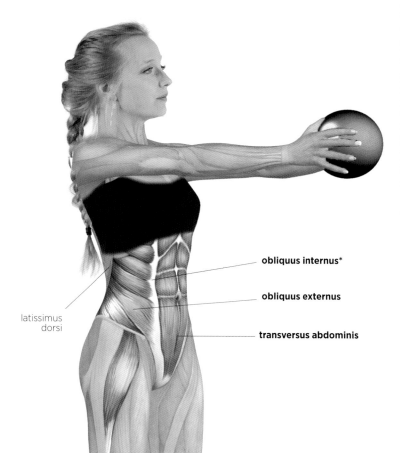

latissimus dorsi

obliquus internus*

obliquus externus

transversus abdominis

Annotation Key

Bold text indicates target muscles
Light text indicates other working muscles
* indicates deep muscles

Swiss Ball Circles

A circular motion is combined here with a balancing element, introduced by using a Swiss ball. Together they create a thorough workout for your core—both front and back.

HOW TO DO IT

- Begin in a plank position with your feet about hip-width apart on the floor and your forearms planted on a Swiss ball, palms pressed together. Elongate your spine, and support your weight with your toes.

- Roll toward all four points of direction, going clockwise. Trace a circle with your elbows, pressing your forearms into the ball during the entire movement. Return to center. A complete circle is one repetition. Repeat for the recommended repetitions.

- Repeat going counterclockwise, for the recommended repetitions.

DO IT RIGHT

- Keep your body as one straight line throughout the movement.
- Avoid excessive speed or momentum.
- Avoid allowing the front of your shoulders to lead or take over the movement.

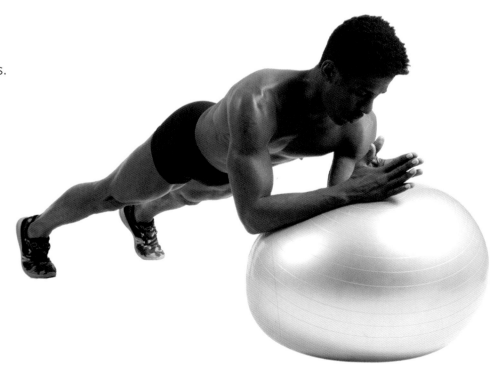

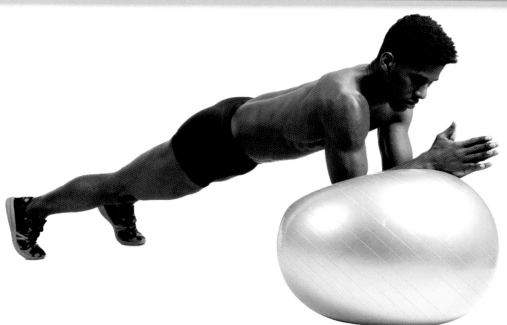

FACT FILE

TARGETS
• Abdominals
• Spinal erector muscles

EQUIPMENT
• Swiss ball

BENEFITS
• Strengthens and stabilizes core

CAUTIONS
• Shoulder issues
• Severe lower-back pain

Annotation Key

Bold text indicates target muscles
Light text indicates other working muscles
* indicates deep muscles

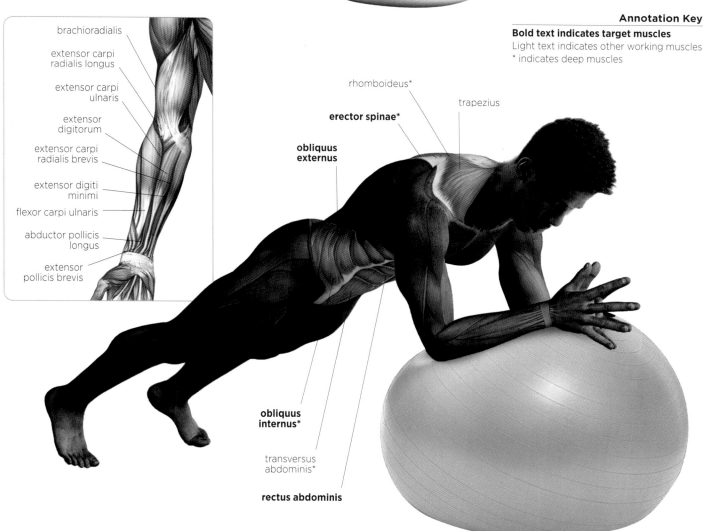

brachioradialis

extensor carpi radialis longus

extensor carpi ulnaris

extensor digitorum

extensor carpi radialis brevis

extensor digiti minimi

flexor carpi ulnaris

abductor pollicis longus

extensor pollicis brevis

rhomboideus*

trapezius

erector spinae*

obliquus externus

obliquus internus*

transversus abdominis*

rectus abdominis

Swiss Ball Atomic Push-Up

Aptly named, the Swiss Ball Atomic Push-Up causes many major muscle groups to fire at the same time. When done correctly, it strengthens your core, works your hip flexors, and generally tones your upper body.

HOW TO DO IT

• Begin on your hands and knees with your fingers facing forward and a Swiss ball placed behind you. Rest your shins on the ball, and straighten your legs so that your body forms a straight line.

• While keeping your back flat, bend your knees to draw the Swiss ball into your core.

• Straighten your legs, moving the ball farther behind you, and then perform a push-up. Repeat for the recommended repetitions.

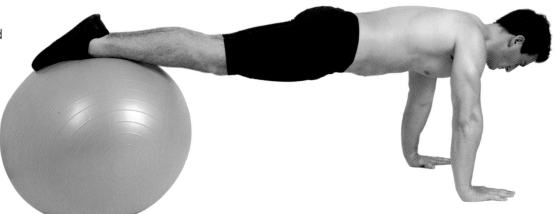

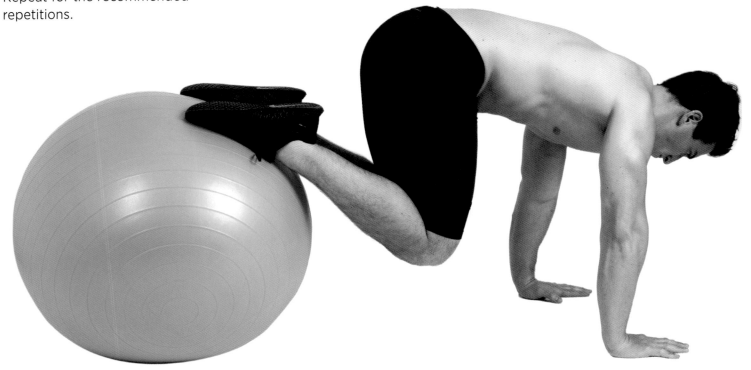

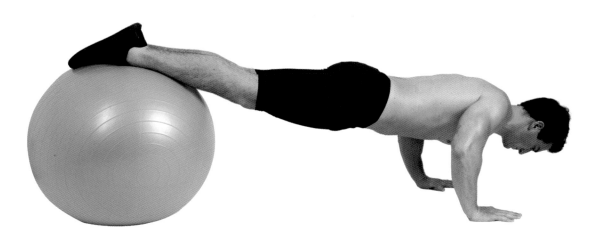

FACT FILE

TARGETS
- Abdominals
- Hip flexors
- Thighs

EQUIPMENT
- Swiss ball

BENEFITS
- Stabilizes core and spine

CAUTIONS
- Lower-back pain
- Wrist pain
- Shoulder issues

DO IT RIGHT
- Keep your hips as level as possible with your torso.
- Avoid either folding your body in on itself in a "pike" or opening out into a wide bridge shape.

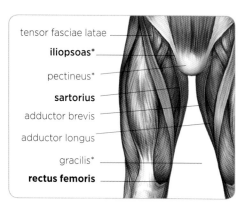

tensor fasciae latae

iliopsoas*

pectineus*

sartorius

adductor brevis

adductor longus

gracilis*

rectus femoris

Annotation Key
Bold text indicates target muscles
Light text indicates other working muscles
* indicates deep muscles

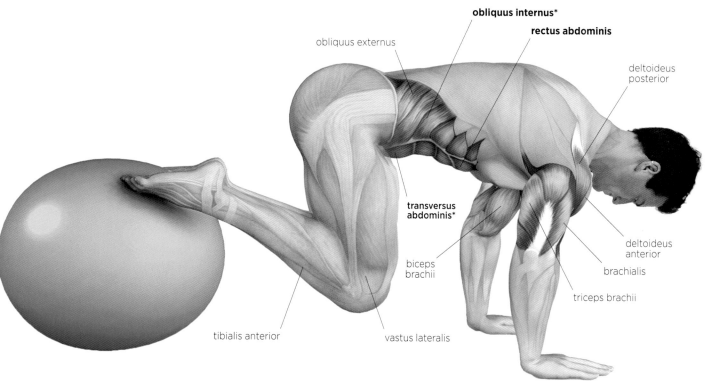

obliquus internus*

obliquus externus

rectus abdominis

deltoideus posterior

transversus abdominis*

biceps brachii

deltoideus anterior

brachialis

triceps brachii

tibialis anterior

vastus lateralis

Swiss Ball Rollout

This exercise scores very highly on the abdominals-strengthening scale. Once again, the Swiss ball proves itself an invaluable aid. Keep strong and stable to get the most from the routine.

HOW TO DO IT

- Kneel with a Swiss ball in front of you, with your hands resting on the ball.

- Use your hands to roll the ball slightly in front of you as you begin to lean forward.

- Leading with your arms and following with your body, roll the ball farther forward.

- Using your abdominals and lower back, roll back to your starting position. Repeat for the recommended repetitions.

DO IT RIGHT

- Keep your upper body elongated.
- Keep your lower legs and feet anchored to the floor throughout the exercise.
- Maintain a flat back.
- Keep your abs pulled in.
- Move smoothly and with control.
- Avoid allowing your hips to sag.

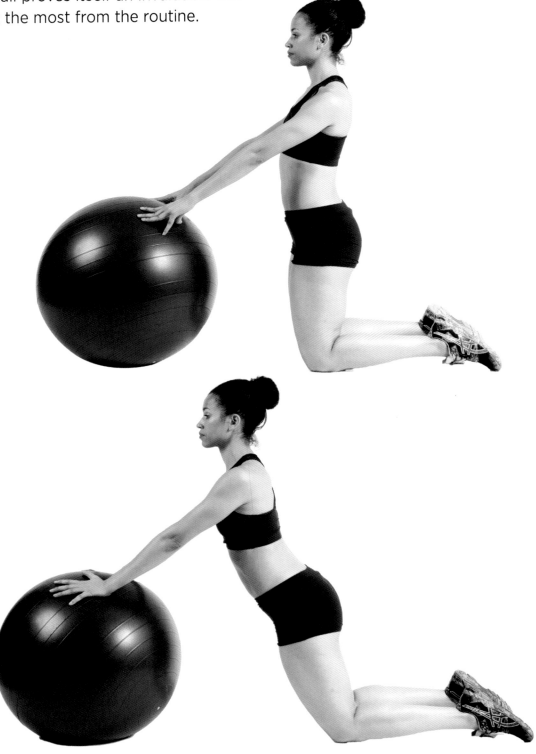

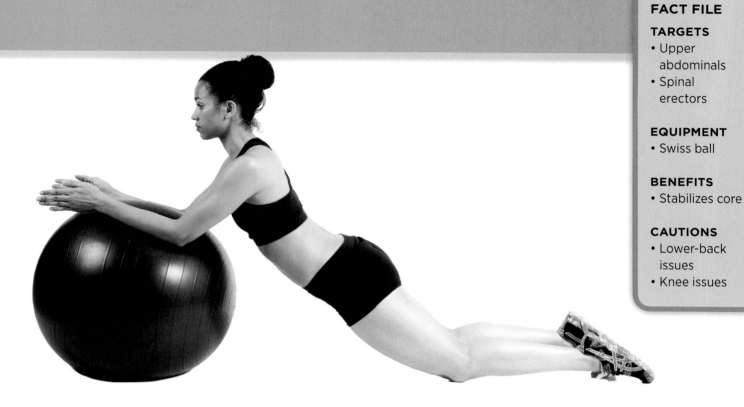

Annotation Key

Bold text indicates target muscles
Light text indicates other working muscles
* indicates deep muscles

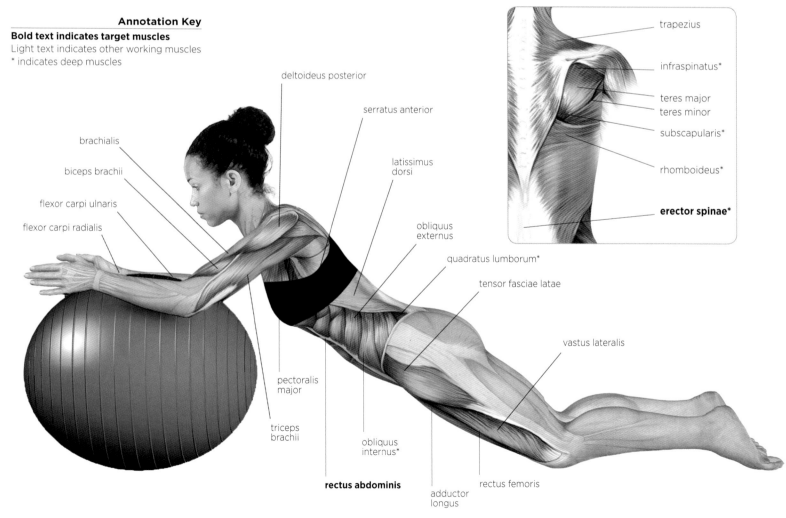

deltoideus posterior

serratus anterior

brachialis

biceps brachii

flexor carpi ulnaris

flexor carpi radialis

latissimus dorsi

obliquus externus

quadratus lumborum*

tensor fasciae latae

vastus lateralis

pectoralis major

triceps brachii

obliquus internus*

rectus abdominis

adductor longus

rectus femoris

trapezius

infraspinatus*

teres major

teres minor

subscapularis*

rhomboideus*

erector spinae*

Balance Push-Up

The Balance Push-Up is a challenging and dynamic upper-body exercise. Mastering it correctly will reward you with a properly strengthened, well-stabilized core.

HOW TO DO IT

- Assume a push-up position with your hands balanced on a Swiss ball, shoulder-width apart.

- Keeping your body in a straight line, bend your arms and lower your chest until it is nearly touching the Swiss ball.

- Straighten your arms, pushing to full extension, and repeat for the recommended repetitions.

DO IT RIGHT

- Keep your hands planted on the ball.
- Try to keep the ball as still as possible.
- Keep your heels lifted so that you are balancing on your toes.
- Avoid arching your back.
- Avoid rushing.

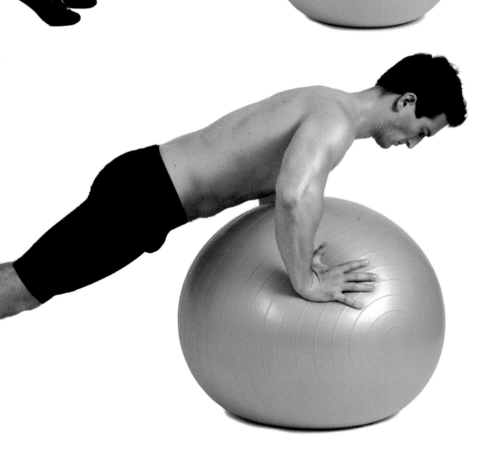

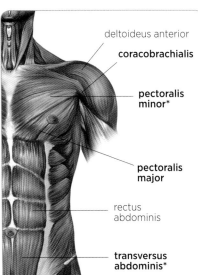

FACT FILE

TARGETS
- Transverse abdominals
- Pectorals
- Triceps
- Shoulder joint mobilizers

EQUIPMENT
- Swiss ball

BENEFITS
- Stabilizes and strengthens core
- Builds general upper-body strength and stability

CAUTIONS
- Lower-back pain
- Wrist pain
- Shoulder issues

rhomboideus*

trapezius

triceps brachii

obliquus externus

obliquus internus*

vastus intermedius*

rectus femoris

deltoideus anterior

coracobrachialis

pectoralis minor*

pectoralis major

rectus abdominis

transversus abdominis*

Annotation Key
Bold text indicates target muscles
Light text indicates other working muscles
* indicates deep muscles

Swiss Ball Russian Twist

The Swiss Ball Russian Twist strengthens your core in a fun way, while also streamlining your waistline. The rotating action means that, although the exercise targets all of your abdominals, it places particular emphasis on your obliques.

HOW TO DO IT

- Sit on your Swiss ball, with feet planted shoulder-width apart. Roll forward until your neck is supported on the ball. Extend your arms fully directly above your chest.

- Turn your left hip out to the side while also turning your torso and your arms in the same direction.

- Return to the center, repeat on the opposite side, and alternate sides for the recommended repetitions.

DO IT RIGHT

- Move slowly and with control.
- Avoid letting your upper back hang off the Swiss ball, unsupported.

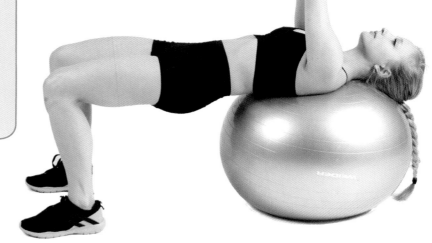

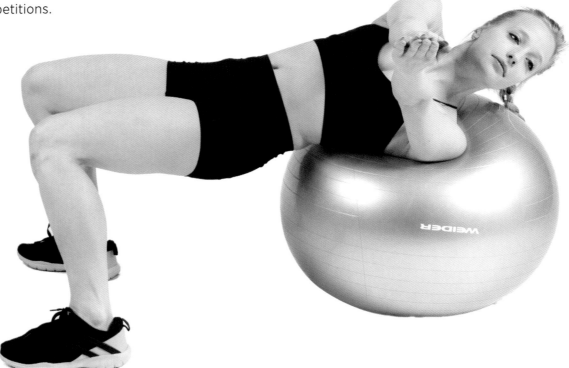

FACT FILE

TARGETS
- Abdominals, especially obliques

EQUIPMENT
- Swiss ball

BENEFITS
- Strengthens core
- Tightens abdominals, especially obliques
- Tones arms and shoulders

CAUTIONS
- Lower-back issues

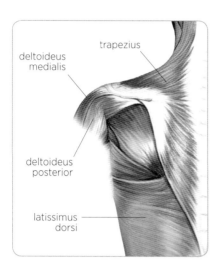

deltoideus medialis

trapezius

deltoideus posterior

latissimus dorsi

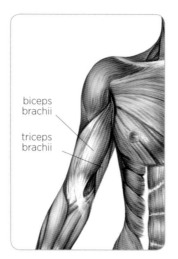

biceps brachii

triceps brachii

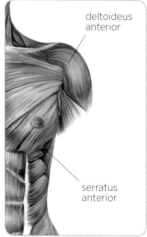

deltoideus anterior

serratus anterior

Annotation Key

Bold text indicates target muscles
Light text indicates other working muscles
* indicates deep muscles

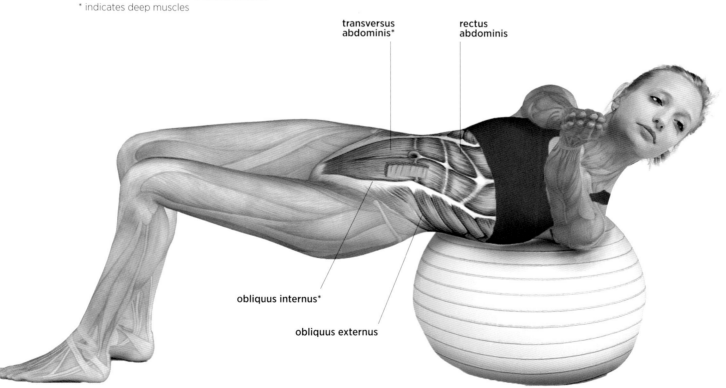

transversus abdominis*

rectus abdominis

obliquus internus*

obliquus externus

Foam Roller Triceps Rollout

As its name suggests, this exercise is great for your triceps. However, it's also a winning routine for core strength—achieved by engaging the abdominals, pecs, and glutes.

HOW TO DO IT

- Kneel on the floor, with the foam roller placed crosswise in front of you. Place your hands on top of the roller, your fingers pointing away from you.

- Maintaining a neutral spine and making sure not to sink your into your shoulders, roll forward on your forearms.

- Continue to roll forward until the roller reaches your elbows. Press into the roller, keeping your hips aligned, and roll back to the starting position. Repeat for the recommended repetitions.

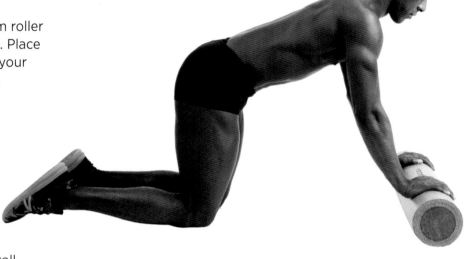

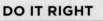

DO IT RIGHT

- Make sure all movement happens at the same time.
- Keep your shoulders relaxed throughout.
- Avoid allowing your shoulders to lift toward your ears.
- Avoid allowing your hips and lower back to drop during the movement.
- Avoid arching your back.

FACT FILE

TARGETS
• Triceps
• Abdominals
• Trunk stabilizers
• Hamstrings

EQUIPMENT
• Foam roller

BENEFITS
• Improves core strength
• Firming core and upper arms enhances shoulder stability

CAUTIONS
• Lower-back pain
• Shoulder pain

semitendinosus

biceps femoris

semimembranosus

Annotation Key
Bold text indicates target muscles
Light text indicates other working muscles
* indicates deep muscles

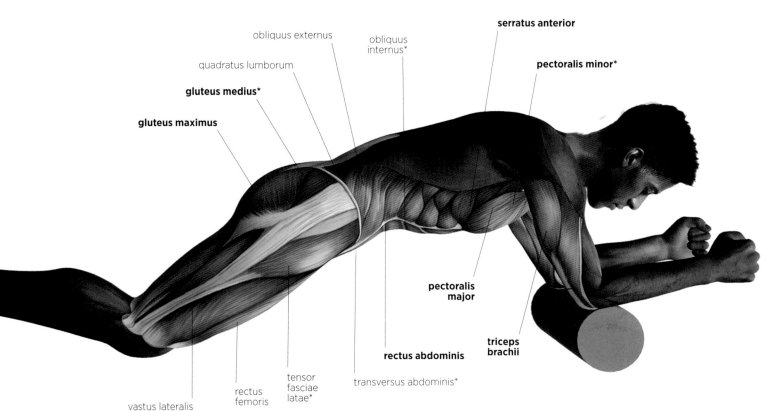

obliquus externus

quadratus lumborum

gluteus medius*

gluteus maximus

obliquus internus*

serratus anterior

pectoralis minor*

pectoralis major

rectus abdominis

transversus abdominis*

tensor fasciae latae*

rectus femoris

vastus lateralis

triceps brachii

Foam Roller Abdominal Rollback

This is such a great exercise. It's easy and quick to do, and it fires up so much of your core while also targeting your quads and shoulders.

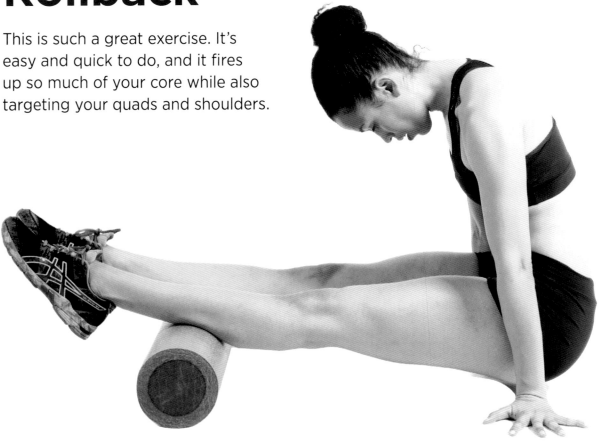

HOW TO DO IT

- Sit on the floor. Position the foam roller beneath your knees, and place your hands on the floor by your sides, palms down.

- Keeping your legs firm, press your hands into the floor as you slowly raise your hips until they are about level with your knees. This is your starting position.

- Draw your hips backward through your arms, rolling your legs over the roller. Drop your head slightly so that your gaze is directed toward your thighs.

- Moving slowly and with control, roll back to your starting position. Keep your hips lifted off the floor. Repeat for the recommended repetitions.

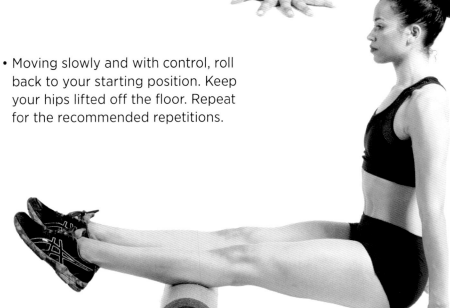

TARGETS
• Abdominals
• Shoulders
• Quads

EQUIPMENT
• Foam roller

BENEFITS
• Strengthens and stabilizes core, pelvis, and shoulders
• Works triceps
• Boosts performance in all sports, especially those requiring balance

CAUTIONS
• Wrist pain
• Shoulder pain

DO IT RIGHT

• Keep your torso upright and facing forward.
• Keep your abdominal muscles engaged.
• Keep your arms anchored to the floor, as stable as possible.
• Avoid twisting to either side.
• Avoid letting your abs bulge outward.
• Avoid twisting your neck.

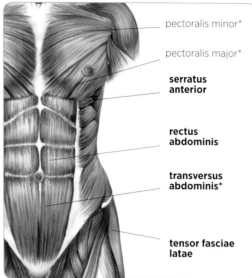

pectoralis minor*

pectoralis major*

serratus anterior

rectus abdominis

transversus abdominis*

tensor fasciae latae

Annotation Key
Bold text indicates target muscles
Light text indicates other working muscles
* indicates deep muscles

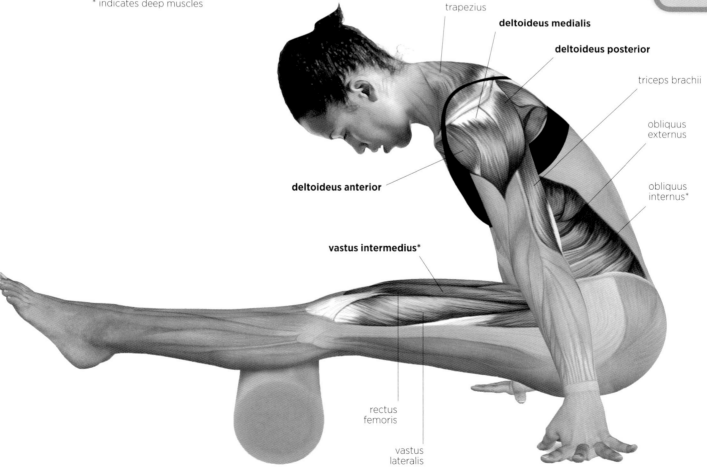

trapezius

deltoideus medialis

deltoideus posterior

triceps brachii

obliquus externus

obliquus internus*

deltoideus anterior

vastus intermedius*

rectus femoris

vastus lateralis

Foam Roller Diagonal Crunch

The Foam Roller Diagonal Crunch, with its crunching and stretching, involves a large array of muscles. It helps to strengthen much of your core and the front of your torso, and improves stability and flexion around your shoulders, hips, and pelvis.

HOW TO DO IT

- Lie on your back, lengthwise, along a foam roller so that it follows the line of your spine. Your buttocks and shoulders should both be in contact with the roller.

- With your legs straight and your feet pressed firmly into the floor, extend your arms over your head.

- Raise your head and upper body, as if to do a crunch. Leave your left leg and right arm down on the ground, using your hand for support. Raise your right leg and left arm, and reach for your ankle.

- Slowly roll down the roller, dropping your raised arm and leg, and repeat on the opposite leg and arm. Alternate sides for the recommended repetitions

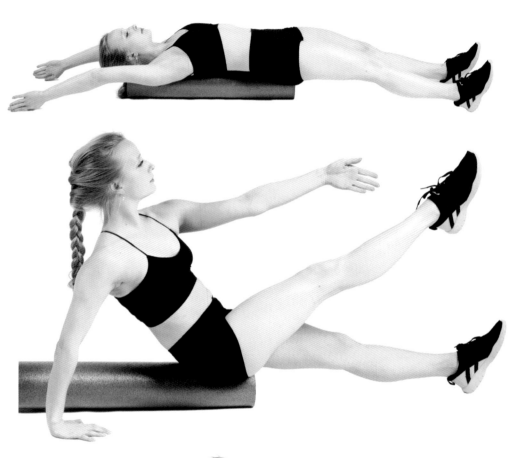

DO IT RIGHT

- Keep your legs firm throughout.
- Keep your buttocks and shoulders in contact with the roller throughout.
- Avoid allowing your shoulders to lift toward your ears.
- Avoid bending your knees.

MODIFICATION

HARDER: Keep one leg on the floor for support, and reach both arms toward your raised leg as you crunch up.

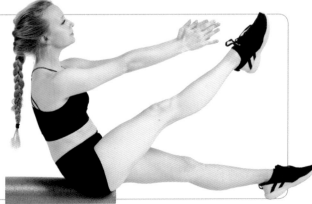

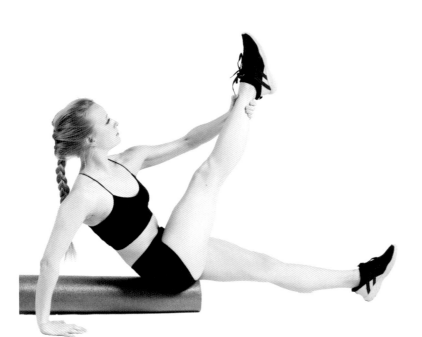

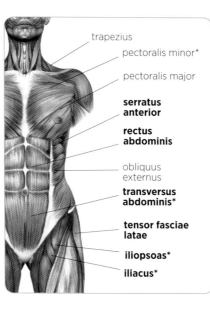

TARGETS
- Abdominals
- Chest
- Shoulder and hip stabilizers and flexors
- Quads

EQUIPMENT
- Foam roller

BENEFITS
- Strengthens core
- Improves core, pelvic, and shoulder stability

CAUTIONS
- Back pain
- Neck pain

trapezius

pectoralis minor*

pectoralis major

serratus anterior

rectus abdominis

obliquus externus

transversus abdominis*

tensor fasciae latae

iliopsoas*

iliacus*

Annotation Key

Bold text indicates target muscles
Light text indicates other working muscles
* indicates deep muscles

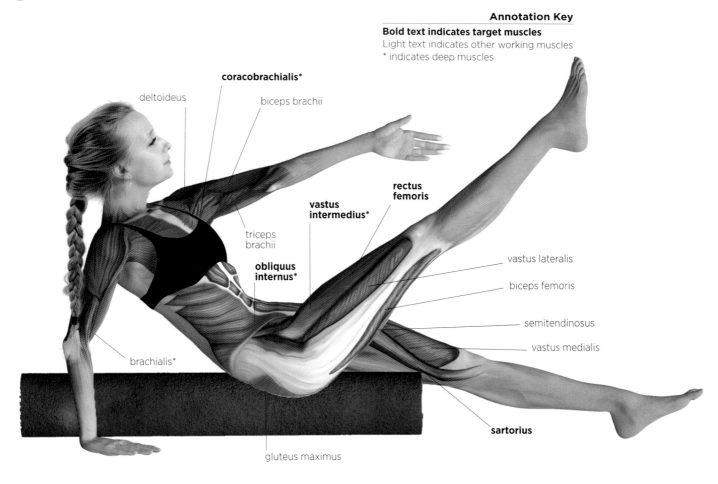

deltoideus

coracobrachialis*

biceps brachii

triceps brachii

rectus femoris

vastus intermedius*

obliquus internus*

vastus lateralis

biceps femoris

semitendinosus

vastus medialis

brachialis*

sartorius

gluteus maximus

Quadruped Knee Pull-In

This calls on your abdominal strength—as well as that of your triceps.
At the same time it helps to balance your pelvis and works your quads.

HOW TO DO IT

- Place a foam roller on the floor.
  Kneel on the roller with your
  hands placed on the floor in front
  of you. Your hands should be
  slightly in front of your torso, and
  your hips lifted off your heels.
  This is your starting position.

- Round out your torso as you
  pull your knees toward your
  hands, allowing the roller to
  move toward your feet.

- Bend your elbows into a push-up,
  straighten, and then roll slowly to
  the starting position. Repeat for
  the recommended repetitions.

DO IT RIGHT

- Round your back as you
  draw your knees inward.
- Keep your head relaxed.
- Ensure you make smooth
  transitions.
- Avoid allowing your
  shoulders to lift toward
  your ears.
- Avoid moving your head
  forward.

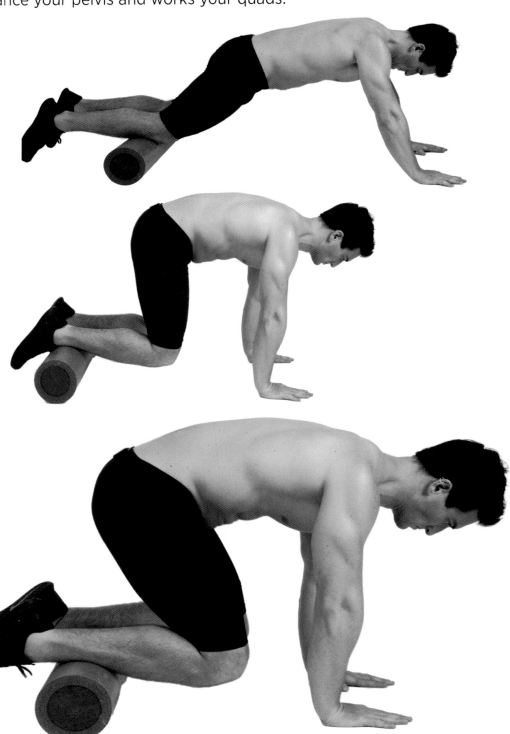

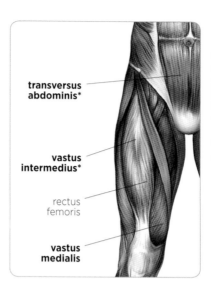

transversus abdominis*

vastus intermedius*

rectus femoris

vastus medialis

Annotation Key
Bold text indicates target muscles
Light text indicates other working muscles
* indicates deep muscles

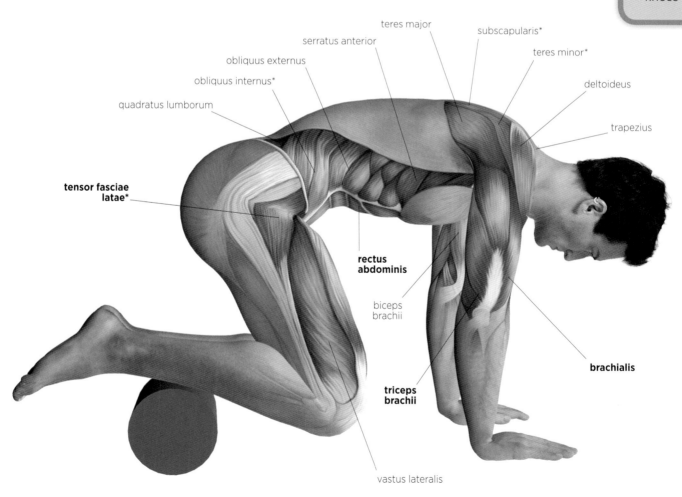

teres major

subscapularis*

serratus anterior

teres minor*

obliquus externus

obliquus internus*

deltoideus

quadratus lumborum

trapezius

tensor fasciae latae*

rectus abdominis

biceps brachii

brachialis

triceps brachii

vastus lateralis

Resistance Band Squat

Using a resistance band is a great way of getting more from your squats—and of learning just how a squat should be done. The band helps you to maintain good, precise squatting form and not get messy with your movements.

HOW TO DO IT

• Stand with your feet shoulder-width apart and your arms at your sides. Position the resistance band beneath both feet. Grasp the handles in both hands, palms facing away from you.

• Bend your knees to lower your body as you bend your elbows, bringing the resistance band up toward your chest, palms facing you.

• Push through your heels as you straighten your legs and bring your arms back to your starting position. Repeat for the recommended repetitions.

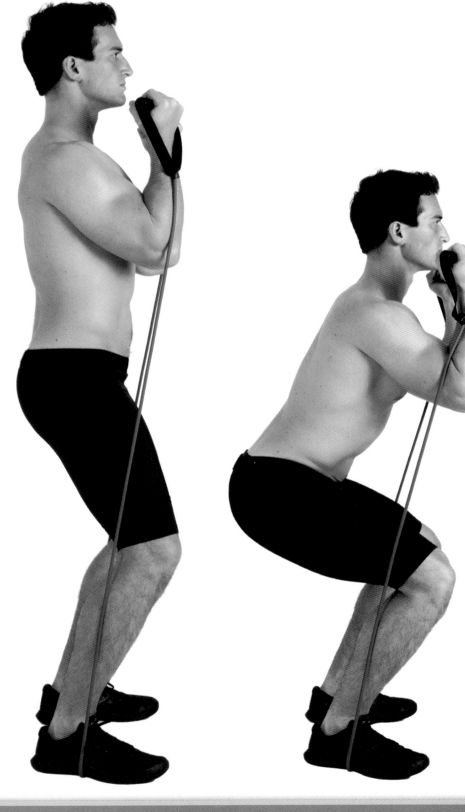

TARGETS
- Glutes
- Quads

EQUIPMENT
- Resistance band

BENEFITS
- Strengthens and tones thighs and buttocks

CAUTIONS
- Lower-back issues

DO IT RIGHT

- Maintain a straight back.
- Push your buttocks slightly outward as you descend.
- Keep your hips square.
- Keep your upper arms stable.
- Gaze forward.
- Avoid arching your back or slumping forward.
- Avoid twisting your torso.
- Avoid lifting one arm higher, or at a faster rate, than the other.

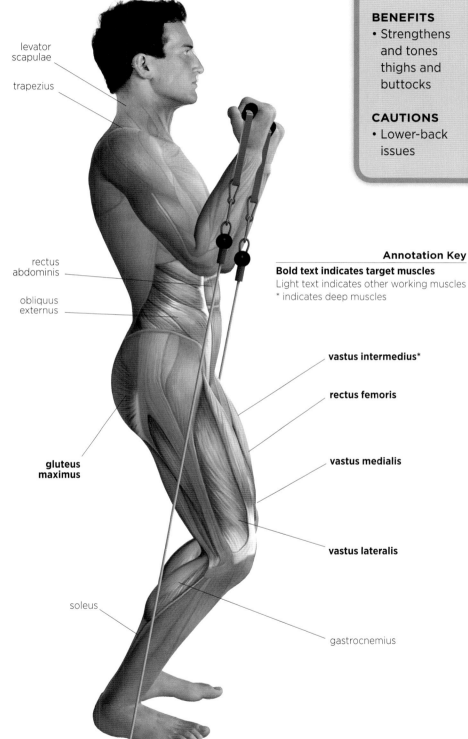

levator scapulae

trapezius

rectus abdominis

obliquus externus

gluteus maximus

soleus

Annotation Key

Bold text indicates target muscles
Light text indicates other working muscles
* indicates deep muscles

vastus intermedius*

rectus femoris

vastus medialis

vastus lateralis

gastrocnemius

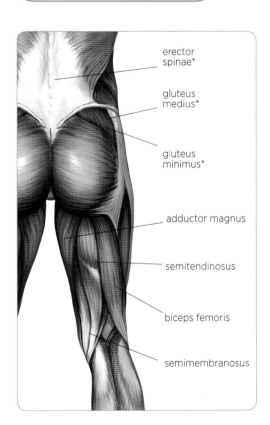

erector spinae*

gluteus medius*

gluteus minimus*

adductor magnus

semitendinosus

biceps femoris

semimembranosus

Resistance Band Lunge

This exercise is another one that's good for your buttocks and thighs. As well as adding resistance, using a band for the lunge action will help you to improve your balancing skills.

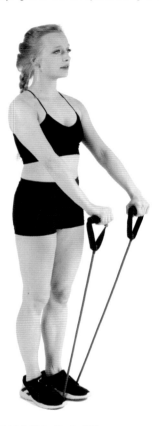

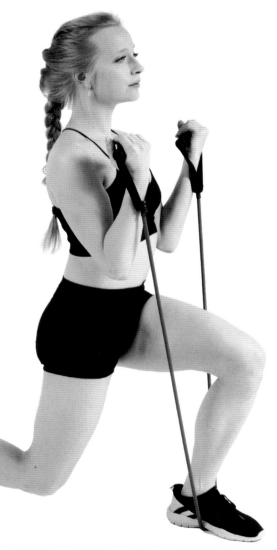

HOW TO DO IT

- Position a resistance band beneath your left foot, grasping both handles. This is your starting position.

- Keeping your head up and your spine neutral, take a big step forward with your left foot.

- Drop your back, right, knee toward the floor, bending both legs until your front, left, thigh is parallel to the ground. At the same time, bring the resistance band closer to your body with palms facing your shoulders.

- Slowly and with control, straighten your legs as you raise your body, lower your arms, and return to your starting position. Repeat, with the left leg going forward, for the recommended repetitions and then repeat with the opposite leg.

FACT FILE

TARGETS
- Glutes
- Quads

EQUIPMENT
- Resistance band

BENEFITS
- Strengthens and tones thighs and buttocks

CAUTIONS
- Knee injury
- Shoulder issues

Annotation Key

Bold text indicates target muscles
Light text indicates other working muscles
* indicates deep muscles

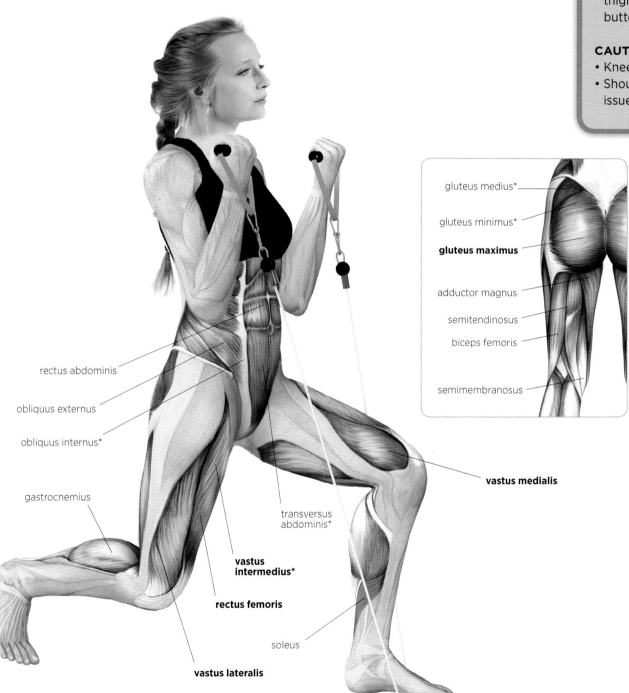

gluteus medius*

gluteus minimus*

gluteus maximus

adductor magnus

semitendinosus

biceps femoris

semimembranosus

vastus medialis

rectus abdominis

obliquus externus

obliquus internus*

gastrocnemius

transversus abdominis*

vastus intermedius*

rectus femoris

soleus

vastus lateralis

Swiss Ball Loop Extension

Strengthen your calves, hamstrings, and glutes with this band-and-ball routine. The Swiss Ball Loop Extension is an all-around winner that will also work your core, shoulders, arms, and quads.

HOW TO DO IT

- With a resistance band looped around your ankles, lie facedown on a Swiss ball, with your hips over the center of the ball as you support your weight on your arms. Your hands should be directly below your shoulders and your toes on the floor.

- Keeping your abs tight, squeeze your gluteal muscles to raise your right leg, lengthening your body as your weight transfers from your arms to your left foot, stretching through your heel.

- Return your right foot to the floor, and repeat for the recommended repetitions raising that leg. Repeat with the opposite leg for the recommended repetitions.

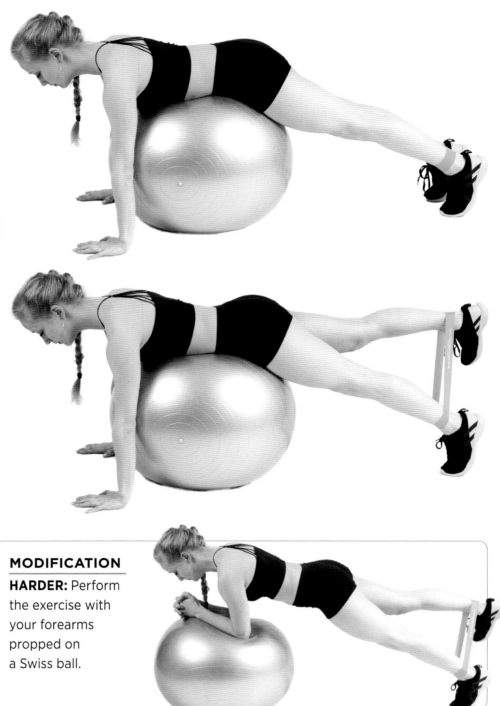

DO IT RIGHT

- Hold a straight plank position throughout, with your hips in line with your shoulders and ankles to achieve optimal weight distribution.
- Keep your neck elongated and relaxed.
- Keep your core tight and your back flat.
- Avoid allowing your shoulders to sink.

MODIFICATION

HARDER: Perform the exercise with your forearms propped on a Swiss ball.

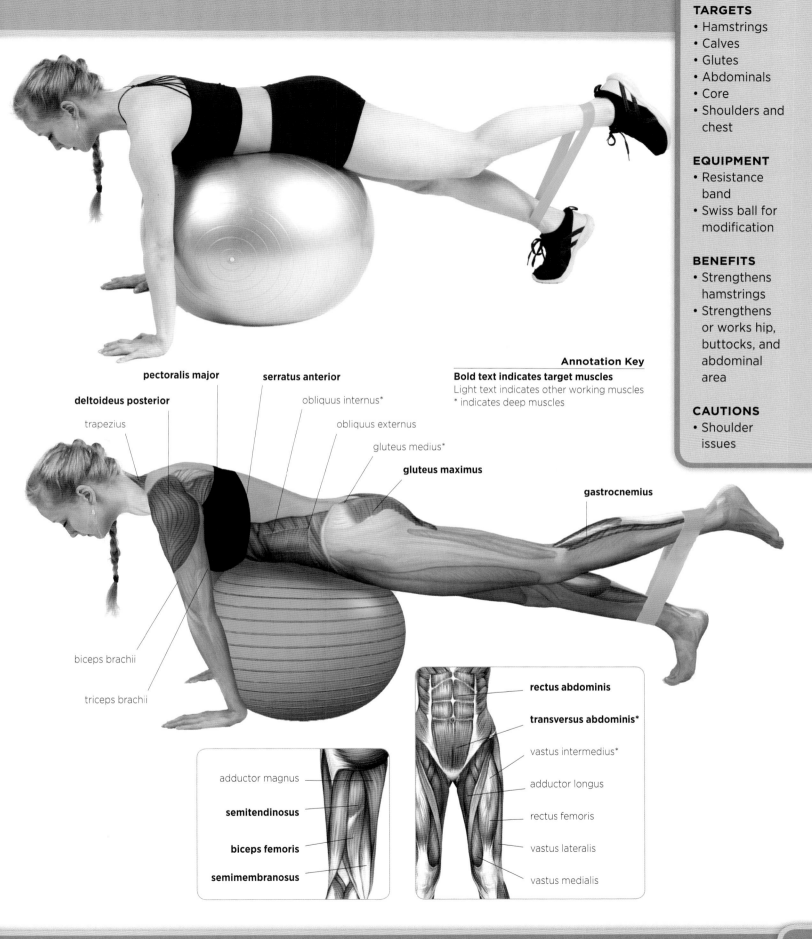

TARGETS
- Hamstrings
- Calves
- Glutes
- Abdominals
- Core
- Shoulders and chest

EQUIPMENT
- Resistance band
- Swiss ball for modification

BENEFITS
- Strengthens hamstrings
- Strengthens or works hip, buttocks, and abdominal area

CAUTIONS
- Shoulder issues

Annotation Key

Bold text indicates target muscles
Light text indicates other working muscles
* indicates deep muscles

pectoralis major

serratus anterior

deltoideus posterior

trapezius

obliquus internus*

obliquus externus

gluteus medius*

gluteus maximus

gastrocnemius

biceps brachii

triceps brachii

rectus abdominis

transversus abdominis*

vastus intermedius*

adductor longus

rectus femoris

vastus lateralis

vastus medialis

adductor magnus

semitendinosus

biceps femoris

semimembranosus

Swiss Ball Bridge

Work on your hamstrings and rectus femoris quad muscle with this Swiss Ball Bridge exercise. Your glutes will also get in on the act, as will your abdominals and back—so, a good one for your core.

HOW TO DO IT

• Lie faceup on the floor with your arms at your sides and your lower legs resting on a Swiss ball.

• Press your palms into the floor and, keeping your arms on the floor too, engage your abdominal muscles as you lift your upper body off the floor. Your ody should form a diagonal line. If desired, hold for just a moment.

• Slowly and with control, lower back to your starting position. Repeat for the recommended repetitions.

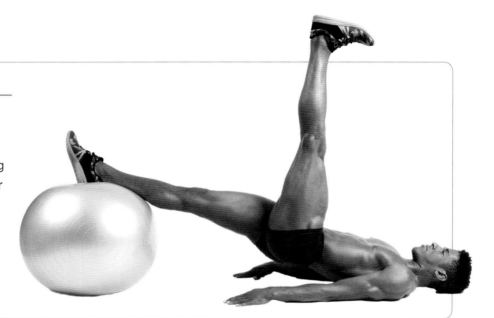

MODIFICATION

HARDER: In the raised position, lift one leg off the ball, extending it upward while maintaining your form. Return to your starting position. Repeat on the opposite side, keeping both legs straight and your back neutral as you move.

TARGETS
- Hamstrings
- Rectus femoris quad

Equipment
- Swiss ball

Benefits
- Strengthens hamstrings and quads
- Stabilizes pelvis and core
- Boosts performance in all field sports

Cautions
- Back issues
- Shoulder issues

Annotation Key

Bold text indicates target muscles

Light text indicates other working muscles

* indicates deep muscles

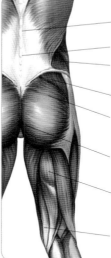

erector spinae*

multifidus spinae*

quadratus lumborum*

gluteus medius*

gluteus minimus*

piriformis*

semitendinosus

semimembranosus

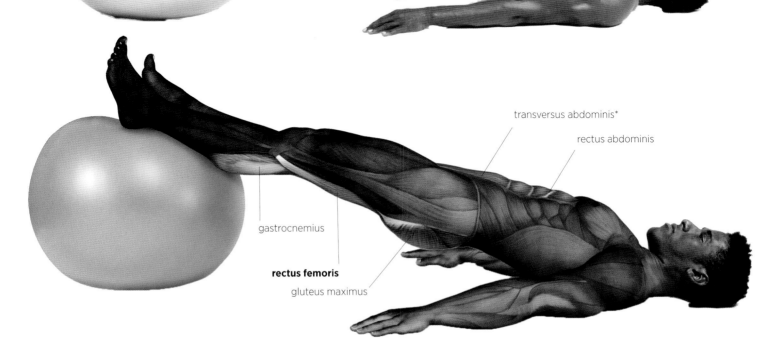

transversus abdominis*

rectus abdominis

gastrocnemius

rectus femoris

gluteus maximus

Swiss Ball Split Squat

This is an advanced leg exercise that involves more than just your legs. To perform Swiss Ball Split Squat correctly requires drawing on a solid core, which gives your entire body a good workout.

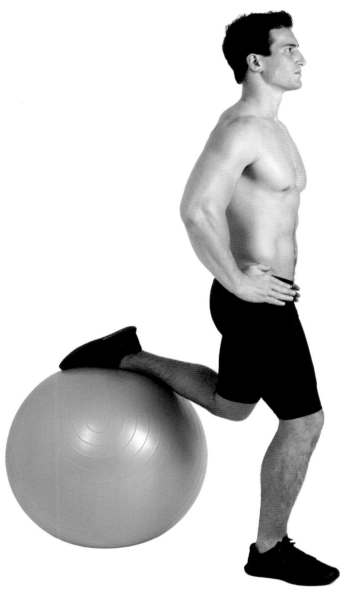

HOW TO DO IT

- Stand with a Swiss ball behind you. Place your hands on your hips.

- Bend your left leg to rest your ankle and the top of your left foot on the ball.

- Bend the knee of your front, right, leg until the thigh is nearly parallel to the floor while simultaneously bending your back, left, leg.

- Straighten both legs to return to a standing position. Repeat with the left leg back for the recommended repetitions. Then repeat with the opposite leg back for the recommended repetitions.

DO IT RIGHT

- Keep a firm bend in both legs.
- Keep your torso as upright as possible.
- Avoid allowing your front knee to hyperextend past your toes.
- Avoid twisting your torso.
- Avoid arching your back or slouching forward.

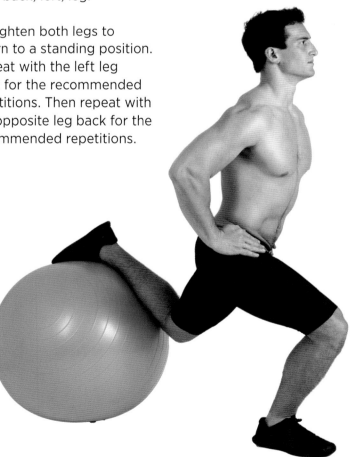

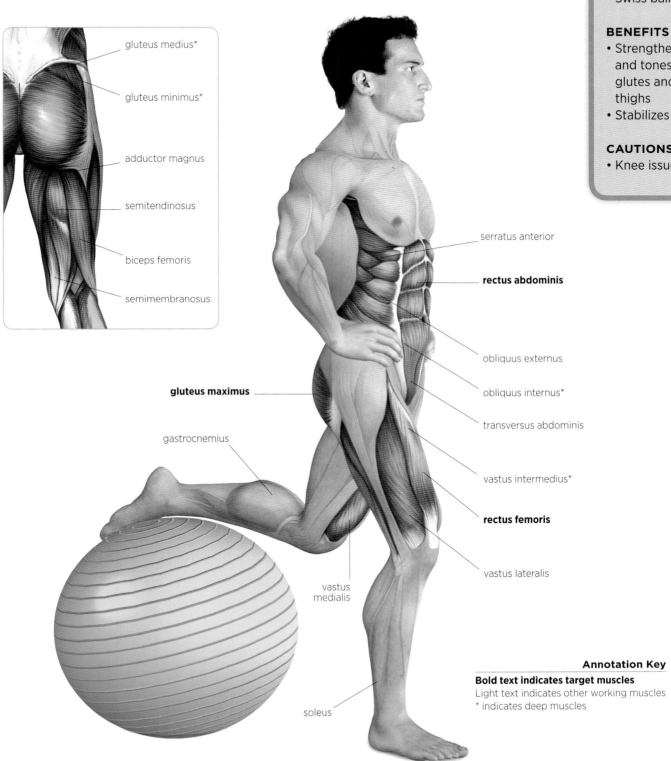

FACT FILE

TARGETS
- Thigh adductors
- Quads
- Glutes

EQUIPMENT
- Swiss ball

BENEFITS
- Strengthens and tones glutes and thighs
- Stabilizes core

CAUTIONS
- Knee issues

gluteus medius*

gluteus minimus*

adductor magnus

semitendinosus

biceps femoris

semimembranosus

serratus anterior

rectus abdominis

obliquus externus

obliquus internus*

transversus abdominis

vastus intermedius*

rectus femoris

vastus lateralis

gluteus maximus

gastrocnemius

vastus medialis

soleus

Annotation Key
Bold text indicates target muscles
Light text indicates other working muscles
* indicates deep muscles

Hamstrings Pull-In

The Hamstrings Pull-in is particularly effective at building endurance in your hamstrings, as the name suggests. In addition, it benefits your glutes and your whole leg, including the thigh adductors that pull your legs toward your body.

HOW TO DO IT

- Lie on your back on the floor, arms by your sides, palms facing down, foam roller under your feet, and your knees bent up.

- Raise your body into a Bridge position (pages 96–97), lifting your hips to form a straight line down to your shoulders.

- Squeeze your buttocks, and pull your calves in and out as you roll the roller back and forth under your feet.

- Repeat for the recommended repetitions.

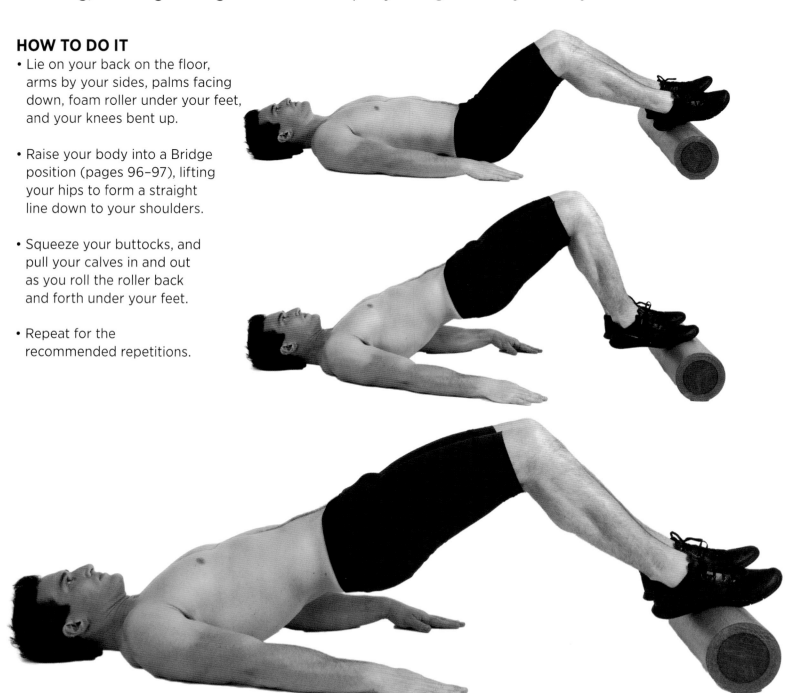

DO IT RIGHT

- Keep your shoulders relaxed throughout.
- Keep your body in a straight line from shoulder to knee.
- Avoid allowing your hips and lower back to drop as you move the roller.
- Avoid arching your back.

Annotation Key

Bold text indicates target muscles
Light text indicates other working muscles
* indicates deep muscles

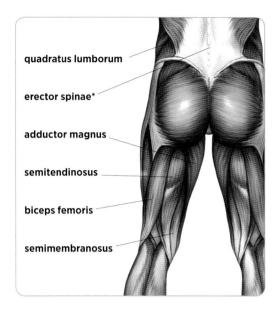

quadratus lumborum

erector spinae*

adductor magnus

semitendinosus

biceps femoris

semimembranosus

TARGETS
- Hamstrings
- Quads
- Thigh adductors
- Calf muscles
- Glutes
- Lower back

EQUIPMENT
- Foam roller

BENEFITS
- Increases hamstring strength and endurance
- Strengthens glutes and pelvic stabilizers
- Increases thigh mobilization

CAUTIONS
- Hamstring injury
- Lower-back pain
- Ankle pain

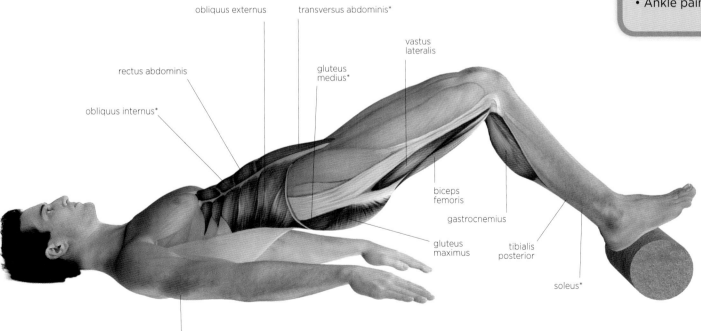

obliquus externus

transversus abdominis*

vastus lateralis

rectus abdominis

gluteus medius*

obliquus internus*

biceps femoris

gastrocnemius

gluteus maximus

tibialis posterior

soleus*

triceps brachii

Box Jumps

Spring into action—literally—by jumping between boxes or platforms to power both the back and front of your thighs. Try to jump in a streamlined way.

HOW TO DO IT

- Stand with two plyo (plyometric) boxes or platforms, placed about 3 feet apart from each other, facing you. Step up to stand on top of the one closest to you.

- Jump off the plyo box; be sure to land between the two boxes on the balls of your feet. Use your arms to increase your speed if you wish.

- As soon as your feet hit the ground, spring up onto the other box.

- As soon as you land on the second box, turn around and start again. Repeat for the recommended repetitions.

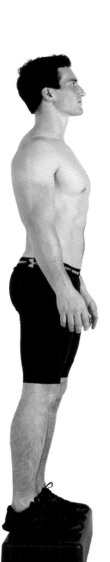

> **DO IT RIGHT**
> - Maintain an erect posture throughout.
> - Avoid landing on your toes or heels.

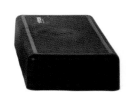
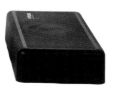
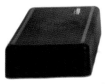

TARGETS
- Quads
- Hamstrings

Equipment
- Two plyo boxes or platforms

Benefits
- Strengthens thighs
- Improves speed, power, and athleticism

Cautions
- Ankle issues

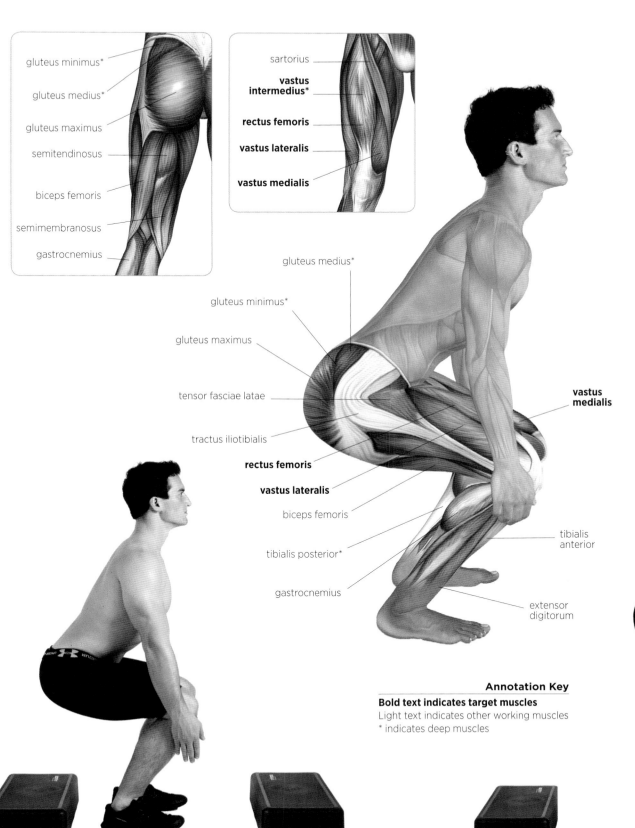

gluteus minimus*

gluteus medius*

gluteus maximus

semitendinosus

biceps femoris

semimembranosus

gastrocnemius

sartorius

vastus intermedius*

rectus femoris

vastus lateralis

vastus medialis

gluteus medius*

gluteus minimus*

gluteus maximus

tensor fasciae latae

tractus iliotibialis

rectus femoris

vastus lateralis

biceps femoris

tibialis posterior*

gastrocnemius

vastus medialis

tibialis anterior

extensor digitorum

Annotation Key
Bold text indicates target muscles
Light text indicates other working muscles
* indicates deep muscles

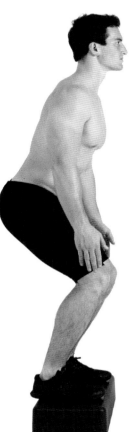

Step-Down

For such a simple step-down movement, this exercise achieves a great amount. Strengthening your thighs and glutes, it also improves movement range in your hips and pelvis while stabilizing your core.

HOW TO DO IT

- Stand facing forward on a plyo box or platform.

- Bend your right leg. Simultaneously step your left leg downward, flexing the foot. Bring the heel of your left foot to rest on the floor.

- Without rotating your torso or knee, press upward through your right leg to return to your starting position. Alternate sides for the recommended repetitions.

DO IT RIGHT

- Hold the wall or a rail for support if desired.
- Move slowly and with control.
- Focus on maintaining good form.
- Avoid letting your knee twist inward; keep it in line with your middle toe.
- Avoid rushing.

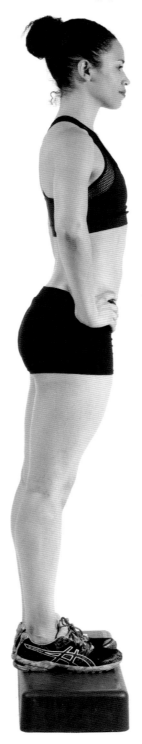
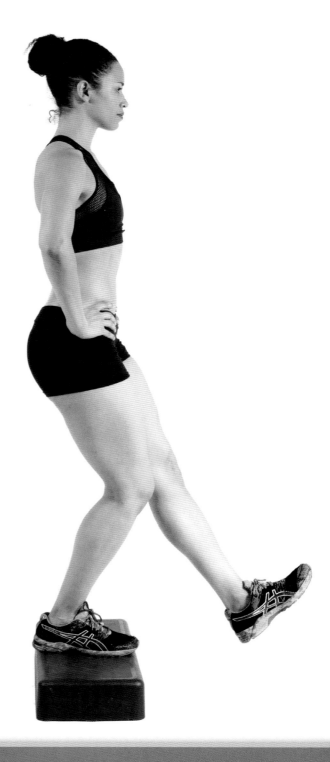

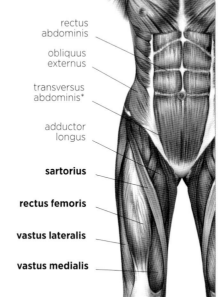

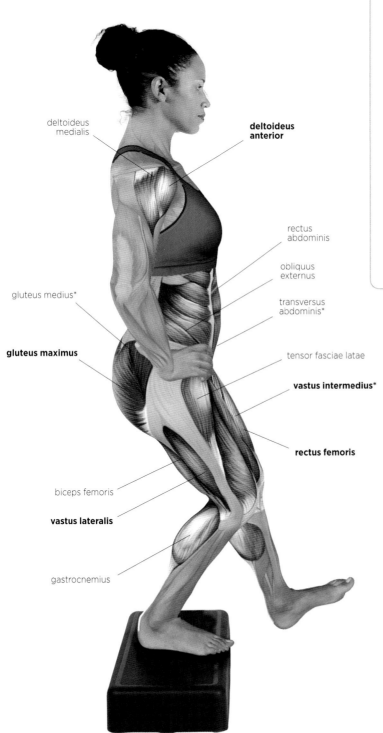

deltoideus medialis

deltoideus anterior

rectus abdominis

obliquus externus

transversus abdominis*

gluteus medius*

gluteus maximus

tensor fasciae latae

vastus intermedius*

rectus femoris

biceps femoris

vastus lateralis

gastrocnemius

rectus abdominis

obliquus externus

transversus abdominis*

adductor longus

sartorius

rectus femoris

vastus lateralis

vastus medialis

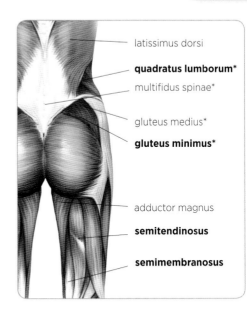

latissimus dorsi

quadratus lumborum*

multifidus spinae*

gluteus medius*

gluteus minimus*

adductor magnus

semitendinosus

semimembranosus

Annotation Key

Bold text indicates target muscles
Light text indicates other working muscles
* indicates deep muscles

Step-Up

The Step-Up strengthens, tones, and sculpts your quads, glutes, hip flexors, and hamstrings. At the same time this balance movement improves pelvic and leg stability while adding a cardio benefit.

HOW TO DO IT

- Stand in front of a step, bench, or other stable platform.

- Step onto the bench with your right leg, making sure your foot is flat against the bench.

- Lean forward slightly and push yourself upward through the heel of your right foot, so that your left leg comes up onto the bench too.

- Step down with your right leg, and then repeat the same sequence with the opposite leg. Continue stepping up and down, alternating sides, for the recommended repetitions.

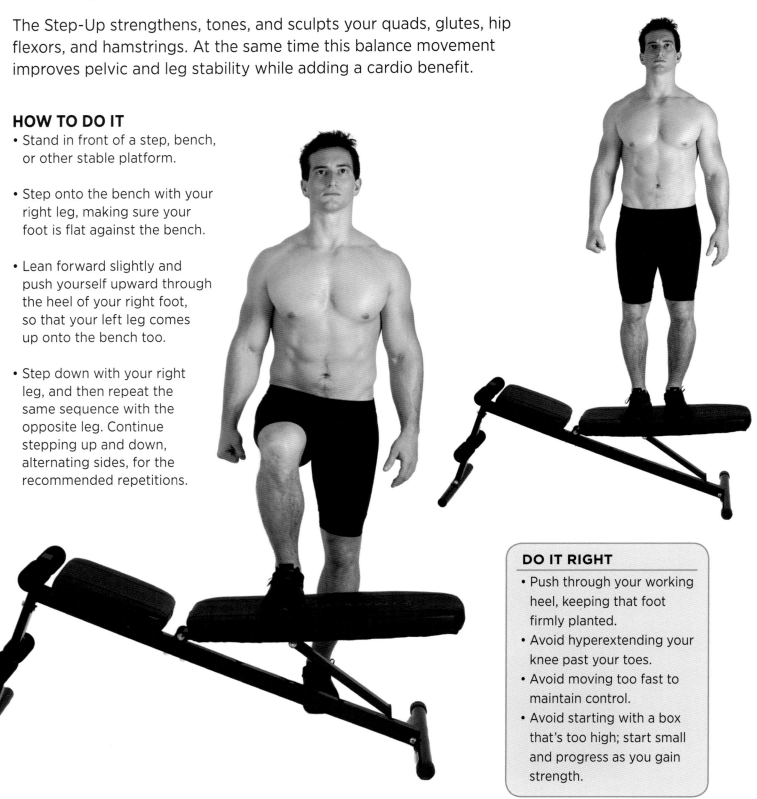

DO IT RIGHT

- Push through your working heel, keeping that foot firmly planted.
- Avoid hyperextending your knee past your toes.
- Avoid moving too fast to maintain control.
- Avoid starting with a box that's too high; start small and progress as you gain strength.

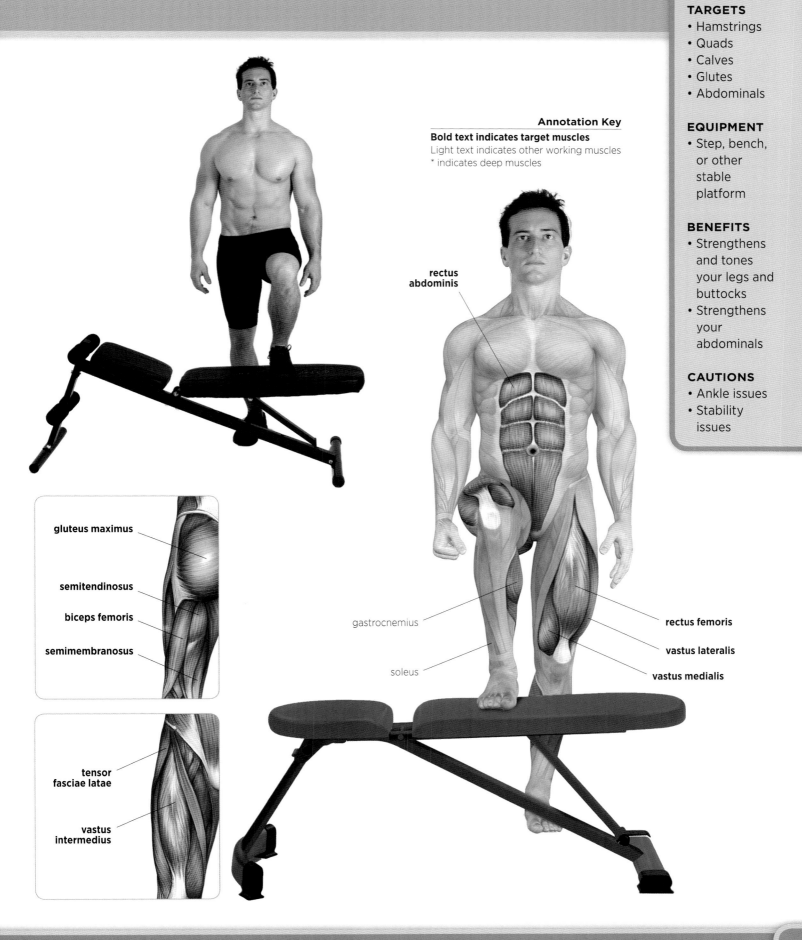

TARGETS
- Hamstrings
- Quads
- Calves
- Glutes
- Abdominals

EQUIPMENT
- Step, bench, or other stable platform

BENEFITS
- Strengthens and tones your legs and buttocks
- Strengthens your abdominals

CAUTIONS
- Ankle issues
- Stability issues

Annotation Key

Bold text indicates target muscles
Light text indicates other working muscles
* indicates deep muscles

rectus abdominis

gluteus maximus

semitendinosus

biceps femoris

semimembranosus

tensor fasciae latae

vastus intermedius

gastrocnemius

soleus

rectus femoris

vastus lateralis

vastus medialis

Push-Up Hand Walk-Over

Keep a stable position to get the most from this side-to-side routine.
It will reward you with a really effective total-body workout.

HOW TO DO IT

- Start in a Plank position (pages 114–115) with your left hand on the floor and your right on a box, platform, or step between 4 and 6 inches high.

- Keeping your torso rigid and your legs straight, bend your elbows into a Push-Up position (pages 68–69).

- Push back up, straightening your elbows to return to your starting position.

- Lift your left hand off the floor, and place it beside your right on the top of the box.

- Lift your right hand off the box, placing it on the floor some way to the right.

- Bend your elbows to perform another push-up, this time on the other side of the box.

- Return to the top of the box and repeat. Alternate sides for the recommended repetitions.

DO IT RIGHT

- Keep your hands aligned under your shoulders.
- Avoid dipping your shoulders to one side.
- Avoid craning your neck.

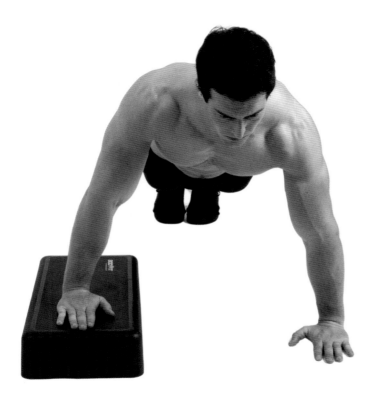
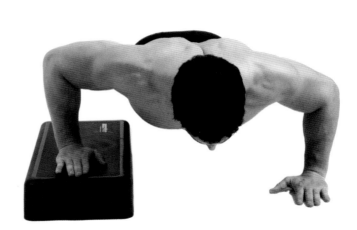

TARGETS
- Lats
- Abdominals
- Thighs
- Triceps
- Trapezius

EQUIPMENT
- Box, platform, or step

BENEFITS
- Total-body strengthening and stabilization
- Strengthens pelvic, trunk, and shoulder stabilizers

CAUTIONS
- Shoulder pain
- Back pain
- Neck pain

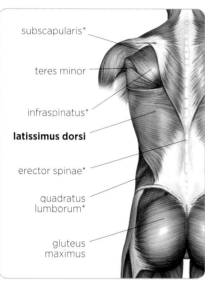

subscapularis*

teres minor

infraspinatus*

latissimus dorsi

erector spinae*

quadratus lumborum*

gluteus maximus

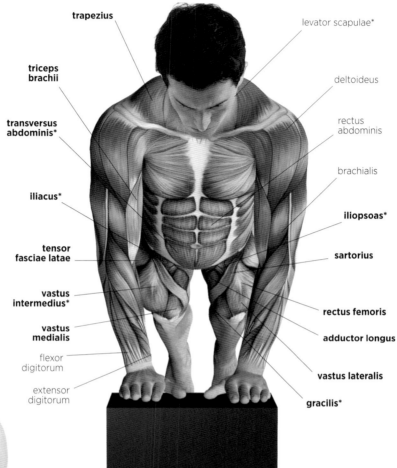

trapezius

levator scapulae*

triceps brachii

deltoideus

transversus abdominis*

rectus abdominis

brachialis

iliacus*

iliopsoas*

tensor fasciae latae

sartorius

vastus intermedius*

vastus medialis

flexor digitorum

rectus femoris

adductor longus

extensor digitorum

vastus lateralis

gracilis*

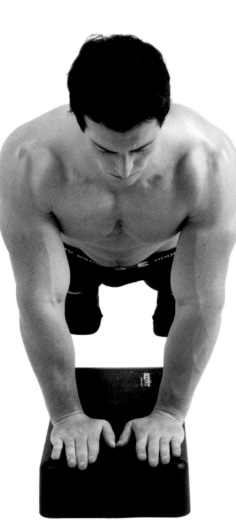

Annotation Key
Bold text indicates target muscles
Light text indicates other working muscles
* indicates deep muscles

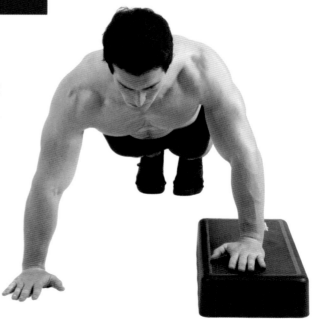

Foam Roller Push-Up

This straightforward rolling Push-Up tones and strengthens much of your upper body, arms, and thighs. Practice in order to perfect a smooth, flowing action.

HOW TO DO IT

- Kneel on the floor with a foam roller placed crosswise in front of you. Place your hands on the roller with your fingers pointed away from you.

- Press down and rise up into a Plank position, lifting your knees and straightening your legs.

- Keeping your hips as level with your shoulders as possible, and without letting your shoulders sink, bend your elbows and lower your chest to the roller. Avoid any roller movement throughout the motion.

- Return to your starting position by pressing upward, straightening your elbows, and maintaining a straight spine. Repeat for the recommended repetitions.

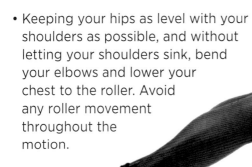
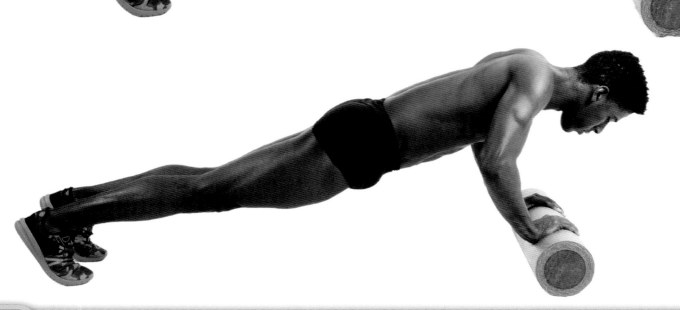

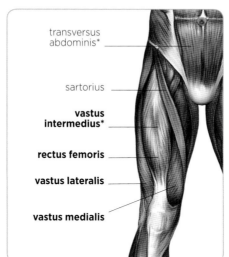

FACT FILE

TARGETS
- Triceps and biceps
- Shoulder stabilizers
- Abdominals

EQUIPMENT
- Foam roller

BENEFITS
- Improves core, pelvic, and shoulder strength and stability

CAUTIONS
- Wrist pain
- Shoulder pain
- Lower-back pain

DO IT RIGHT

- Aim for a single plane of movement; your body should form a straight line from shoulders to ankles.
- Keep your neck and shoulders relaxed throughout.
- Avoid letting your shoulders lift toward your ears.
- Avoid bending your knees.
- Avoid raising or lowering your body in segments.

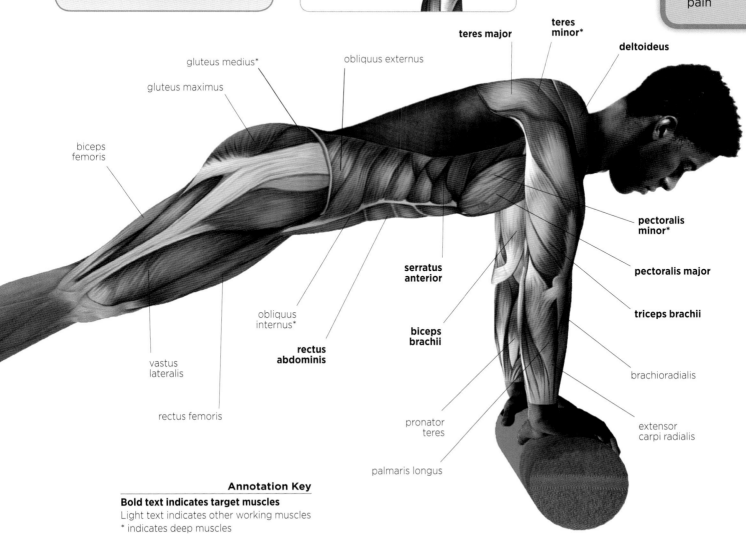

Annotation Key
Bold text indicates target muscles
Light text indicates other working muscles
* indicates deep muscles

Swiss Ball Plank with Leg Lift

Your core will really gain strength from this Swiss Ball Plank, which uses a leg lift to work leg muscles and glutes too. This is a good exercise to promote a more stable back and shoulder girdle.

HOW TO DO IT

- Kneel on your hands and knees, with a Swiss ball behind you. Your hands should be planted on the floor, with your arms straight.

- One at a time, place your feet on the ball so that your legs are fully extended behind you and your body forms a line from head to toe. Find your balance.

- Slowly and with control, raise your right foot off the ball. Hold for as long as you can, starting with around 10 to 15 seconds and working your way up to 1 minute.

- Lower your foot to the ball, repeat the raise with the opposite leg, and keep alternating sides for the recommended repetitions.

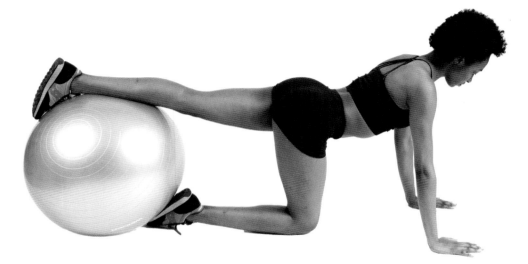

DO IT RIGHT
- Keep your abs tight.
- Keep your body in a straight line.
- Keep your neck straight and your gaze downward.
- Engage your whole body as you work to keep the ball in place.
- Avoid allowing your back to sag.
- Avoid arching your neck.
- Avoid lifting your legs so high that you can't maintain your form or keep the rest of your body stable.

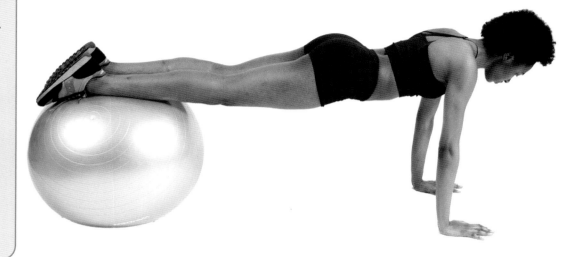

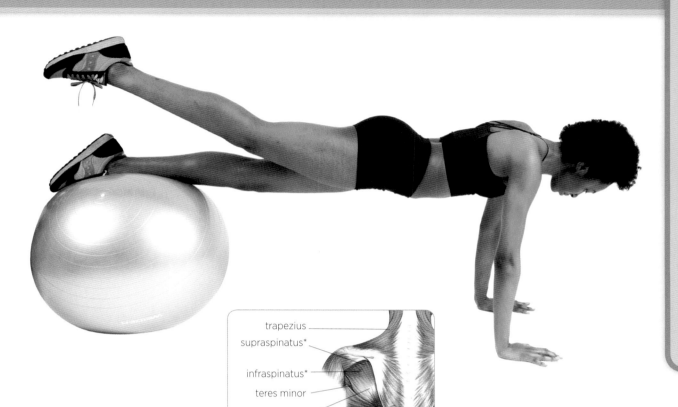

FACT FILE

TARGETS
- Abdominals, including obliques
- Back
- Glutes

EQUIPMENT
- Swiss ball

BENEFITS
- Strengthens and stabilizes core, buttocks, and back

CAUTIONS
- Shoulder injury
- Wrist pain
- Lower-back issues

trapezius

supraspinatus*

infraspinatus*

teres minor

subscapularis*

rhomboideus*

erector spinae*

Annotation Key

Bold text indicates target muscles
Light text indicates other working muscles
* indicates deep muscles

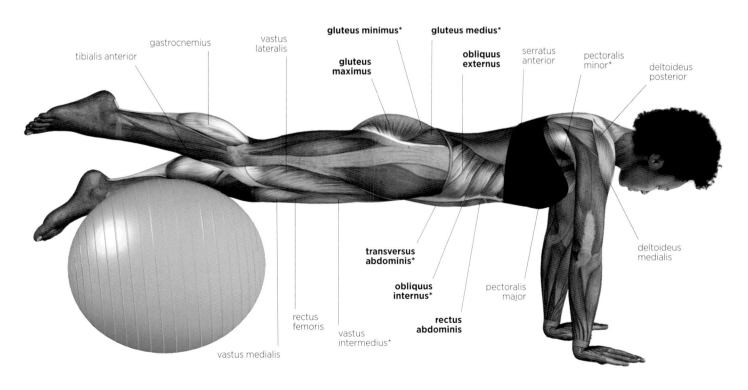

gluteus minimus*

gluteus medius*

gastrocnemius

vastus lateralis

tibialis anterior

gluteus maximus

obliquus externus

serratus anterior

pectoralis minor*

deltoideus posterior

deltoideus medialis

transversus abdominis*

obliquus internus*

pectoralis major

rectus abdominis

rectus femoris

vastus intermedius*

vastus medialis

Swiss Ball Lateral Roll

Swiss Ball Lateral Roll relies on your balance and stability to achieve the subtle movements required for this dynamic exercise. It offers a unique way to achieve core strength and stability, driven by full engagement of your core.

HOW TO DO IT

- Lie faceup on a Swiss ball, with your upper back firmly supported. Plant your feet shoulder-width apart or a little wider. Your hips and thighs should be parallel to your torso; if necessary, raise your hips to achieve this alignment.

- Extend your arms out to the sides.

- Take "baby steps" as you move toward the right side of the ball.

- Take equally small steps back to the center of the ball.

- Repeat on the opposite side, and continue alternating sides for the recommended repetitions.

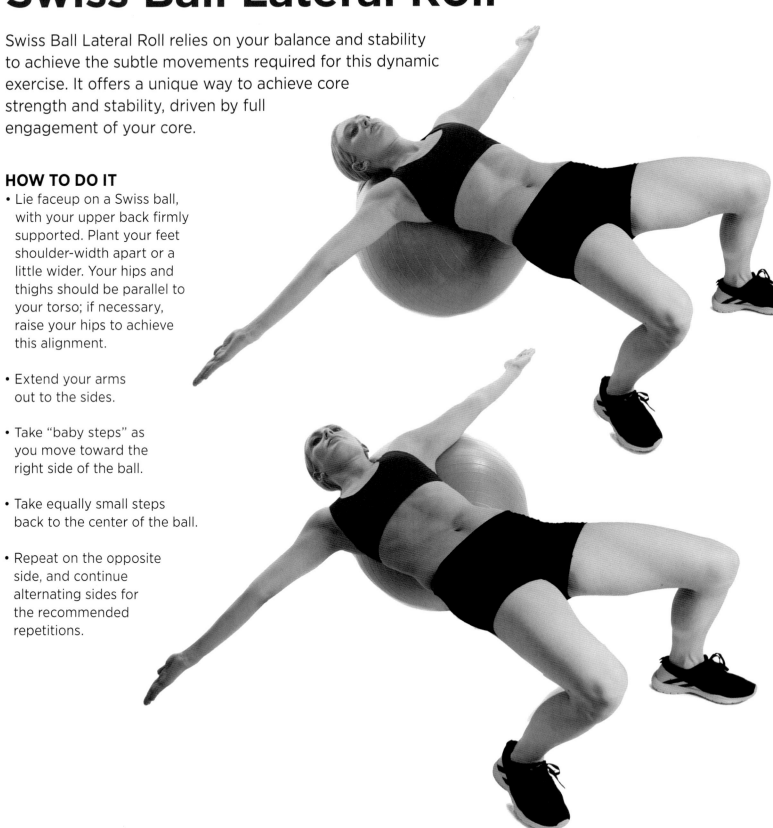

FACT FILE

TARGETS
- Abdominals
- Quads
- Upper leg/hip mobilizers

EQUIPMENT
- Swiss ball

BENEFITS
- Strengthens abdominals and quads
- Stabilizes core

CAUTIONS
- Lower-back issues
- Neck issues

DO IT RIGHT

- Keep your core braced.
- Keep your hips raised.
- Keep both arms extended.
- Avoid dropping your hips.
- Avoid moving to the side too quickly.

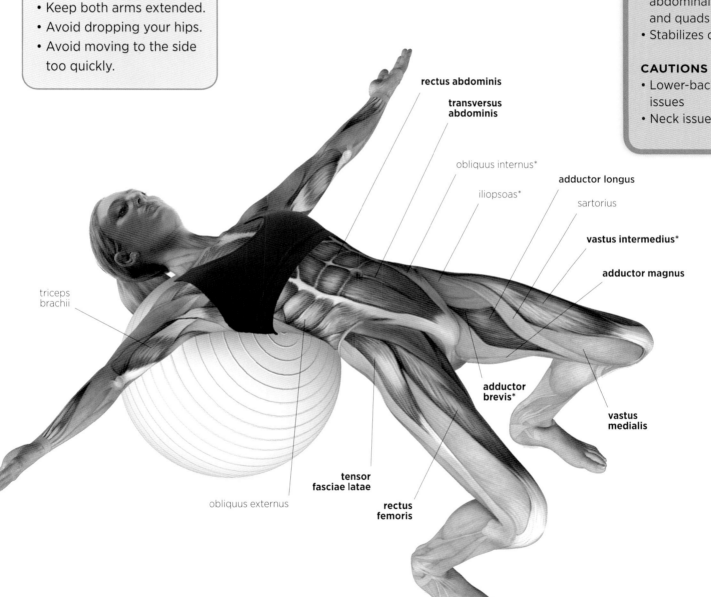

rectus abdominis

transversus abdominis

obliquus internus*

iliopsoas*

adductor longus

sartorius

vastus intermedius*

adductor magnus

triceps brachii

adductor brevis*

vastus medialis

tensor fasciae latae

rectus femoris

obliquus externus

Annotation Key
Bold text indicates target muscles
Light text indicates other working muscles
* indicates deep muscles

Medicine Ball Slam

This is another dynamic routine, and one that targets the abdominals—specifically the rectus abdominis muscle. However, it also works pretty much most of your upper body and thighs.

HOW TO DO IT
- Stand with your feet about shoulder-width apart, holding a medicine ball above your head with arms outstretched.

- Keeping your back straight, lean forward at the waist and forcefully throw the ball on to the floor. Pick up the ball and repeat for the recommended repetitions.

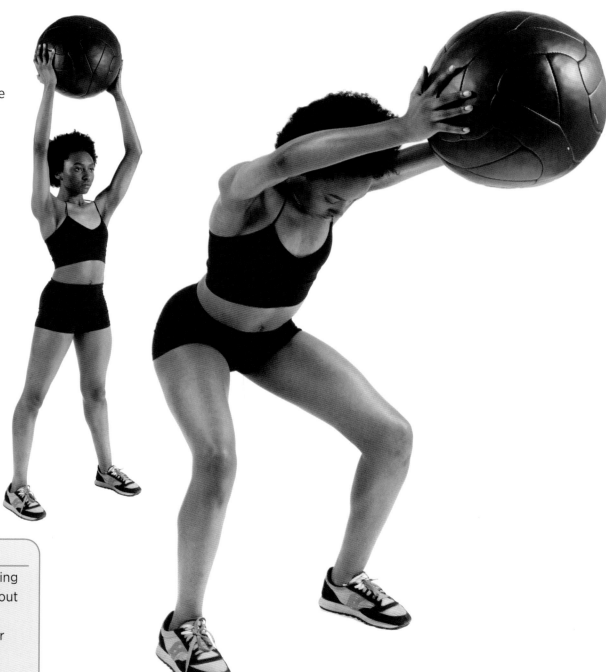

DO IT RIGHT
- Keep your torso facing straight on throughout the movement.
- Avoid rounding your back excessively.

TARGETS
• Abdominals

EQUIPMENT
• Medicine ball

BENEFITS
• Engages, strengthens, and readies the frontal core

CAUTIONS
• Back issues
• Shoulder issues

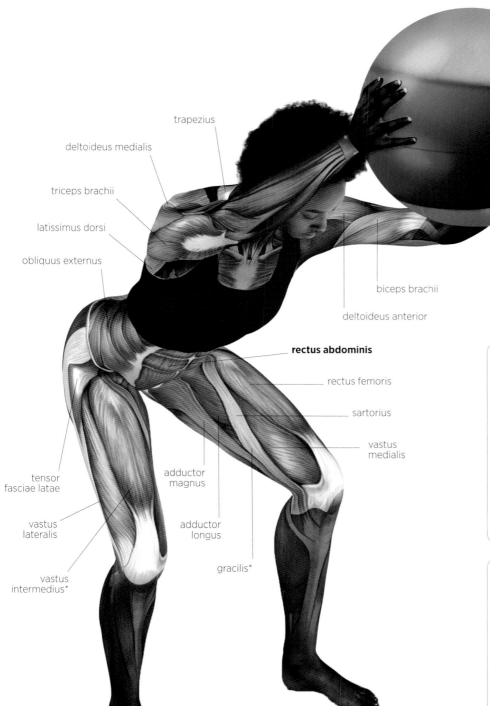

trapezius

deltoideus medialis

triceps brachii

latissimus dorsi

obliquus externus

biceps brachii

deltoideus anterior

rectus abdominis

rectus femoris

sartorius

vastus medialis

tensor fasciae latae

adductor magnus

vastus lateralis

adductor longus

vastus intermedius*

gracilis*

Annotation Key

Bold text indicates target muscles
Light text indicates other working muscles
* indicates deep muscles

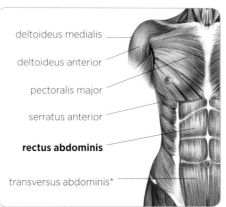

deltoideus medialis

deltoideus anterior

pectoralis major

serratus anterior

rectus abdominis

transversus abdominis*

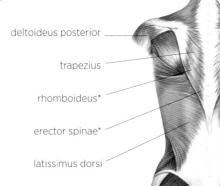

deltoideus posterior

trapezius

rhomboideus*

erector spinae*

latissimus dorsi

Medicine Ball Squat to Press

Medicine Ball Squat to Press provides a strengthening workout for various different areas of your body. It does this by engaging a spectrum of muscles at the same time. Plus it offers you a cardio element too.

HOW TO DO IT

- Stand, holding the medicine ball in front of your chest. Plant your feet shoulder-width apart, and stick out your buttocks slightly.

- Lower toward the floor until your thighs are parallel to the floor.

- Push evenly through your heels to an upright position, and extend your arms overhead.

- Lower your arms, assume your starting position, and repeat for the recommended repetitions.

DO IT RIGHT

- Keep your head up and your chest out so your body forms a straight line.
- Avoid allowing your knees to hyperextend past your feet.

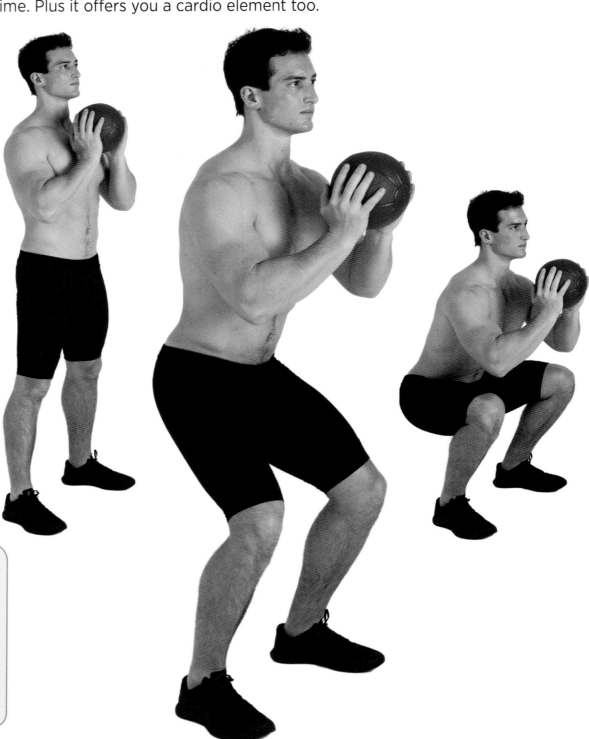

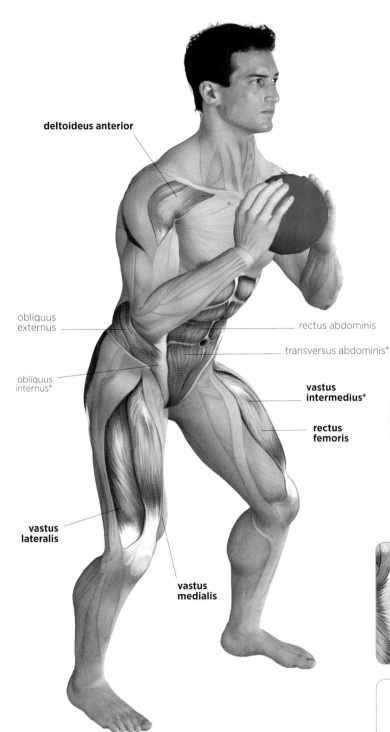

FACT FILE

TARGETS
- Glutes
- Deltoids
- Quads

EQUIPMENT
- Medicine ball

BENEFITS
- Strengthens and tones glutes and quads
- Improves coordination
- Helps maintain a sound cardiovascular system

CAUTIONS
- Lower-back issues
- Knee issues

deltoideus anterior

obliquus externus

obliquus internus*

rectus abdominis

transversus abdominis*

vastus intermedius*

rectus femoris

vastus lateralis

vastus medialis

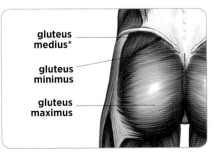

serratus anterior

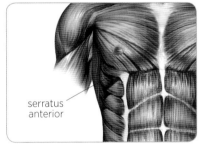

deltoideus posterior

deltoideus medialis

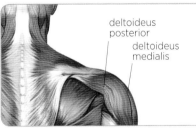

gluteus medius*

gluteus minimus

gluteus maximus

Annotation Key

Bold text indicates target muscles
Light text indicates other working muscles
* indicates deep muscles

CHAPTER FIVE

WORKOUT ROUTINES

This chapter offers a varied choice of routines created from exercises featured in the book. It is divided into three sections. The first targets specific body areas; the second contains performance boosters for sports; the third offers workouts for everything from balance to posture. There's something for all levels, and remember—you can switch things down or up by changing the repetitions or times, or by following modification suggestions in the book.

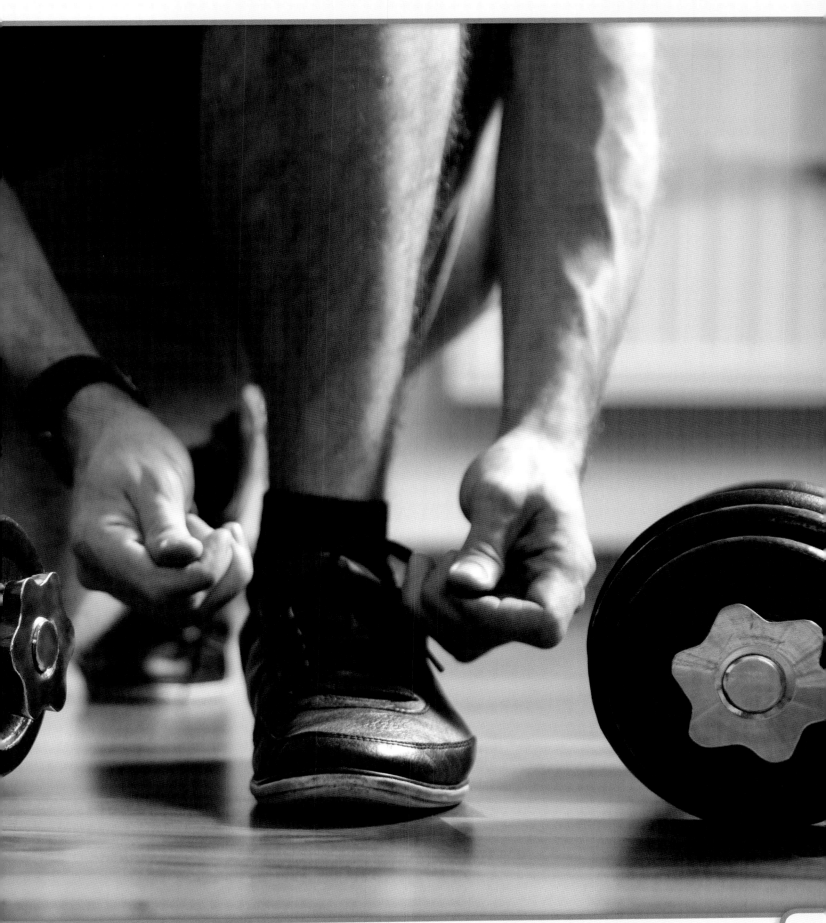

Shoulder Routine

This routine is designed as an all-encompassing shoulder workout. It will develop mass, strength, and quality in the three-headed musculature that forms your deltoids.

1 SHOULDER PRESS

page 152–153
• Perform 10 repetitions

2 ALTERNATING KETTLEBELL PRESS

pages 166–167
• Perform 8–10 repetitions per arm

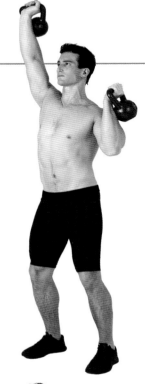

3 BOTTOM-UP KETTLEBELL CLEAN

pages 168–169
• Perform 8–10 repetitions per arm

4 LATERAL SHOULDER RAISE

pages 156–157
• Perform 8–10 repetitions

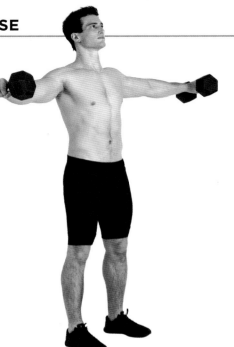

5 RESISTANCE BAND LATERAL RAISE

pages 240–241
• Perform 8–10 repetitions

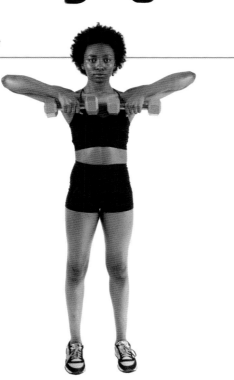

6 DUMBBELL SHRUG

pages 134–135
• Perform 10–12 repetitions

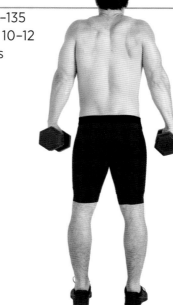

7 DUMBBELL UPRIGHT ROW

pages 138–139
• Perform 15 repetitions

8 BENT-OVER CABLE RAISE

pages 236–237
• Perform 10–12 repetitions per arm

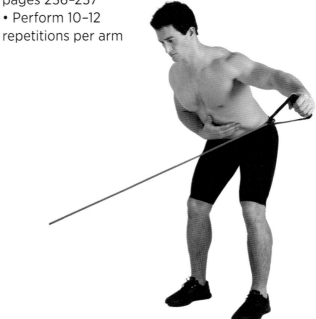

Arm Routine

Designed as an all-around arm workout, this routine will really strengthen and build your upper arms. It targets the three-headed musculature of your triceps and the two-headed muscles of your biceps.

1 TRICEPS DIP

pages 66–67
• Perform 10–12 repetitions

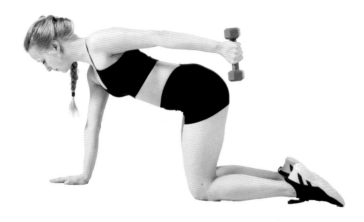

2 TRICEPS PUSH-UP

pages 72–73
• Perform 10–12 repetitions

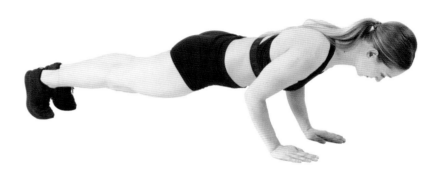

3 DUMBBELL TRICEPS KICKBACK

pages 164–165
• Perform 12–15 repetitions per arm

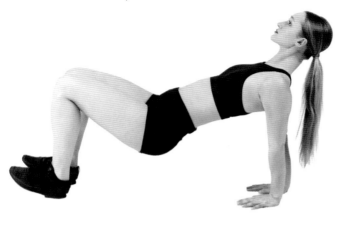

4 PLANK-UP

pages 116–117
• Perform 4–12 repetitions per arm

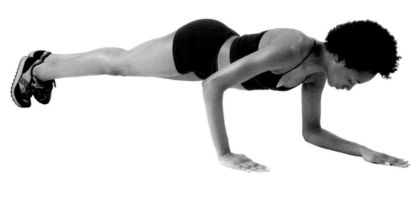

FACT FILE

TARGETS
• Arms

EQUIPMENT
• Barbell
• Dumbbells

BENEFITS
• Strengthens arms

5 BARBELL CURL

pages 172–173
• Perform 8–10 repetitions

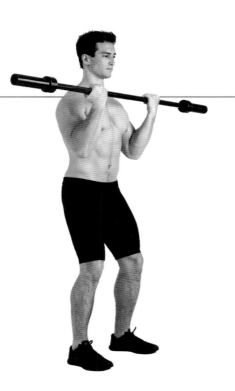

6 BALLET BICEPS

pages 158–159
• Perform 6–10 repetitions

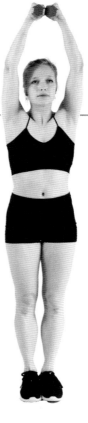

7 ALTERNATING HAMMER CURL

pages 160–161
• Perform 8–10 repetitions per arm

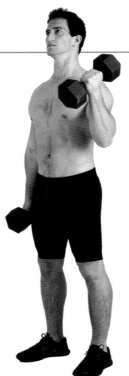

8 SINGLE-ARM CONCENTRATION CURL

pages 162–163
• Perform 10–12 repetitions per arm

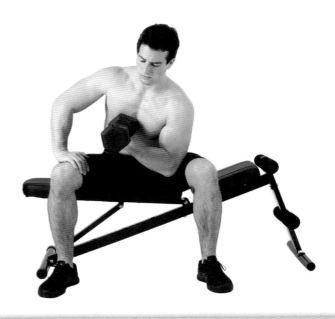

Chest Routine

This routine will lend mass, strength, and quality to the pectoral musculature that forms your chest. Work on your chest helps develop the stable torso needed for so many fitness routines.

1 HAMMER-GRIP PRESS

pages 176–177
• Perform 8–10 repetitions

2 ALTERNATING CHEST PRESS

pages 256–257
• Perform 15 repetitions per arm

3 SWISS BALL PUSH-UP

pages 260–261
• Perform 10 repetitions

4 DUMBBELL FLY

pages 180–181
• Perform 10–12 repetitions

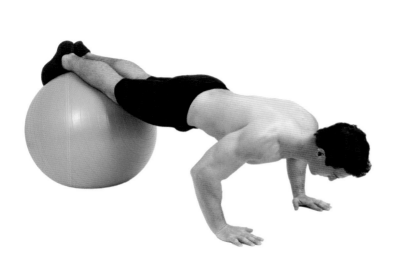

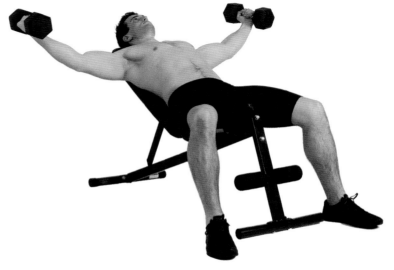

FACT FILE

TARGETS
- Chest

EQUIPMENT
- Resistance band
- Cable machine
- Dumbbells
- Incline bench/ similar
- Swiss ball

BENEFITS
- Strengthens chest

5 ZIPPER

pages 174–175
- Perform 10–20 repetitions

6 CABLE FLY

pages 250–251
- Perform 12–15 repetitions

7 CABLE CROSSOVER FLY

pages 254–255
- Perform 12–15 repetitions

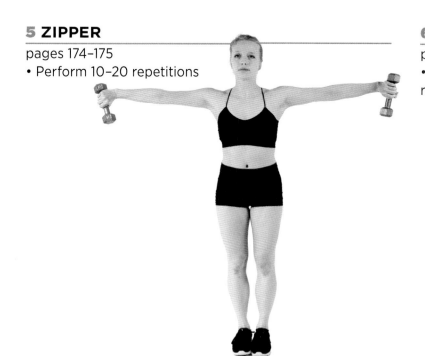

8 RESISTANCE BAND STANDING FLY

pages 258–259
- Perform 12–15 repetitions

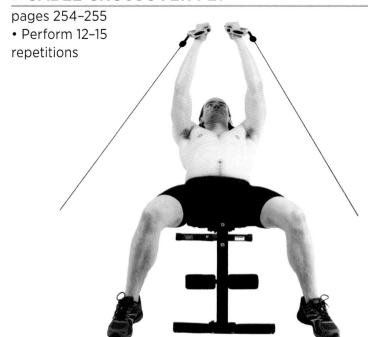

Back Routine

This back routine will build width, strength, and quality in the complex musculature of your back. A strong back is essential for all-around optimal fitness.

1 REVERSE-GRIP PULL-UP

pages 226–227
• Perform 10 repetitions

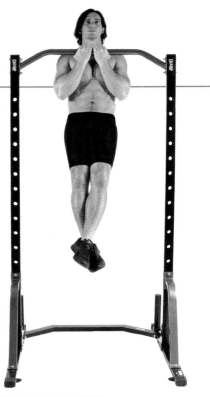

2 WIDE-GRIP PULL-UP

pages 224–225
• Perform 20 repetitions

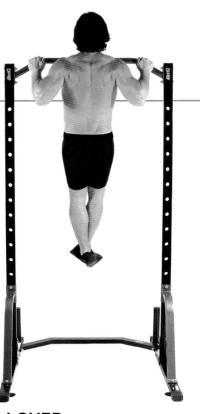

3 ALTERNATING FLOOR ROW

pages 142–143
• Perform 15 repetitions per arm

4 SWISS BALL PULLOVER

pages 144–145
• Perform 10–12 repetitions

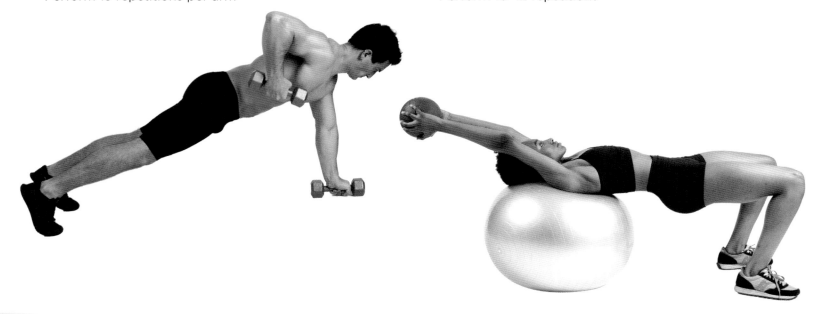

FACT FILE

TARGETS
• Back

EQUIPMENT
• Barbell
• Dumbbells
• Kettlebells
• Medicine ball
• Pull-up bar
• Swiss ball

BENEFITS
• Strengthens back

5 SINGLE-ARM T-ROW

pages 188–189
• Perform 10–12 repetitions per arm

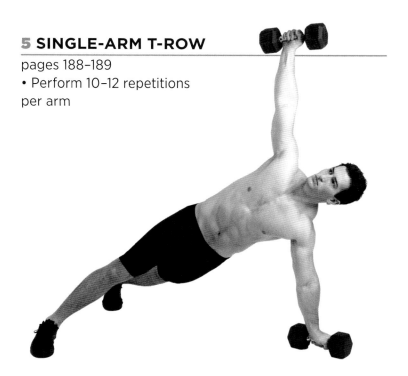

6 ALTERNATING KETTLEBELL ROW

pages 146–147
• Perform 8–10 repetitions per arm

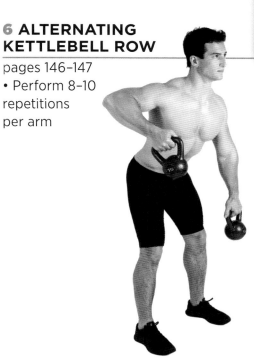

7 BARBELL DEADLIFT

pages 148–149
• Perform 6–8 repetitions

8 LOWER-BACK EXTENSION

pages 150–151
• Perform 10 repetitions

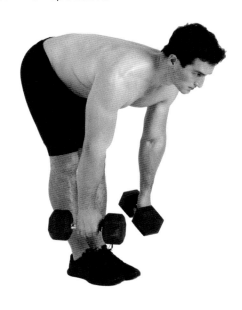

Functional Chest/Back Routine

This is a combination chest/back workout. It has been devised to focus on creating functional mass, strength, and quality in specific muscles: the pectoralis and latissimus dorsi.

1 COBRA STRETCH

pages 36–37
• Hold for 15–30 seconds

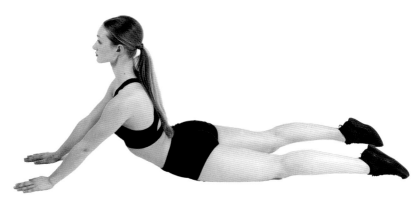

2 HALF-KNEELING ROTATION

pages 40–41
• Perform 10 repetitions per side

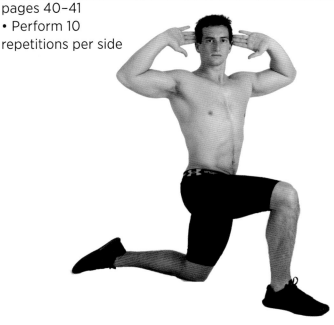

3 BACK BURNER

pages 56–57
• Perform 10 repetitions

4 BREAST STROKE

pages 54–55
• Perform 10 repetitions

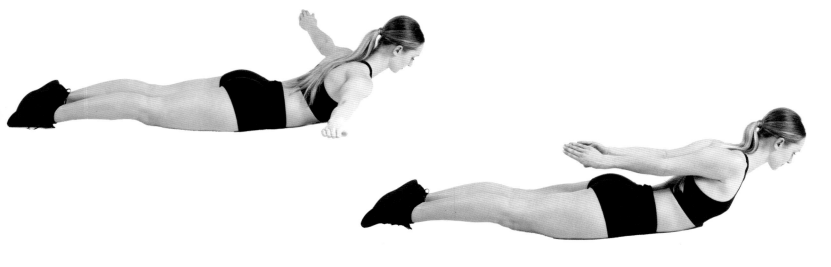

FACT FILE

TARGETS
• Chest and back

EQUIPMENT
• Dumbbells
• Flat bench/similar
• Kettlebells
• Swiss ball

BENEFITS
• Strengthens chest and back

5 PUSH-UP

pages 68–69
• Perform 12 repetitions

6 SWISS BALL FLY

pages 182–183
• Perform 15 repetitions

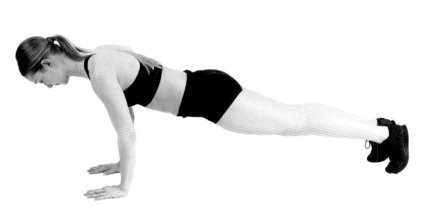

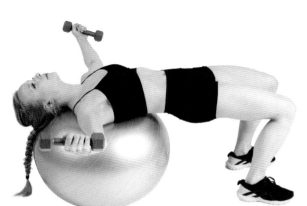

7 ALTERNATING RENEGADE ROW

pages 190–191
• Perform 8–10 repetitions per arm

8 BENT-ARM DUMBBELL PULLOVER

pages 178–179
• Perform 15 repetitions

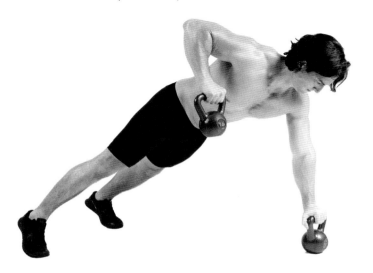

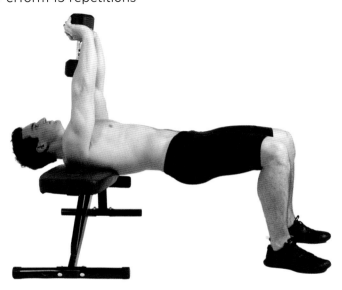

Rectus Abdominis Routine

Performing this routine will provide a great general workout for the abdominal muscles. However, it especially promotes strength and quality in the pronounced musculature of the rectus abdominis.

1 CRUNCH
pages 76–77
• Perform 25 repetitions

2 REVERSE CRUNCH
pages 78–79
• Perform 20 repetitions

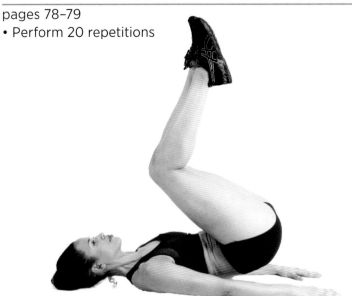

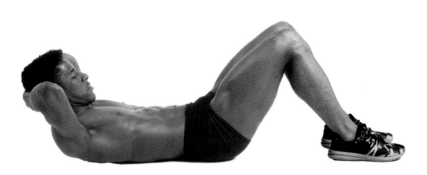

3 SCISSORS
pages 84–85
• Perform 12–15 repetitions per leg

4 LEG LEVELERS
pages 86–87
• Perform 25 repetitions

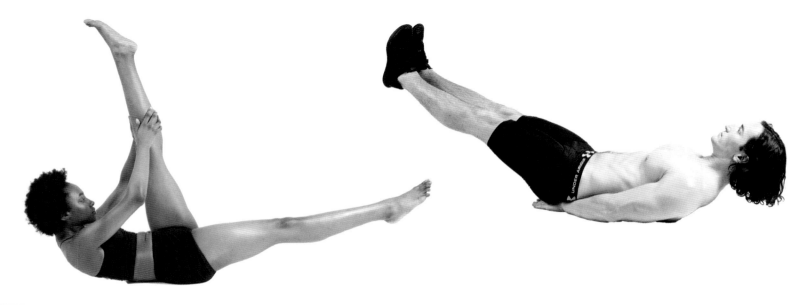

5 BODY SAW

pages 88–89
• Perform 20 repetitions

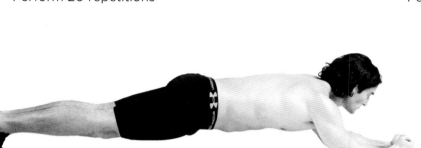

6 THIGH ROCK-BACK

pages 90–91
• Perform 5 repetitions

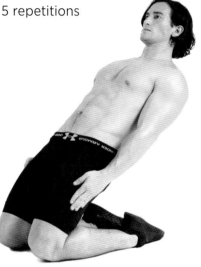

7 PLANK

pages 114–115
• Hold for 60 seconds

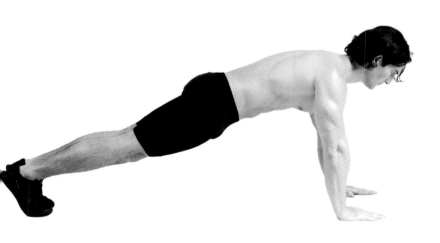

8 UP-DOWN

pages 128–129
• Perform 10 repetitions

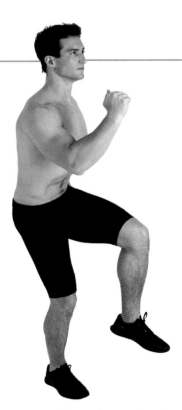

Obliques Routine

Choose this routine if you want to target your obliques. These muscles are a vital part of your abdominal musculature, and of your core strength.

1 SIDE PLANK
pages 120–121
• Hold for 30–60 seconds per side

2 SIDE PLANK WITH REACH-UNDER
pages 122–123
• Perform 15 repetitions per side

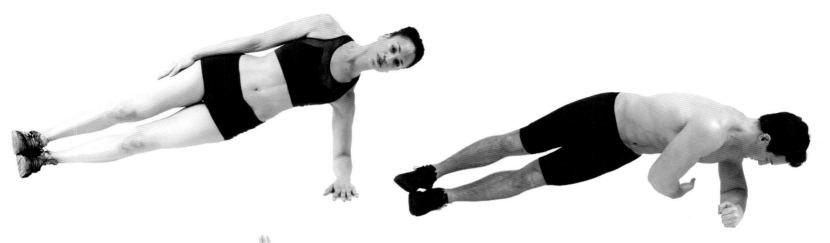

3 T-STABILIZATION
pages 124–125
• Hold for 30–60 seconds per side

4 SWISS BALL RUSSIAN TWIST
pages 276–277
• Perform 15 repetitions per side

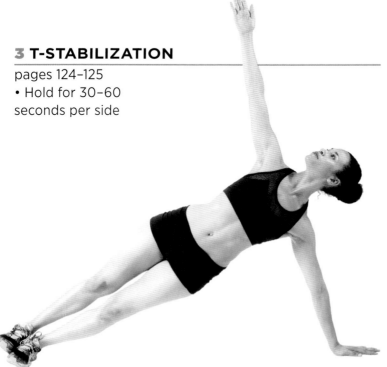

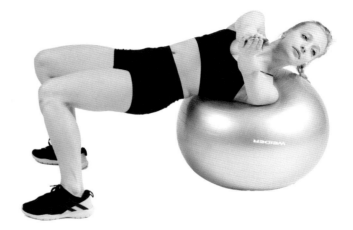

FACT FILE

TARGETS
• Obliques

EQUIPMENT
• Dumbbells
• Medicine ball
• Swiss ball

BENEFITS
• Strengthens
  obliques

5 SEATED DUMBBELL RUSSIAN TWIST

pages 184–185
• Perform 12–15 repetitions per side

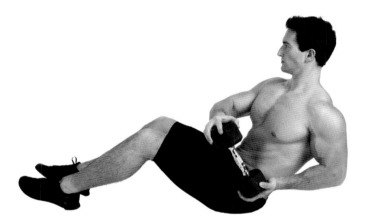

6 DIAGONAL CRUNCH WITH MEDICINE BALL

pages 264–265
• Perform 15 repetitions per side

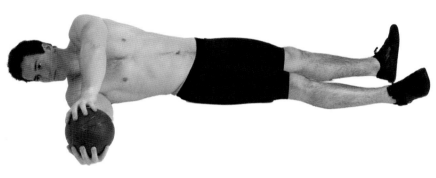

7 MEDICINE BALL STANDING RUSSIAN TWIST

pages 266–267
• Perform 20
repetitions per side

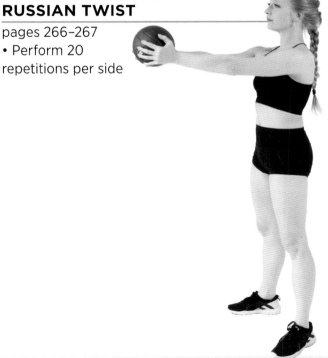

8 SWISS BALL ATOMIC PUSH-UP

pages 270–271
• Perform 12–15 repetitions

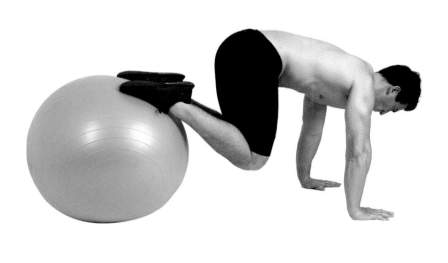

Thighs and Glutes Routine

Your quads and glutes get all the attention in this routine, which develops both size and strength. But other body areas get to work out here too.

1 BARBELL SQUAT

pages 208–209
• Perform 6–8 repetitions

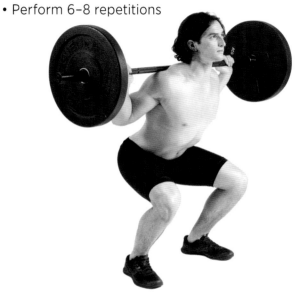

2 SUMO SQUAT

pages 204–205
• Perform 15 repetitions

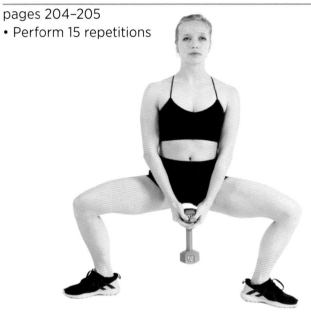

3 GOBLET SQUAT

pages 206–207
• Perform 8–10 repetitions

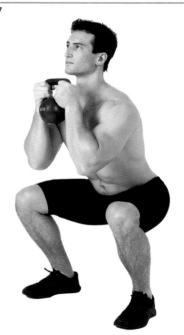

4 DUMBBELL LYING HIP ABDUCTION

pages 196–197
• Perform 10 repetitions per side

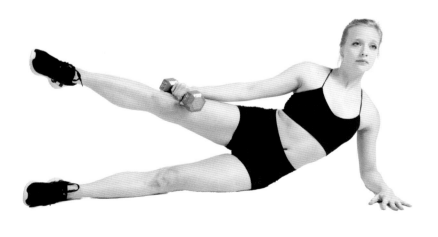

FACT FILE

TARGETS
• Thighs and glutes

EQUIPMENT
• Barbell
• Dumbbells
• Kettlebells
• Resistance band
• Swiss ball

BENEFITS
• Strengthens thighs and glutes

5 DUMBBELL LUNGE

pages 198–199
• Perform 12 repetitions per leg

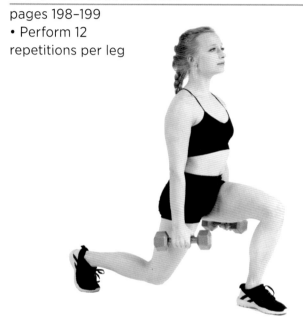

6 DUMBBELL WALKING LUNGE

pages 200–201
• Perform 12 repetitions per leg

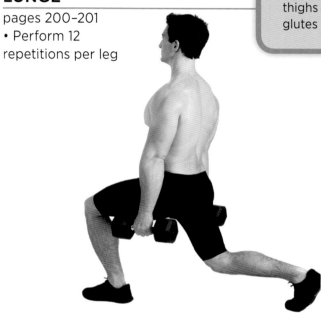

7 RESISTANCE BAND LUNGE

pages 288–289
• Perform 15 repetitions per leg

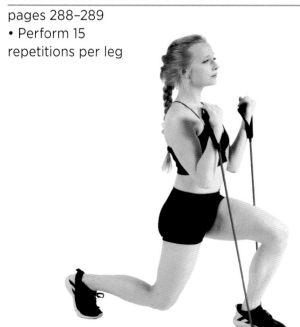

8 SWISS BALL SPLIT SQUAT

pages 294–295
• Perform 15 repetitions per leg

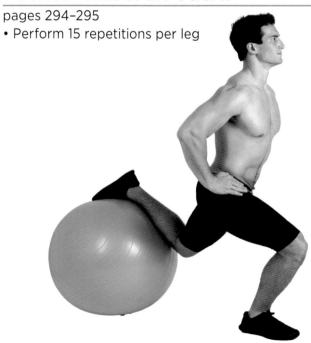

Shapely Glutes Routine

This workout has been compiled with health and aesthetics in mind. You will not only improve mass and strength in your glutes but also acquire a toned shape.

1 STIFF-LEGGED DUMBBELL DEADLIFT

pages 136–137
• Perform 15 repetitions

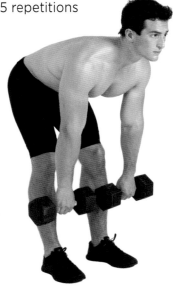

2 STEP-DOWN

pages 300–301
• Perform 20 repetitions per leg

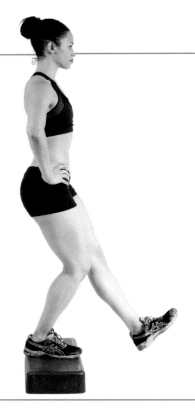

3 STEP-UP

pages 302–303
• Perform 15 repetitions per side

4 BOX JUMPS

pages 298–299
• Perform 15 repetitions

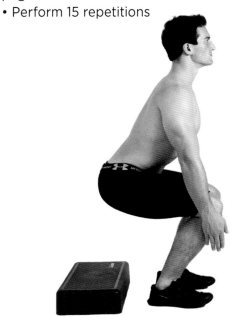

FACT FILE

TARGETS
• Glutes

EQUIPMENT
• Dumbbells
• 2 plyo boxes/
  similar
• Step/bench/
  platform

BENEFITS
• Strengthens
  and tones
  glutes

5 BUTT KICK

pages 110–111
• Perform for
30–60 seconds

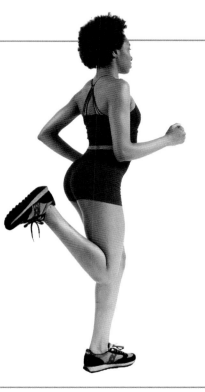

6 SINGLE-LEG GLUTEAL LIFT

pages 108–109
• Perform 15
repetitions per leg

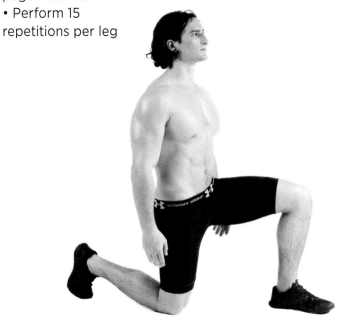

7 SQUAT

pages 106–107
• Perform 15
repetitions

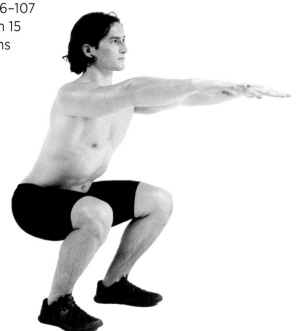

8 LUNGE

pages 100–101
• Perform 15
repetitions per leg

Full-Body Routine

This full-body routine will bring unified strength, stability, and quality to a wide range of your muscles. Getting different muscles to work together well promotes excellent physical health.

1 CLEAN-AND-PRESS

pages 210–211
• Perform 10 repetitions

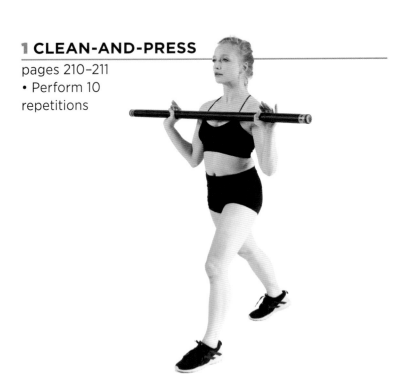

2 BARBELL POWER CLEAN AND JERK

pages 216–217
• Perform 6–8 repetitions

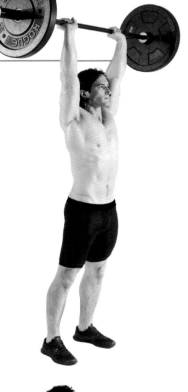

3 CURLING STEP-AND-RAISE

pages 212–213
• Perform 10 repetitions per side

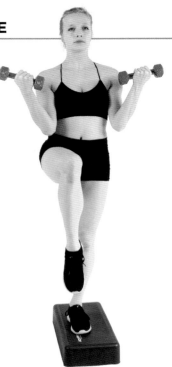

4 KNEE RAISE WITH LATERAL EXTENSION

pages 214–215
• Perform 5–10 repetitions per leg

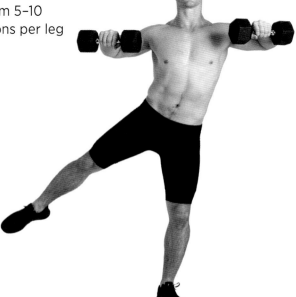

FACT FILE

TARGETS
• Whole body

EQUIPMENT
• Barbell
• Body bar
• Dumbbells
• Medicine ball
• Step/box/
  platform
• Swiss ball

BENEFITS
• Strengthens
  whole body

5 PUSH-UP HAND WALK-OVER

pages 304–305
• Perform 5 repetitions per side

6 SWISS BALL PLANK WITH LEG LIFT

pages 308–309
• Hold for 10–60 seconds per leg

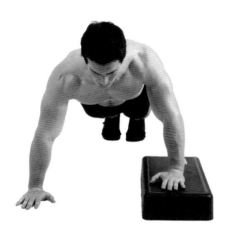

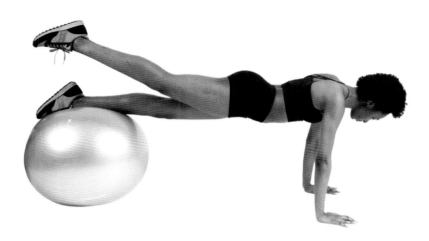

7 MEDICINE BALL SLAM

pages 312–313
• Perform 20 repetitions

8 MEDICINE BALL SQUAT TO PRESS

pages 314–315
• Perform 15 repetitions

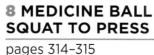

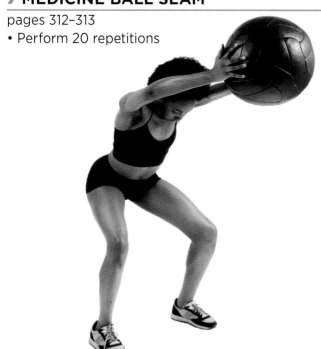

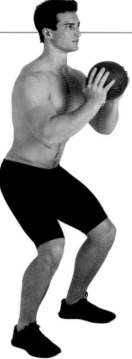

Baseball Routine

Build the elements of speed and strong agility into your performance in this set of exercises that have been combined specifically to improve your play on the baseball field.

1 SINGLE-ARM BAND PULL

pages 232–233
• Perform 15 repetitions per arm

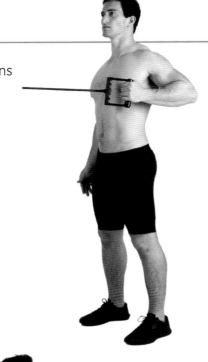

2 PYRAMID CABLE PRESS

pages 234–235
• Perform 12 repetitions

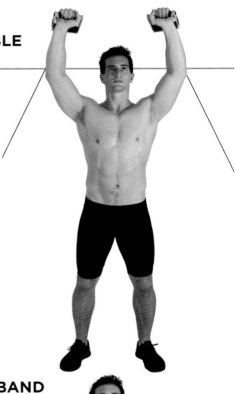

3 SHOULDER FLEXING

pages 154–155
• Perform 25 repetitions

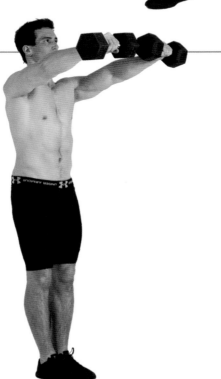

4 RESISTANCE BAND BICEPS CURL

pages 242–243
• Perform 15 repetitions

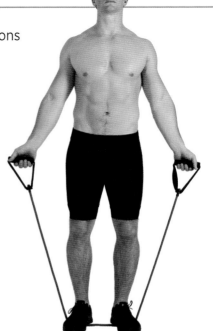

TARGETS
• Whole body

EQUIPMENT
• Cable machine
• Dumbbells
• Foam roller
• Resistance band

BENEFITS
• Strengthens whole body

5 FOAM ROLLER DIAGONAL CRUNCH

pages 282–283
• Perform 15 repetitions per side

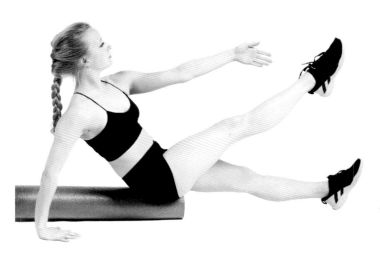

6 T-STABILIZATION

pages 124–125
• Hold for 30–60 seconds per side

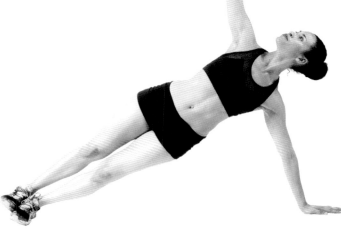

7 BUTT KICK

pages 110–111
• Perform for 30–60 seconds

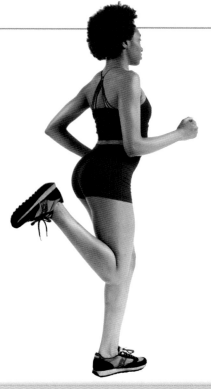

8 PENGUIN CRUNCH

pages 80–81
• Perform 25 repetitions per side

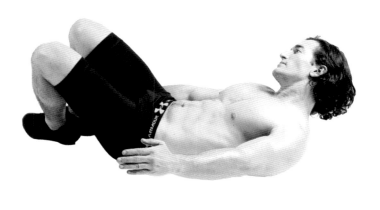

Cycling Routine

Riding a bicycle calls for strength, stamina, and unified coordination. This routine will work on specific muscle sets to build up these qualities and really improve your performance.

1 THREAD THE NEEDLE

pages 48–49
• Perform 15 repetitions per side

2 SWIMMER

pages 52–53
• Perform 6–8 repetitions per side

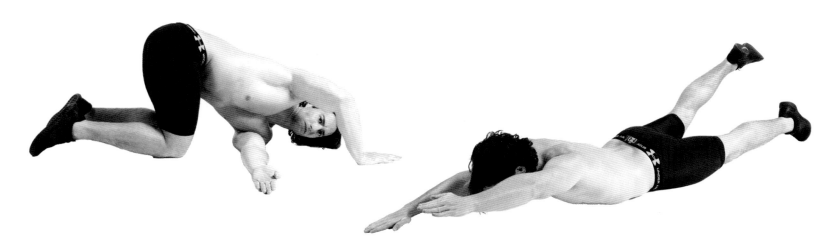

3 HIP CROSSOVER

pages 50–51
• Perform 15 repetitions per side

4 HAMSTRINGS PULL-IN

pages 296–297
• Perform 15 repetitions

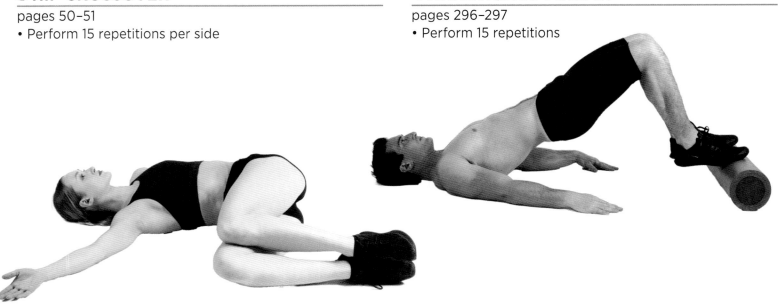

FACT FILE

TARGETS
• Lower body

EQUIPMENT
• Body bar
• Foam roller
• Dumbbells for
  modification
• Kettlebells
• Swiss ball

BENEFITS
• Strengthens
  lower body

5 LATERAL-EXTENSION REVERSE LUNGE

pages 102–103
• Perform 10
  repetitions per side

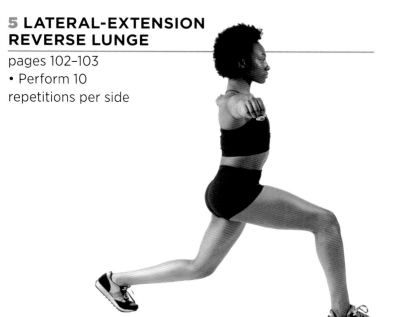

6 CLEAN-AND-PRESS

pages 210–211
• Perform 10
  repetitions

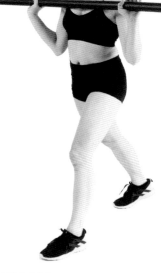

7 ALTERNATING KETTLEBELL ROW

pages 146–147
• Perform 8–10
  repetitions per arm

8 BICYCLE CRUNCH

pages 82–83
• Perform 25 repetitions per side

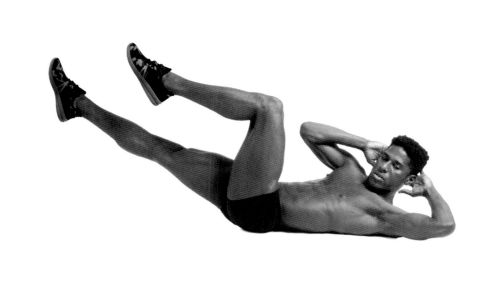

Dance Routine

Dancing is demanding on the body—and a good workout in itself. It requires coordination skills and accuracy, and this routine will help you deliver on both fronts.

1 MOUNTAIN CLIMBER

pages 126–127
• Perform for 30–60 seconds

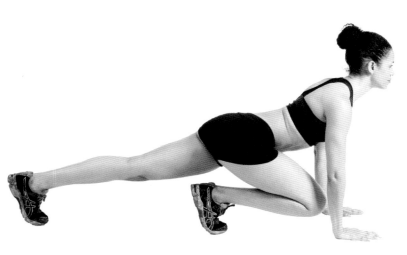

2 SKATER'S LUNGE

pages 104–105
• Perform for 45–60 seconds

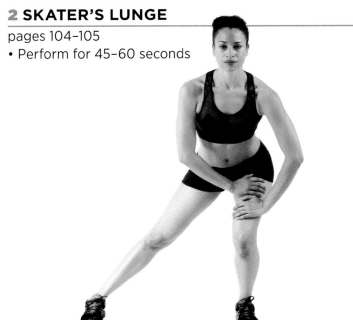

3 SINGLE-LEG GLUTEAL LIFT

pages 108–109
• Perform 5 repetitions per leg

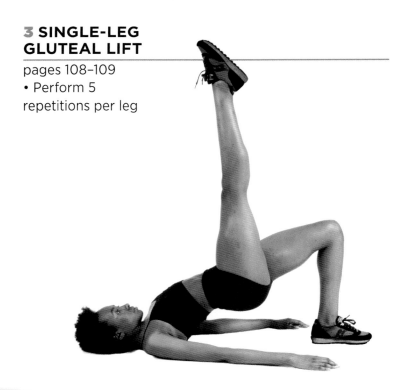

4 DUMBBELL WALKING LUNGE

pages 200–201
• Perform 15 repetitions per leg

FACT FILE

TARGETS
• Lower body

EQUIPMENT
• Dumbbells
• Kettlebells for modification

BENEFITS
• Strengthens lower body

5 DUMBBELL LYING HIP ABDUCTION

pages 196–197
• Perform 10 repetitions per side

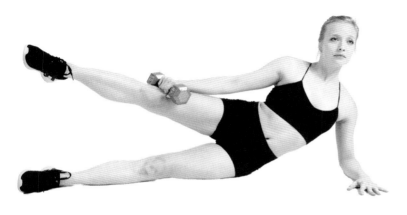

6 STANDING QUADRICEPS STRETCH

page 30
• Perform for 30 seconds per leg

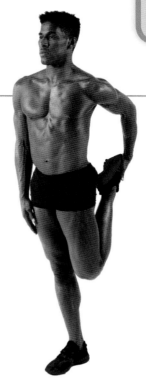

7 STANDING HAMSTRINGS STRETCH

page 31
• Perform for 30 seconds per leg

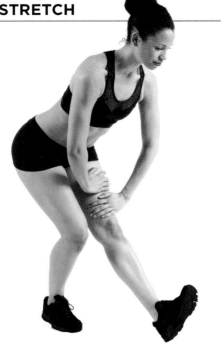

8 ILIOTIBIAL BAND STRETCH

pages 32–33
• Perform for 15 seconds per side

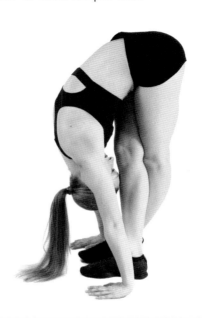

Football Routine

Power and energy are needed for football, as well as strength. Follow this workout to build all these qualities and see your game gather momentum.

1 WIDE PUSH-UP

pages 70–71
• Perform 10–12 repetitions

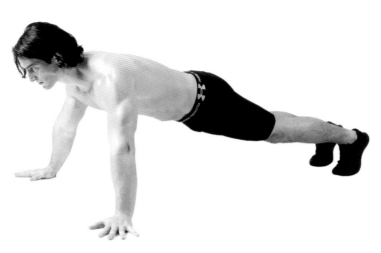

2 STANDING BARBELL ROW

pages 170–171
• Perform 8–10 repetitions

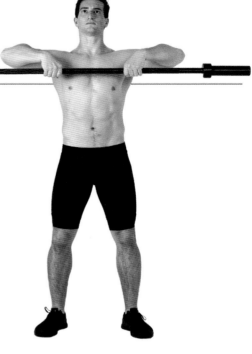

3 DUMBBELL SHRUG

pages 134–135
• Perform 12–15 repetitions

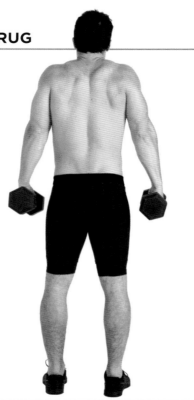

4 SHOULDER FLEXING

pages 154–155
• Perform 25 repetitions

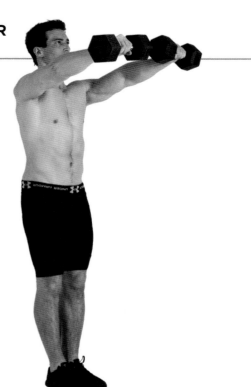

FACT FILE

TARGETS
• Whole body

EQUIPMENT
• Barbell
• Dumbbells
• Kettlebells
• Resistance band

BENEFITS
• Strengthens whole body

5 RESISTANCE BAND SINGLE-ARM ROW

pages 244–245
• Perform 20 repetitions per side

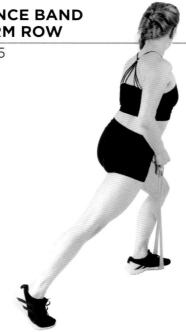

6 HIP CROSSOVER

pages 50–51
• Perform 15 repetitions per side

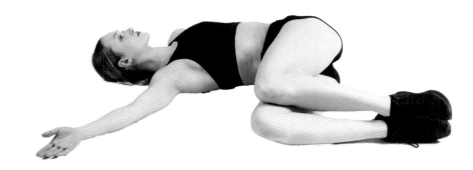

7 ALLIGATOR CRAWL

pages 58–59
• Perform for 60 seconds

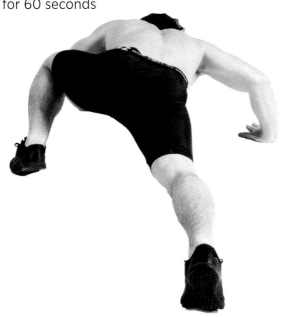

8 GOBLET SQUAT

pages 206–207
• Perform 8–10 repetitions

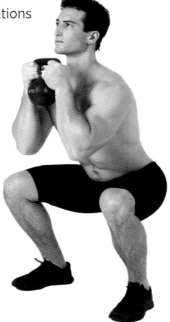

Marathon Running Routine

Marathon running calls on different, very specific qualities compared to sprinting. This routine has been specially designed to develop stamina, longevity, and improved output.

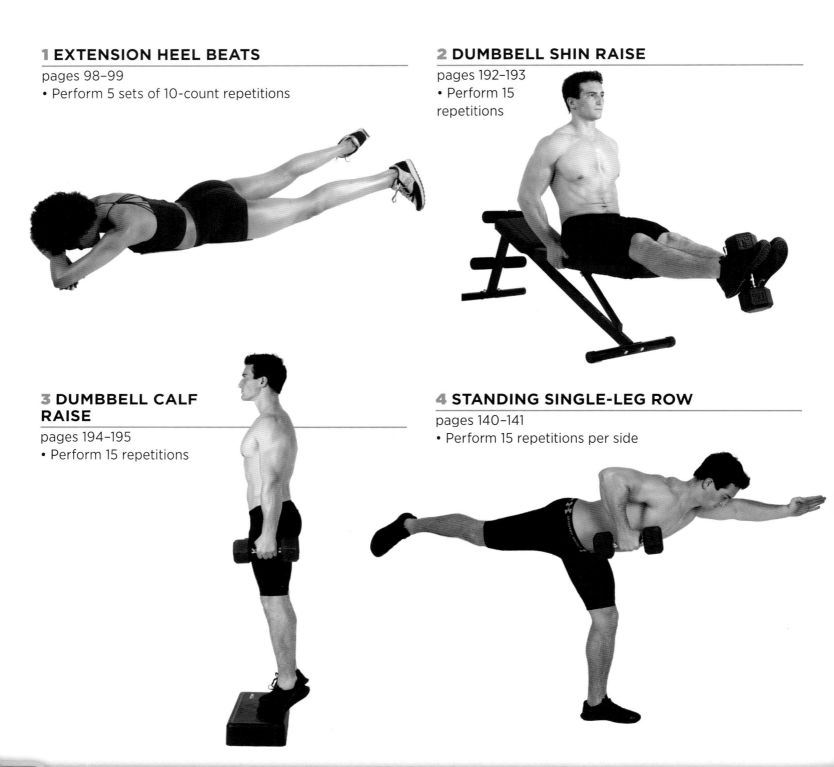

1 EXTENSION HEEL BEATS
pages 98–99
• Perform 5 sets of 10-count repetitions

2 DUMBBELL SHIN RAISE
pages 192–193
• Perform 15 repetitions

3 DUMBBELL CALF RAISE
pages 194–195
• Perform 15 repetitions

4 STANDING SINGLE-LEG ROW
pages 140–141
• Perform 15 repetitions per side

FACT FILE

TARGETS
• Lower body

EQUIPMENT
• Dumbbells
• Flat bench/
  similar
• Medicine ball
• Platform/
  step/block
• Swiss ball for
  modification

BENEFITS
• Strengthens
  lower body

5 DUMBBELL WALKING LUNGE

pages 200–201
• Perform 15
repetitions per leg

6 MEDICINE BALL SQUAT TO PRESS

pages 314–315
• Perform 15
repetitions

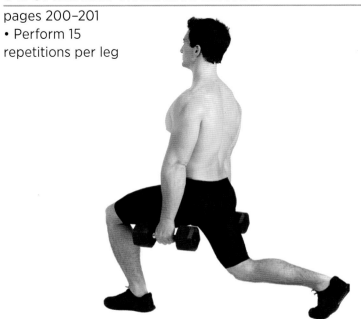

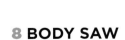

7 SCISSORS

pages 84–85
• Perform 12–15 repetitions per leg

8 BODY SAW

pages 88–89
• Perform 20 repetitions

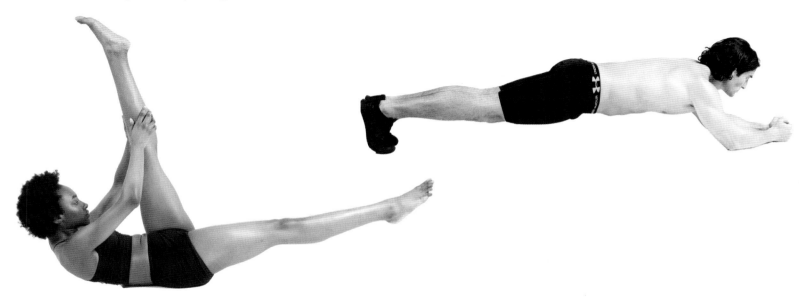

Sprinting Routine

This sprinter's routine will help you to develop better explosiveness, speed, and power—just what the sprinter needs. It should also build muscle durability.

1 EXTENSION HEEL BEATS

pages 98–99
• Perform 5 sets of 10-count repetitions

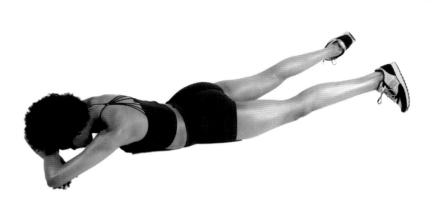

2 DUMBBELL SHIN RAISE

pages 192–193
• Perform 15 repetitions

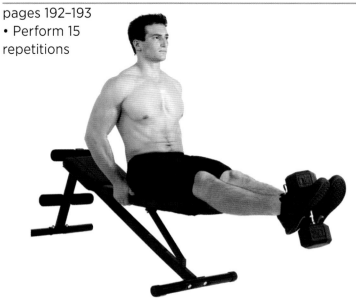

3 DUMBBELL CALF RAISE

pages 194–195
• Perform 15 repetitions

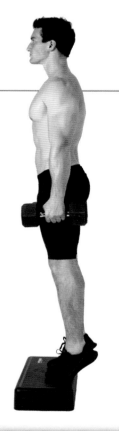

4 MOUNTAIN CLIMBER

pages 126–127
• Perform for 30–60 seconds

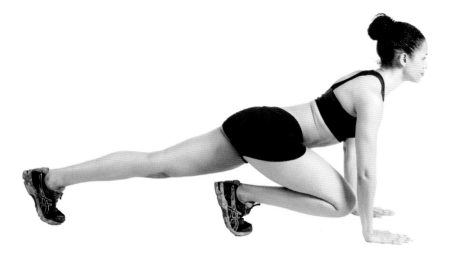

FACT FILE

TARGETS
• Lower body

EQUIPMENT
• Dumbbells
• Flat bench
• Medicine ball
• Platform/
  step/block

BENEFITS
• Strengthens
  lower body

5 SINGLE-LEG V-UP

pages 92–93
• Perform 15 repetitions per leg

6 BURPEE

pages 130–131
• Perform for up to 60 seconds

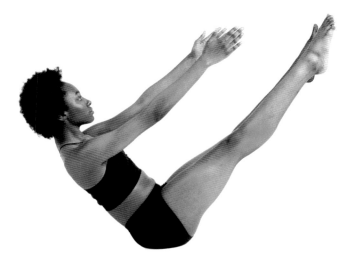

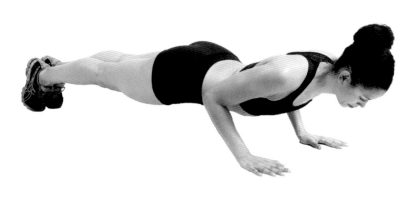

7 MEDICINE BALL SLAM

pages 312–313
• Perform 20 repetitions

8 ALLIGATOR CRAWL

pages 58–59
• Perform for 60 seconds

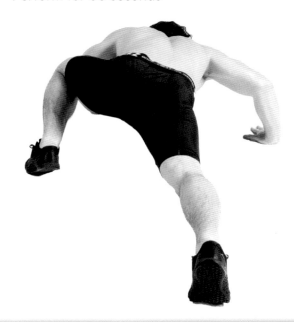

Swimming Routine

Anyone looking to improve swimming form will really benefit from this routine. It addresses strengthening the core, arms, and legs in ways especially relevant to swimmers.

1 SWISS BALL ABDOMINAL STRETCH

pages 44–45
• Perform for 30 seconds

2 SWIMMER

pages 52–53
• Perform 6–8 repetitions per side

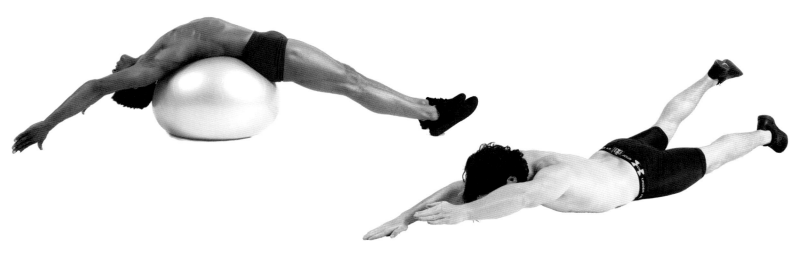

3 BREAST STROKE

pages 54–55
• Perform 10 repetitions

4 SWISS BALL W

pages 246–247
• Perform 12–15 repetitions

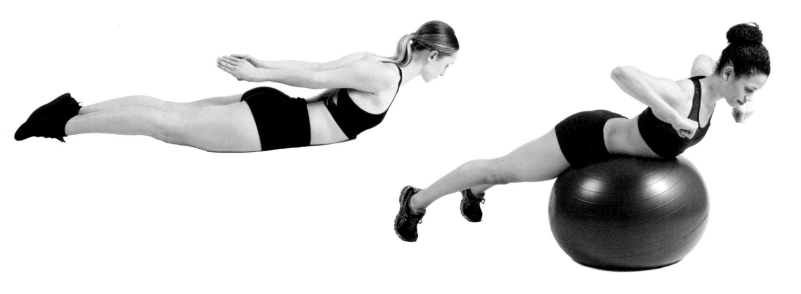

FACT FILE

TARGETS
• Whole body

EQUIPMENT
• Dumbbells
• Foam roller
• Kettlebells
• Swiss ball

BENEFITS
• Strengthens
  whole body

5 MOUNTAIN CLIMBER

pages 126–127
• Perform for 30–60 seconds

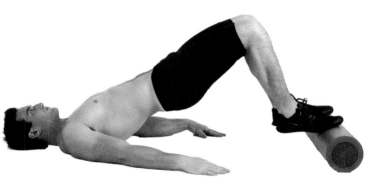

6 HAMSTRINGS PULL-IN

pages 296–297
• Perform 15 repetitions

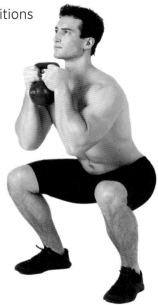

7 SIDE LUNGE AND PRESS

pages 202–203
• Perform 15
repetitions per side

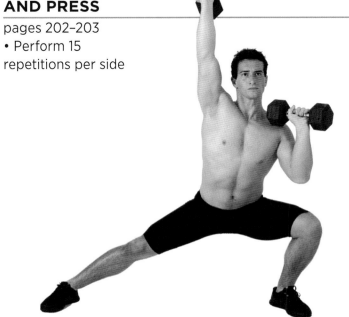

8 GOBLET SQUAT

pages 206–207
• Perform 8–10 repetitions

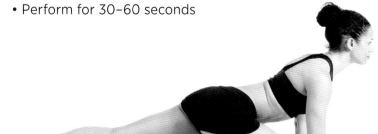

Tennis Routine

Precision, athleticism, and power are important drivers in producing a good tennis player. Strengthen your muscles and your match-playing with this specially tailored routine.

1 SWISS BALL PRONE ROW WITH EXTERNAL ROTATION

pages 228–229
• Perform 15 repetitions

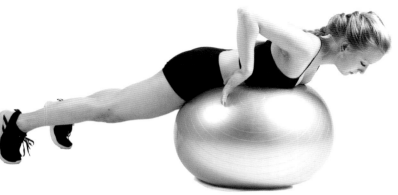

2 SWISS BALL W

pages 246–247
• Perform 12–15 repetitions

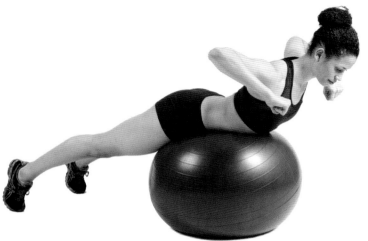

3 SWISS BALL CIRCLES

pages 268–269
• Perform 8–10 repetitions per direction

4 SHOULDER FLEXING

pages 154–155
• Perform 25 repetitions

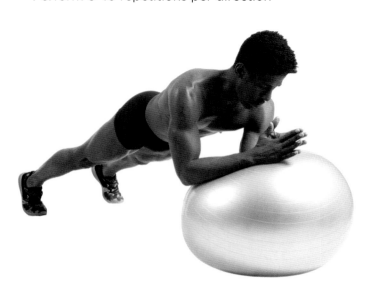

TARGETS
• Whole body

EQUIPMENT
• Dumbbells
• Kettlebells for modification
• Resistance band
• Swiss ball

BENEFITS
• Strengthens whole body

5 RESISTANCE BAND OVERHEAD PRESS

pages 238–239
• Perform 15 repetitions

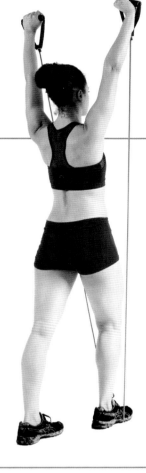

6 SKATER'S LUNGE

pages 104–105
• Perform for 45–60 seconds

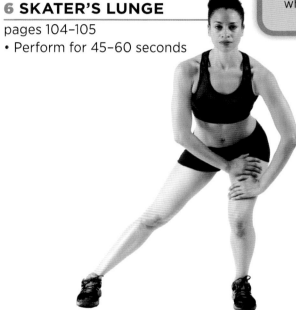

7 PLANK

pages 114–115
• Hold for 60 seconds

8 SIDE PLANK

pages 120–121
• Hold for 30–60 seconds per side

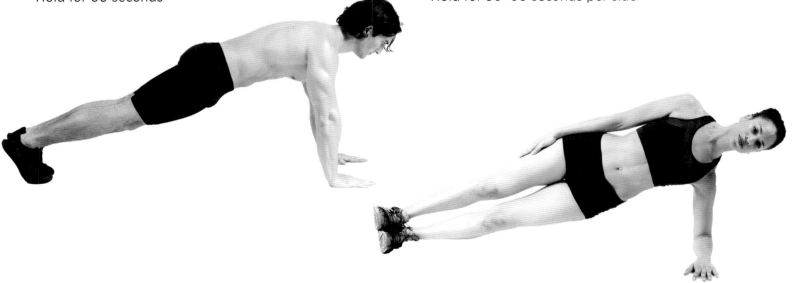

Artillery Routine

The army's artillery units provide firepower, and that's what this all-around routine will do for your muscles. You should feel energized and fit after these exercises.

1 ALTERNATING KETTLEBELL PRESS

pages 166–167
• Perform 8–10 repetitions per arm

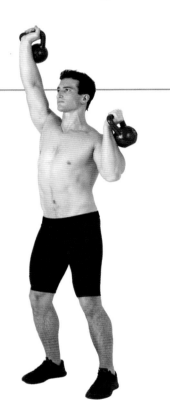

2 BOTTOM-UP KETTLEBELL CLEAN

pages 168–169
• Perform 8–10 repetitions per arm

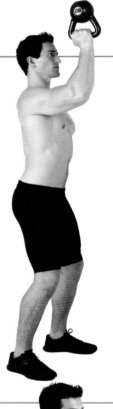

3 ALTERNATING RENEGADE ROW

pages 190–191
• Perform 8–10 repetitions per arm

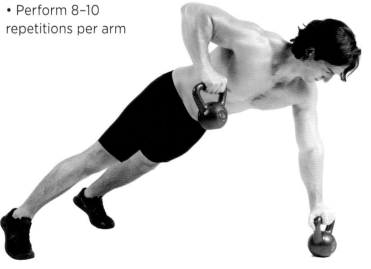

4 ALTERNATING KETTLEBELL ROW

pages 146–147
• Perform 8–10 repetitions per arm

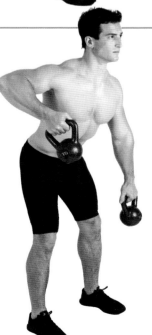

FACT FILE

TARGETS
• Whole body

EQUIPMENT
• Kettlebells

BENEFITS
• Strengthens and energizes whole body

5 GOBLET SQUAT

pages 206–207
• Perform 8–10 repetitions

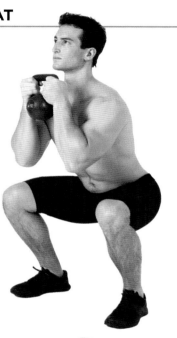

6 BEAR CRAWL

pages 60–61
• Perform for 60 seconds

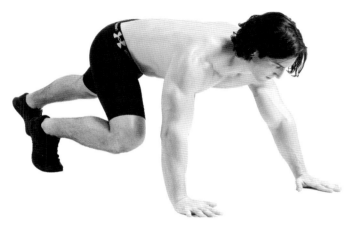

7 POWER PUNCH

page 64
• Perform 10 repetitions per side

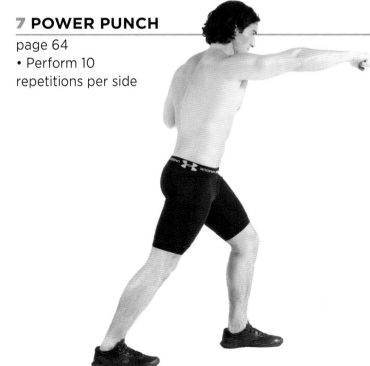

8 UPPERCUT

page 65
• Perform for 30 seconds per side

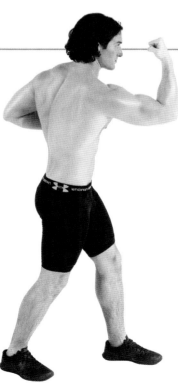

Balance Routine

This all-encompassing balance workout will promote functional strength and improved balance in your body as a whole. Good balance is an essential part of being able to move well.

1 ARM-REACH PLANK
pages 118–119
• Perform for 30–60 seconds per arm

2 BURPEE
pages 130–131
• Perform for up to 60 seconds

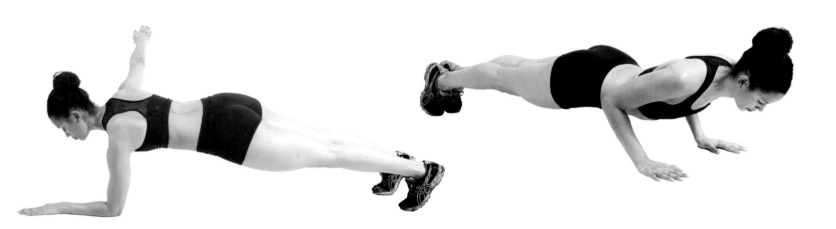

3 SWISS BALL CIRCLES
pages 268–269
• Perform 8–10 repetitions per direction

4 SWISS BALL ROLLOUT
pages 272–273
• Perform 15 repetitions

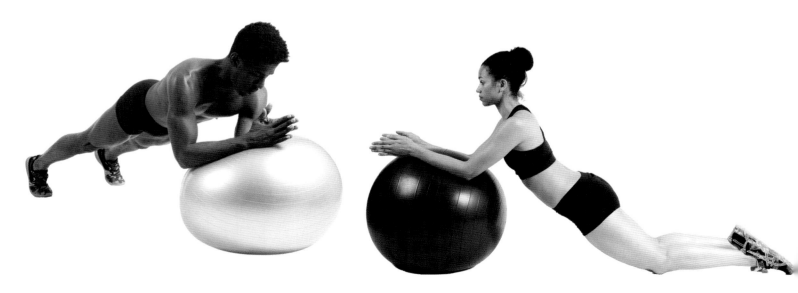

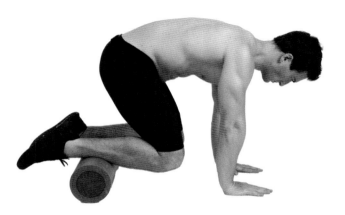
5 BALANCE PUSH-UP

pages 274–275
• Perform 10 repetitions

6 QUADRUPED KNEE PULL-IN

pages 284–285
• Perform 15 repetitions

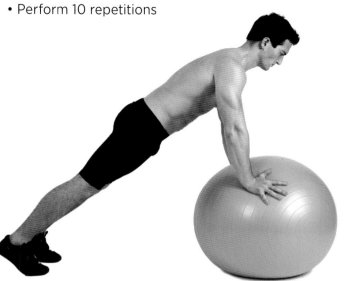

7 C-CURVE ARM CROSS

pages 186–187
• Perform 10 sets of 10 arm-crosses

8 SWISS BALL BACK EXTENSION

pages 230–231
• Perform 12–15 repetitions

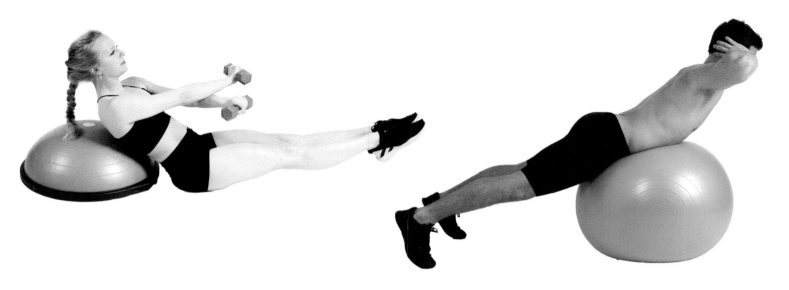

Foam Roller Routine

This full-body workout will develop general functionality, mobility, and performance. The harder Diagonal Crunch version included here is a challenging addition, so just omit it if it's too tough!

1 FOAM ROLLER PUSH-UP

pages 306–307
• Perform 15 repetitions

2 FOAM ROLLER ABDOMINAL ROLLBACK

pages 280–281
• Perform 12–15 repetitions

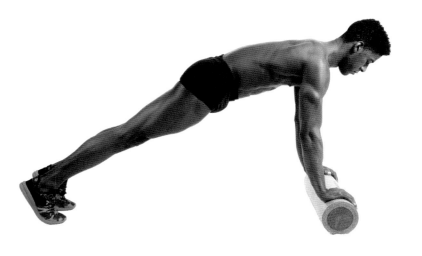

3 FOAM ROLLER TRICEPS DIP

pages 248–249
• Perform 15 repetitions

4 FOAM ROLLER TRICEPS ROLLOUT

pages 278–279
• Perform 15 repetitions

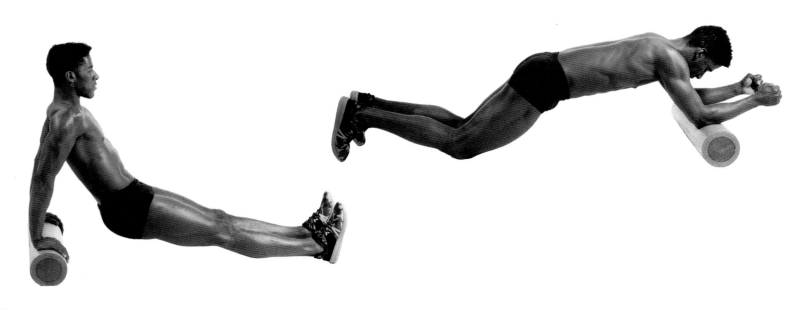

FACT FILE

TARGETS
• Whole body

EQUIPMENT
• Foam roller

BENEFITS
• Strengthens whole body

5 FOAM ROLLER DIAGONAL CRUNCH

pages 282–283
• Perform 12–15 repetitions per side

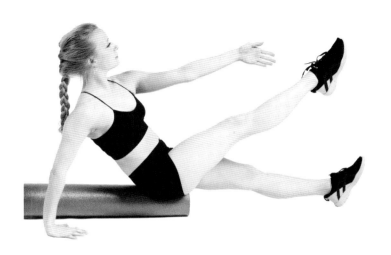

6 FOAM ROLLER DIAGONAL CRUNCH/HARDER MODIFICATION

pages 282–283
• Perform 8–10 repetitions per side

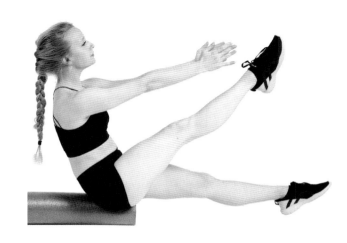

7 QUADRUPED KNEE PULL-IN

pages 284–285
• Perform 15 repetitions

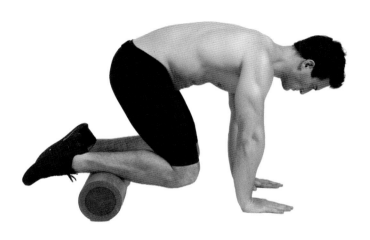

8 HAMSTRINGS PULL-IN

pages 296–297
• Perform 15 repetitions

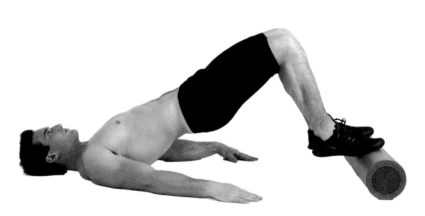

Hero Routine

This "hero" routine will make you a hero in your own life by building general improvements in stamina, strength, and performance. In turn this should boost your general sense of well-being.

1 SWIMMER

pages 52–53
• Perform 6–8 repetitions per side

2 SWISS BALL PRONE ROW WITH EXTERNAL ROTATION

pages 228–229
• Perform 15 repetitions

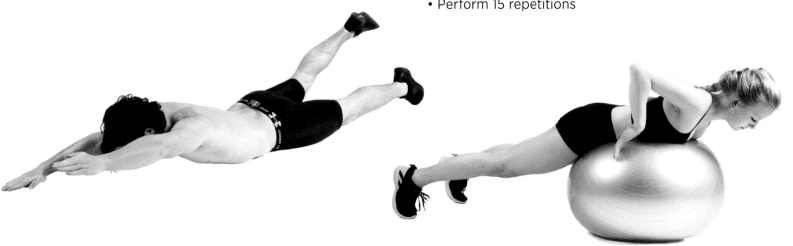

4 BALANCE BALL CRUNCH

pages 262–263
• Perform 25 repetitions

3 CABLE DECLINE FLY

pages 252–253
• Perform 12–15 repetitions

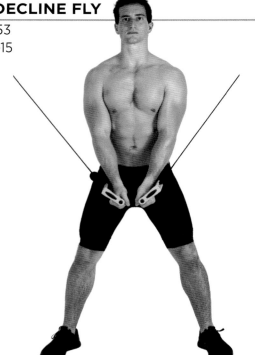

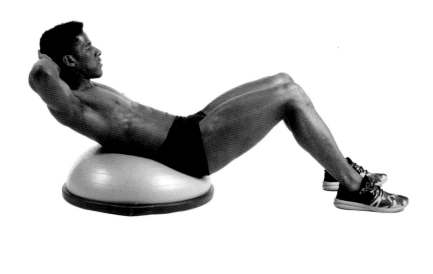

FACT FILE

TARGETS
• Whole body

EQUIPMENT
• Cable machine
• Half-dome balance ball
• Small inflatable ball for modification
• Swiss ball

BENEFITS
• Strengthens whole body

5 FOREARM PLANK

pages 112–113
• Perform for 30 seconds to 2 minutes

6 DIAGONAL REACH

pages 74–75
• Perform 12 repetitions per side

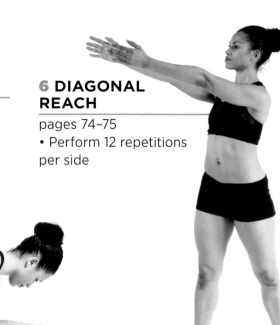

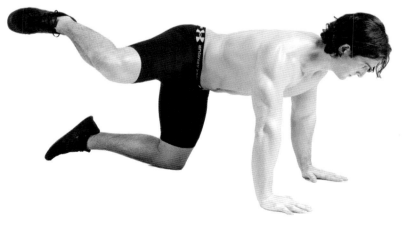

7 FIRE HYDRANT IN-OUT

pages 94–95
• Perform 15 repetitions per side

8 BRIDGE

pages 96–97
• Perform 15 repetitions

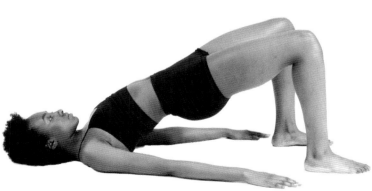

Military Routine Private

Another full-body routine, this routine is at a beginner level but is reasonably taxing. A good challenge for all of the complex musculature of your body!

1 CRAB CRAWL

pages 62–63
• Perform for 60 seconds

2 SWISS BALL CROSSOVER

pages 220–221
• Perform 20 repetitions per side

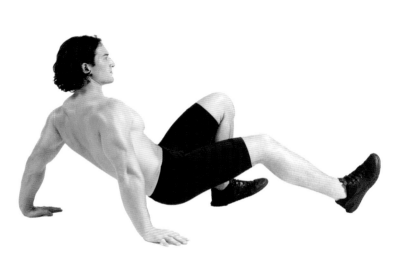

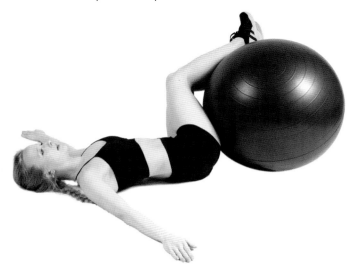

3 LUNGE

pages 100–101
• Perform 15 repetitions per leg

4 SQUAT

pages 106–107
• Perform 15 repetitions

FACT FILE

TARGETS
- Whole body

EQUIPMENT
- Barbell
- Dumbbells for modification
- Swiss ball

BENEFITS
- Strengthens whole body

5 BARBELL POWER CLEAN AND JERK

pages 216–217
- Perform 6–8 repetitions

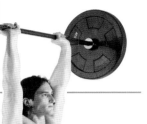

6 SWISS BALL BRIDGE

pages 292–293
- Perform 10 repetitions

7 SWISS BALL LATERAL ROLL

pages 310–311
- Perform 10 repetitions per side

8 EXTENSION HEEL BEATS

pages 98–99
- Perform 5 sets of 10-count repetitions

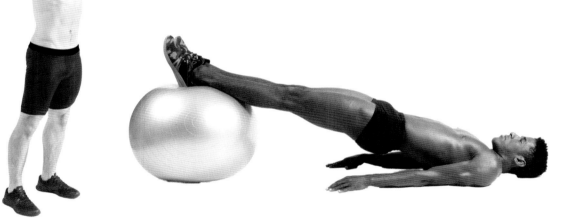

Military Routine Sergeant

The ability required for this routine is midlevel but it is a taxing workout. However, it offers a comprehensive strengthening mini-program for the whole body.

1 WIDE PUSH-UP

pages 70–71
• Perform 10–12 repetitions

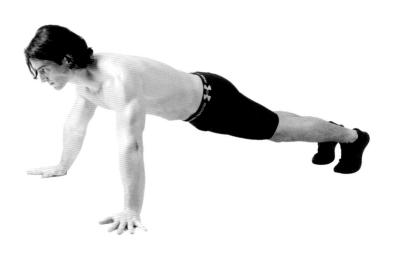

2 BUTT KICK

pages 110–111
• Perform for
30–60 seconds

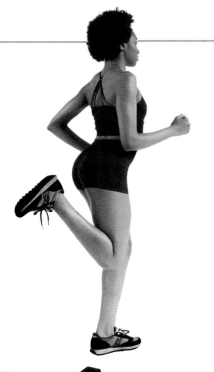

3 LATERAL-EXTENSION REVERSE LUNGE

pages 102–103
• Perform 10
repetitions per side

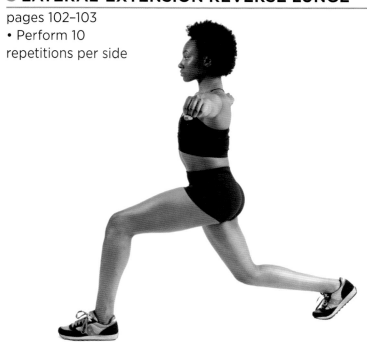

4 SIDE LUNGE AND PRESS

pages 202–203
• Perform 15
repetitions per side

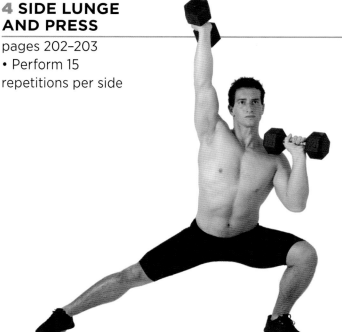

FACT FILE

TARGETS
• Whole body

EQUIPMENT
• Dumbbells
• Foam roller
• Pull-up bar
• Step/bench/
  platform

BENEFITS
• Strengthens
  whole body

5 NEUTRAL-GRIP PULL-UP

pages 222–223
• Perform 10 repetitions

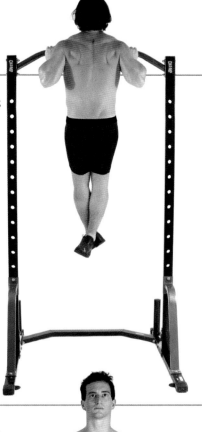

6 FOAM ROLLER TRICEPS DIP

pages 248–249
• Perform 15 repetitions

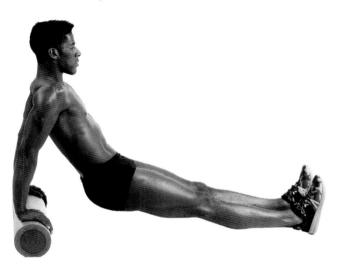

7 STEP-UP

pages 302–303
• Perform 15 repetitions
per side

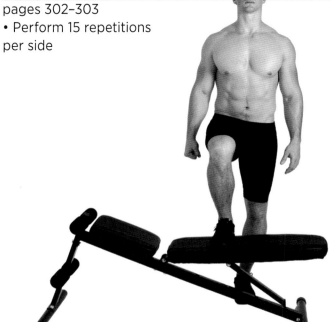

8 HAMSTRINGS PULL-IN

pages 296–297
• Perform 15 repetitions

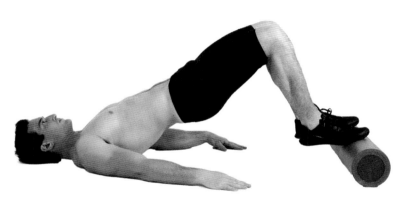

Military Routine General

Moving up a notch from the Sergeant routine, this is another taxing routine but this time at an advanced level. Again it improves strength and functionality in the whole body.

1 ALLIGATOR CRAWL
pages 58–59
• Perform for 60 seconds

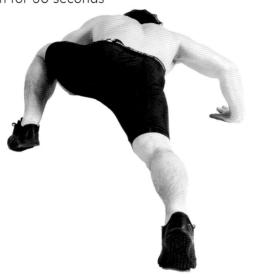

2 SKATER'S LUNGE
pages 104–105
• Perform for 45–60 seconds

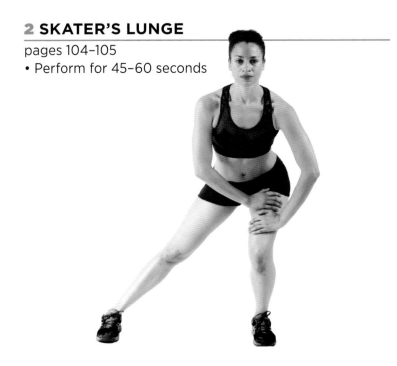

3 BURPEE
pages 130–131
• Perform for up to 60 seconds

4 MOUNTAIN CLIMBER
pages 126–127
• Perform for 30–60 seconds

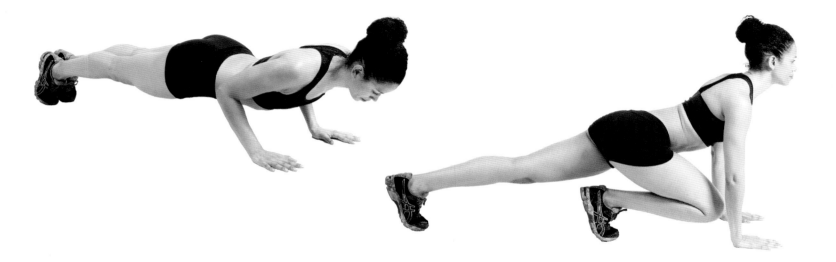

FACT FILE

TARGETS
• Whole body

EQUIPMENT
• Dumbbells
• Kettlebells for modification
• 2 plyo boxes/ similar
• Pull-up bar
• Swiss ball

BENEFITS
• Strengthens whole body

5 WIDE-GRIP PULL-UP

pages 224–225
• Perform 20 repetitions

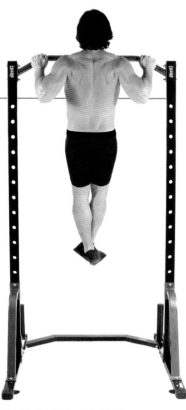
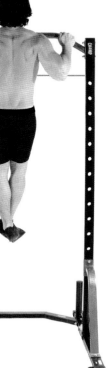

6 ALTERNATING FLOOR ROW

pages 142–143
• Perform 15 repetitions per arm

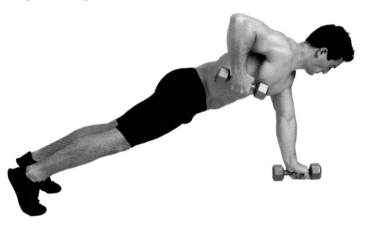

7 SWISS BALL ATOMIC PUSH-UP

pages 270–271
• Perform 12–15 repetitions

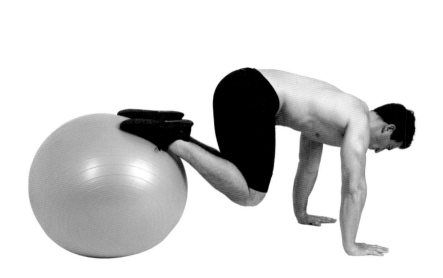

8 BOX JUMPS

pages 298–299
• Perform 15 repetitions

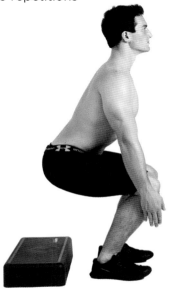

Postural Routine

Posture is such an issue for so many people, producing all kinds of problems. This workout will enhance your posture and general physical alignment.

1 SWISS BALL W

pages 246–247
• Perform 12–15 repetition

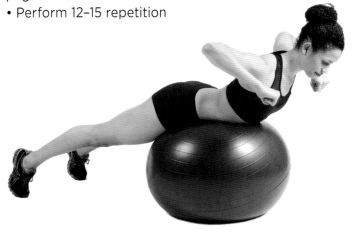

2 T-STABILIZATION

pages 124–125
• Hold for 30–60 seconds per side

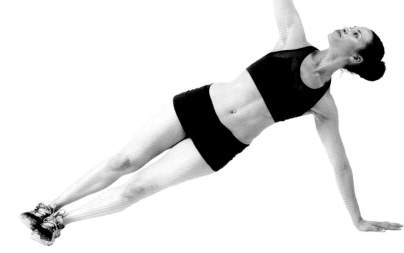

3 ZIPPER

pages 174–175
• Perform 10–20 repetitions

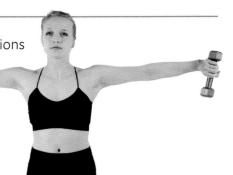

4 C-CURVE ARM CROSS

pages 186–187
• Perform 10 sets of 10 arm-crosses

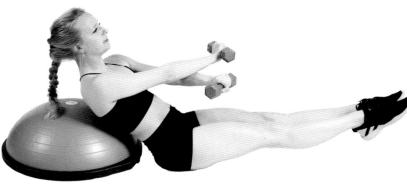

FACT FILE

TARGETS
• Posture

EQUIPMENT
• Dumbbells
• Half-dome
  balance ball
• Pull-up bar
• Swiss ball

BENEFITS
• Improves
  posture

5 SWISS BALL CROSSOVER

pages 220–221
• Perform 20 repetitions per side

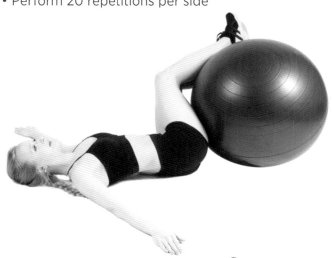

6 SWISS BALL PRONE ROW WITH EXTERNAL ROTATION

pages 228–229
• Perform 15 repetitions

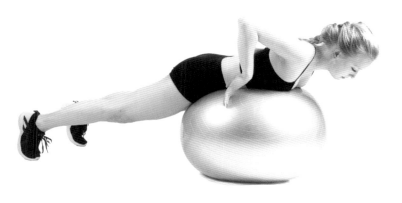

7 REVERSE-GRIP PULL-UP

pages 226–227
• Perform 10
repetitions

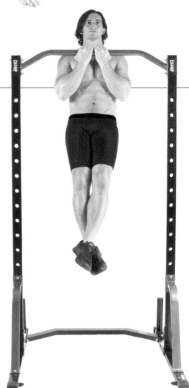

8 SWISS BALL BACK EXTENSION

pages 230–231
• Perform 12–15 repetitions

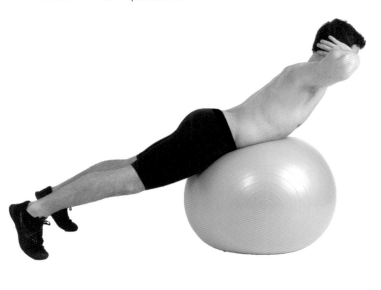

Resistance Routine

Understanding the value of resistance to strength training is an important first principle. This routine will show you how to bring cohesion and quality to your movement.

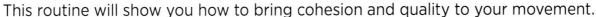

1 RESISTANCE BAND STANDING FLY

pages 258–259
• Perform 15 repetitions

2 RESISTANCE BAND OVERHEAD PRESS

pages 238–239
• Perform 15 repetitions

3 SINGLE-ARM BAND PULL

pages 232–233
• Perform 15 repetitions per arm

4 RESISTANCE BAND SINGLE-ARM ROW

pages 244–245
• Perform 20 repetitions per side

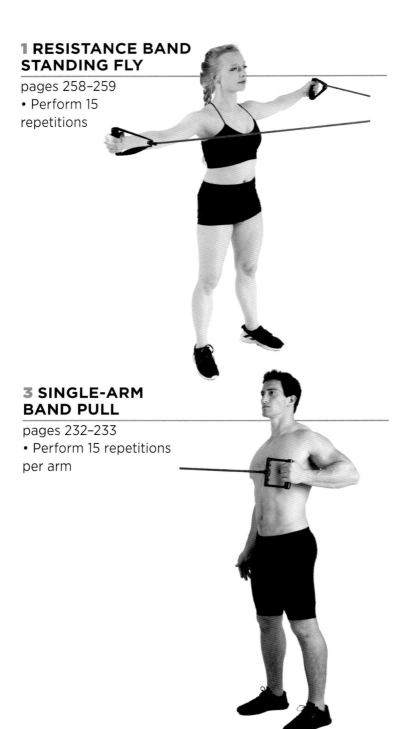
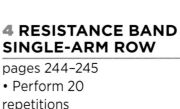

FACT FILE

TARGETS
• Whole body

EQUIPMENT
• Resistance band

BENEFITS
• Strengthens whole body

5 RESISTANCE BAND LATERAL RAISE

pages 240–241
• Perform 8–10 repetitions

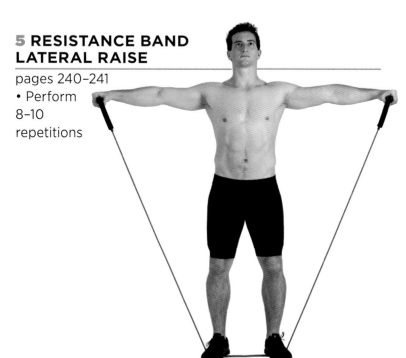

6 RESISTANCE BAND BICEPS CURL

pages 242–243
• Perform 15 repetitions

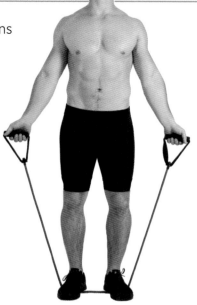

7 RESISTANCE BAND SQUAT

pages 286–287
• Perform 15 repetitions

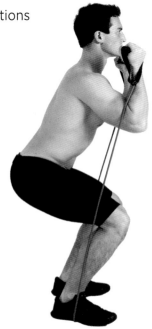

8 RESISTANCE BAND LUNGE

pages 288–289
• Perform 15 repetitions per leg

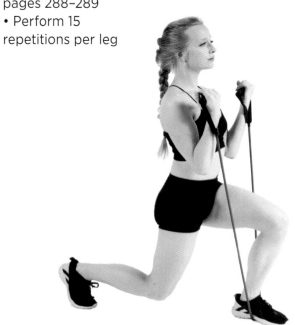

Stretch Routine

Stretching is vital in any fitness regimen. This routine uses your own body weight only—to develop flexibility, posture, and improved mobility in a range of muscles.

1 COBRA STRETCH

pages 36–37
• Hold for 15–30 seconds

2 CAT-TO-COW STRETCH

pages 34–35
• Hold for 30 seconds; perform 3 repetitions

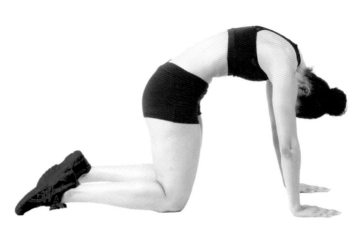

3 BIRDDOG

pages 38–39
• Hold for 15 seconds; perform 5 repetitions per side

4 LATERAL LUNGE STRETCH

pages 28–29
• Perform 3 x 30-second holds per leg

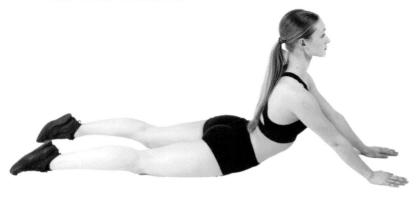

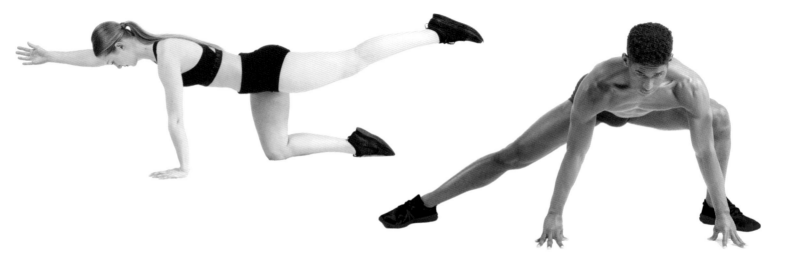

FACT FILE

TARGETS
• Whole body

EQUIPMENT
• Swiss ball for
a modification

BENEFITS
• Stretches
whole body

5 BICEPS-PECS STRETCH

page 27
• Hold for 30 seconds

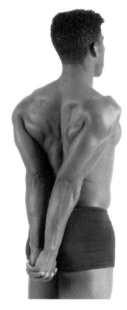

6 TRICEPS STRETCH

page 26
• Perform 3 x
30-second
holds per side

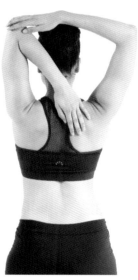

7 HALF-KNEELING ROTATION

pages 40–41
• Perform 10
repetitions per side

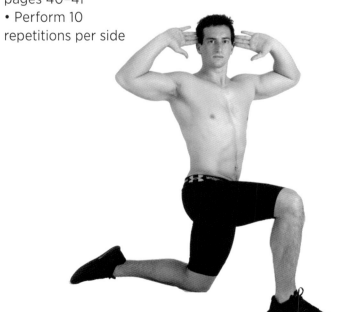

8 SIDE BENDING

pages 42–43
• Perform 5
repetitions per side

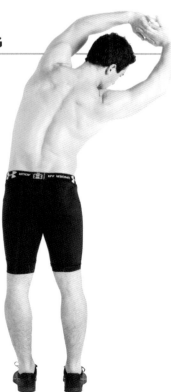

Swiss Ball Routine

A Swiss ball adds a new dimension to many different kinds of exercise. This added extra really helps with flexibility and balance, plus it offers a resistance to work against.

1 SWISS BALL BRIDGE
pages 292–293
• Perform 10 repetitions

2 SWISS BALL LATERAL ROLL
pages 310–311
• Perform 10 repetitions per side

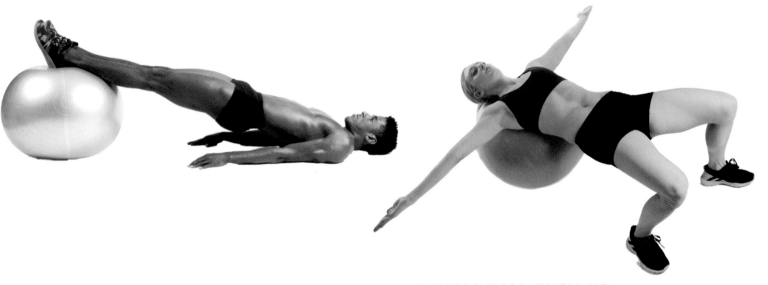

3 SWISS BALL PLANK WITH LEG LIFT
pages 308–309
• Hold for 10–60 seconds per leg

4 SWISS BALL PUSH-UP
pages 260–261
• Perform 10 repetitions

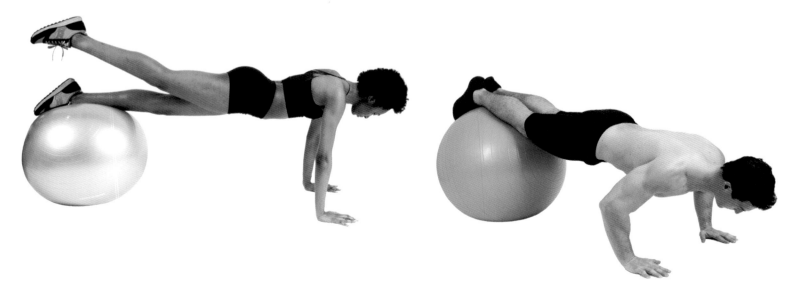

FACT FILE

TARGETS
• Whole body

EQUIPMENT
• Resistance band
• Swiss ball

BENEFITS
• Strengthens whole body

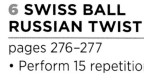

5 SWISS BALL ROLLOUT

pages 272–273
• Perform 15 repetition

6 SWISS BALL RUSSIAN TWIST

pages 276–277
• Perform 15 repetitions per side

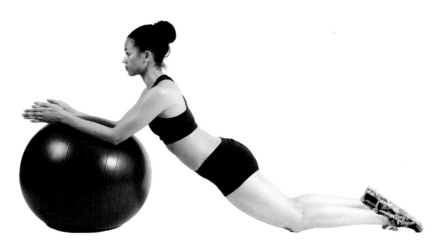

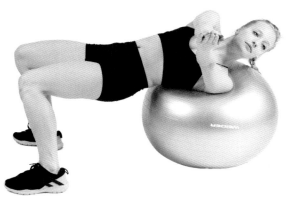

7 SWISS BALL LOOP EXTENSION

pages 290–291
• Perform 10 repetitions per leg

8 SWISS BALL SPLIT SQUAT

pages 294–295
• Perform 15 repetitions per leg

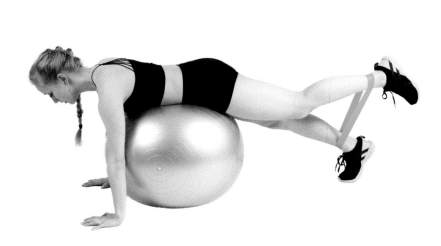

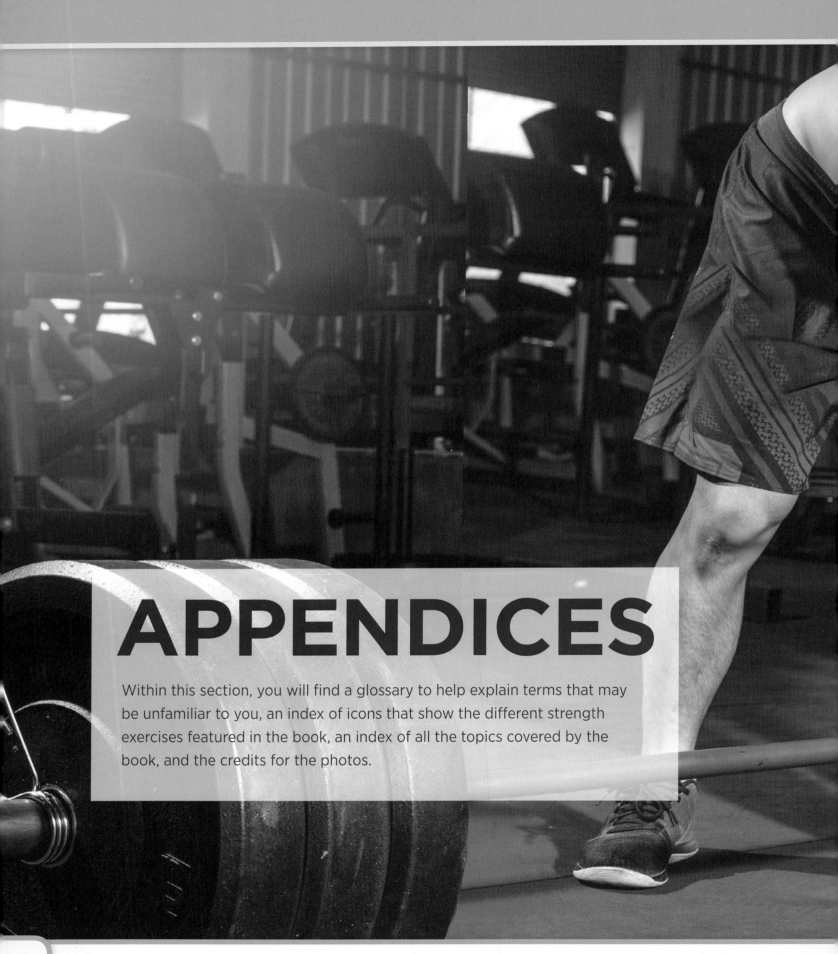

APPENDICES

Within this section, you will find a glossary to help explain terms that may be unfamiliar to you, an index of icons that show the different strength exercises featured in the book, an index of all the topics covered by the book, and the credits for the photos.

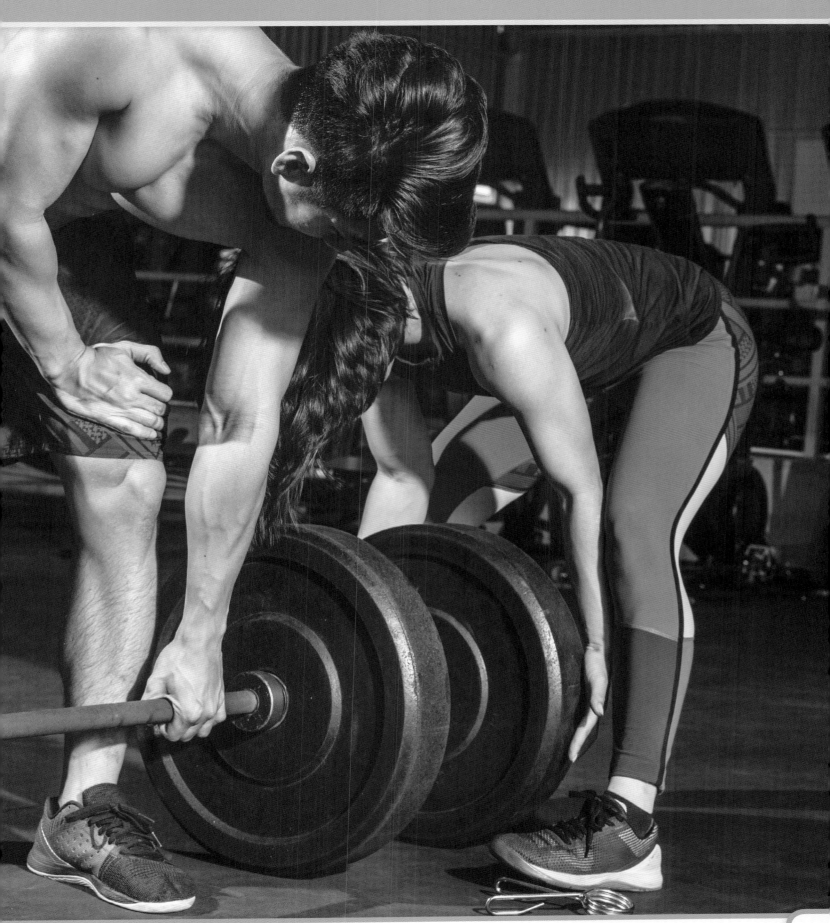

Glossary

GENERAL TERMS

This includes terms used in the book plus others that you may encounter elsewhere.

abduction: Movement away from the body.

adduction: Movement toward the body.

aerobic exercise: An exercise form in which your body uses oxygen for energy.

anaerobic exercise: An exercise form in which your muscles break down glucose (sugar) to use as energy.

anterior: Located in the front.

barbell: A long metal bar to which discs of varying weights are attached at each end.

battle rope: A rope of varying length and width that is anchored to a wall or other secure object and used for strength, agility, and endurance training.

cardiovascular exercise: Any exercise that increases the heart rate, making oxygen and nutrient-rich blood available to working muscles. The term "cardio" is often used to mean aerobic exercise.

clean: Lifting a weight from the floor to a higher "racked" position, typically held close to the body.

clean and jerk: A clean lift followed by powerfully moving the weight overhead in one smooth and powerful motion.

compound exercise: A move that incorporates multiple muscle groups, such as a lunge, deadlift, or squat. Also refers to two moves strung together, such as a power clean and press.

cooldown: An exercise performed at the end of the workout session that works to cool and relax the body.

core: Refers to the deep muscle layers that lie close to the spine and provide structural support for the entire body. The core muscles are divided into two groups: the major and the minor. The major muscles reside on the trunk and include the belly area and the middle and lower back. This area encompasses the pelvic floor muscles (levator ani, pubococcygeus, iliococcygeus, puborectalis, and coccygeus), the abdominals (rectus abdominis, transversus abdominis, obliquus externus, and obliquus internus), the spinal extensors (multifidus spinae, erector spinae, splenius, longissimus thoracis, and semispinalis), and the diaphragm. The minor core muscles include the latissimus dorsi, gluteus maximus, and trapezius. Minor core muscles assist the major muscles when the body engages in activities or movements that require added stability.

core stabilizer: An exercise that calls for resisting motion at the lumbar spine through activation of the abdominal muscles and deep stabilizers; improves core strength and endurance.

core strengthener: An exercise that allows for motion in the lumbar spine, while working the abdominal muscles and deep stabilizers; improves core strength.

crunch: A common abdominal exercise that calls for curling the shoulders toward the pelvis while lying supine with hands at your head and knees bent.

curl: An exercise movement, usually targeting the biceps brachii, that calls for a weight to be moved through an arc, in a "curling" motion.

deadlift: An exercise movement that calls for lifting a weight, such as a dumbbell, off the floor from a stabilized bent-over position.

dumbbell: A basic piece of equipment that consists of a short bar on which plates are secured. A person can use a dumbbell in one or both hands during an exercise. Most gyms offer dumbbells with the weight plates welded on and poundage indicated on the plates, but many intended for home use come with removable plates that allow you to adjust the weight. Especially at the lighter end of the weight scale, there are many dumbbells for gym and home use that have simple all-in-one forms that include weighted ends.

extension: The act of straightening.

extensor muscle: A muscle serving to extend a body part away from the body.

flexed foot: A foot that is at a 90-degree angle to the leg, as opposed to being pointed.

flexion: The bending of a joint.

flexor muscle: A muscle that decreases the angle between two bones, as when bending the arm at the elbow or raising the thigh toward the stomach.

fly: An exercise movement in which the hand and arm move through an arc while the elbow is kept at a constant angle. It works the muscles of the upper body.

foam roller: A tube that comes in a variety of sizes, materials, and densities that can be used for stretching, strengthening, and balance training.

front rack position: A barbell hold in which the bar rests on your clavicles and flexed shoulders.

functional exercise: A group of exercises that help you move in everyday life, often mimicking everyday movements, such as a squat or deadlift.

hammer-grip: Holding something as you would a hammer's handle.

hamstrings: The three muscles of the posterior thigh (the semitendinosus, semimembranosus, and biceps femoris) that work to flex the knee and extend the hip.

head of a muscle: Where a muscle originates. Some muscles have more than one head, such as the biceps, which has two.

hyperextension: An exercise that works the lower back as well as the mid and upper back, specifically the erector spinae, which usually involves raising the torso and/or lower body from the floor while keeping the pelvis firmly anchored.

iliotibial band (ITB): A thick band of fibrous tissue that runs down the outside of the leg, beginning at the hip and extending to the outer side of the tibia just below the knee joint. The band functions in concert with several of the thigh muscles to provide stability to the outside of the knee joint.

internal rotation: The act of moving a body part toward the center of the body.

interval: A period of activity or a period of rest.

isolation exercise: A movement that focuses on just one muscle or muscle group.

kettlebell: A bell-shaped weight of varying poundage used to build strength and endurance, improve cardiovascular health, and increase grip strength.

lateral: Located on, or extending toward, the outside, or the side.

lunge: A group of lower-body exercises in which one leg is positioned forward with knee bent and foot flat on the ground while the other leg is positioned behind.

medial: Located on, or extending toward, the middle.

neutral: Describes the position of the legs, pelvis, hips, or other part of the body that is neither arched nor curved forward.

neutral position: A position in which the natural curve of the spine is maintained, typically adopted when lying on one's back with one or both feet on the floor.

plate: A cast-iron weight placed on a dumbbell. The weight of plates generally starts at 10 pounds and ranges upward to 50 pounds and higher.

plyometrics: Explosive exercises that increase power, such as jumps.

posterior: Located behind.

posterior chain: The glutes, hamstrings, and back.

press: An exercise movement that calls for moving a weight or other resistance away from the body.

push-up: A basic exercise that involves raising and lowering the body using the arms.

quadriceps: A large muscle group (full name: quadriceps femoris) that includes the four prevailing muscles on the front of the thigh: the rectus femoris, vastus intermedius, vastus lateralis, and vastus medialis. It is the great extensor muscle of the knee, forming a large fleshy mass that covers the front and sides of the femur muscle.

range of motion: The distance and direction a joint can move between the flexed and the extended positions.

repetition/"rep": The number of times you repeat a movement or exercise.

resistance: How much weight your muscles are working against to complete a movement, whether your own body weight or added weight, such as dumbbells.

rotator muscle: One of a group of muscles that assist the rotation of a joint, such as the hip or the shoulder.

row: An exercise movement that imitates the movement of rowing a boat. It primarily targets the upper back.

scapula: The protrusion of bone on the mid to upper back, also known as the shoulder blade.

set: Refers to how many times you repeat a given number of repetitions of an exercise.

snatch: A total-body move that brings a weight, such as a kettlebell, from floor to overhead.

split squat: An assisted one-legged squat in which the nonlifting leg is rested on the floor a few steps behind the lifting leg, as if it were a static lunge.

squat: An exercise movement that calls for moving the hips back and bending the knees and hips to lower the torso, and any accompanying weight, and then returning to the upright position. A squat primarily targets the muscles of the thighs, hips, buttocks, and hamstrings.

Swiss ball: A flexible, inflatable PVC ball measuring approximately 12 to 30 inches in circumference that is used for weight training, physical therapy, balance training, and many other exercise regimens. It is also called a "balance ball," "fitness ball," "stability ball," "exercise ball," "gym ball," "physioball," "body ball," "therapy ball," and many other names.

ventral aspect: The front of the body.

warm-up: Any form of light exercise of short duration that prepares the body for more intense exercises.

weight: Refers to the plates or weight stacks, or the actual poundage listed on the bar or dumbbell.

work/rest ratio: The comparison between how much time is spent working and the amount spent resting.

LATIN TERMS

The following glossary explains the Latin scientific terminology used to describe the muscles of the human body. Certain words are derived from Greek, which is indicated in each instance.

CHEST

coracobrachialis: Greek *korakoeidés*, "ravenlike," and *brachium*, "arm"

pectoralis (major and minor): *pectus*, "breast"

ABDOMEN

obliquus (externus and internus): *obliquus*, "slanting"

rectus abdominis: *rego*, "straight, upright," and *abdomen*, "belly"

serratus anterior: *serra*, "saw," and *ante*, "before"

transversus abdominis: *transversus*, "moving across," and *abdomen*, "belly"

NECK

scalenus: Greek *skalénós*, "unequal"

semispinalis: *semi*, "half," and *spinae*, "spine"

splenius: Greek *spléníon*, "plaster, patch"

sternocleidomastoideus: Greek *stérnon*, "chest," Greek *kleís*, "key," and Greek *mastoeidés*, "breastlike"

BACK

erector spinae: *erectus*, "straight," and *spina*, "thorn"

latissimus dorsi: *latus*, "wide," and *dorsum*, "back"

multifidus spinae: *multifid*, "to cut into divisions," and *spinae*, "spine"

quadratus lumborum: *quadratus*, "square, rectangular," and *lumbus*, "loin"

rhomboideus: Greek *rhembesthai*, "to spin"

trapezius: Greek *trapezion*, "small table"

SHOULDERS

deltoideus (anterior, medialis, and posterior): Greek *deltoeidés*, "delta-shaped"

infraspinatus: *infra*, "under," and *spina*, "thorn"

levator scapulae: *levare*, "to raise," and *scapulae*, "shoulder [blades]"

subscapularis: *sub*, "below," and *scapulae*, "shoulder [blades]"

supraspinatus: *supra*, "above," and *spina*, "thorn"

teres (major and minor): *teres*, "rounded"

UPPER ARM

biceps brachii: *biceps*, "two-headed," and *brachium*, "arm"

brachialis: *brachium*, "arm"

triceps brachii: *triceps*, "three-headed," and *brachium*, "arm"

LOWER ARM

anconeus: Greek *anconad*, "elbow"

brachioradialis: *brachium*, "arm," and *radius*, "spoke"

extensor carpi radialis: *extendere*, "to extend," Greek *karpós*, "wrist," and *radius*, "spoke"

extensor digitorum: *extendere*, "to extend," and *digitus*, "finger, toe"

flexor carpi pollicis longus: *flectere*, "to bend," Greek *karpós*, "wrist," *pollicis*, "thumb," and *longus*, "long"

flexor carpi radialis: *flectere*, "to bend," Greek *karpós*, "wrist," and *radius*, "spoke"

flexor carpi ulnaris: *flectere*, "to bend," Greek *karpós*, "wrist," and *ulnaris*, "forearm"

flexor digitorum: *flectere*, "to bend," and *digitus*, "finger, toe"

palmaris longus: *palmaris*, "palm," and *longus*, "long"

pronator teres: *pronate*, "to rotate," and *teres*, "rounded"

HIPS

gemellus (inferior and superior): *geminus*, "twin"

gluteus maximus: Greek *gloutós*, "rump," and *maximus*, "largest"

gluteus medius: Greek *gloutós*, "rump," and *medialis*, "middle"

gluteus minimus: Greek *gloutós*, "rump," and *minimus*, "smallest"

iliopsoas: *ilium*, "groin," and Greek *psoa*, "groin muscle"

obturator externus: *obturare*, "to block," and *externus*, "outward"

obturator internus: *obturare*, "to block," and *internus*, "within"

pectineus: *pectin*, "comb"

piriformis: *pirum*, "pear," and *forma*, "shape"

quadratus femoris: *quadratus*, "square, rectangular," and *femur*, "thigh"

UPPER LEG

adductor longus: *adducere*, "to contract," and *longus*, "long"

adductor magnus: *adducere*, "to contract," and *magnus*, "major"

biceps femoris: *biceps*, "two-headed," and *femur*, "thigh"

gracilis: *gracilis*, "slim, slender"

rectus femoris: *rego*, "straight, upright," and *femur*, "thigh"

sartorius: *sarcio*, "to patch" or "to repair"

semimembranosus: *semi*, "half," and *membrum*, "limb"

semitendinosus: *semi*, "half," and *tendo*, "tendon"

tensor fasciae latae: *tenere*, "to stretch," *fasciae*, "band," and *latae*, "laid down"

vastus intermedius: *vastus*, "immense, huge," and *intermedius*, "between"

vastus lateralis: *vastus*, "immense, huge," and *lateralis*, "side"

vastus medialis: *vastus*, "immense, huge," and *medialis*, "middle"

LOWER LEG

adductor digiti minimi: *adducere*, "to contract," *digitus*, "finger, toe," and *minimum*, "smallest"

adductor hallucis: *adducere*, "to contract," and *hallex*, "big toe"

extensor digitorum longus: *extendere*, "to extend," *digitus*, "finger, toe," and *longus*, "long"

extensor hallucis longus: *extendere*, "to extend," *hallex*, "big toe," and *longus*, "long"

flexor digitorum longus: *flectere*, "to bend," *digitus*, "finger, toe," and *longus*, "long"

flexor hallucis longus: *flectere*, "to bend," *hallex*, "big toe," and *longus*, "long"

gastrocnemius: Greek *gastroknémía*, "calf [of the leg]"

peroneus: *peronei*, "of the fibula"

plantaris: *planta*, "the sole"

soleus: *solea*, "sandal"

tibialis (anterior and posterior): *tibia*, "reed pipe"

Icon Index

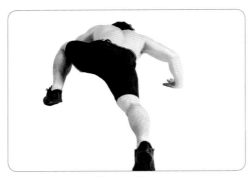

Alligator Crawl
pages 58–59

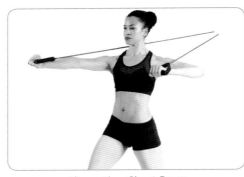

Alternating Chest Press
pages 256–257

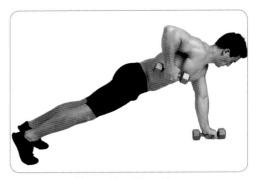

Alternating Floor Row
pages 142–143

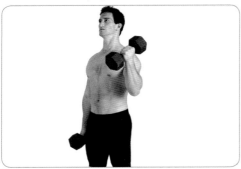

Alternating Hammer Curl
pages 160–161

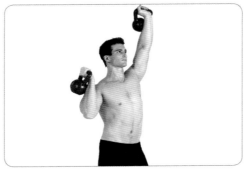

Alternating Kettlebell Press
pages 166–167

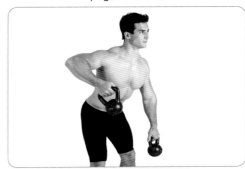

Alternating Kettlebell Row
pages 146–147

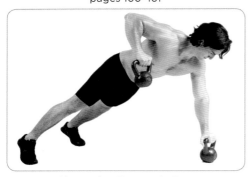

Alternating Renegade Row
pages 190–191

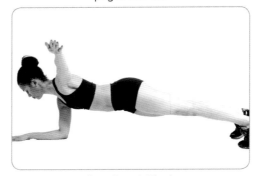

Arm-Reach Plank
pages 118–119

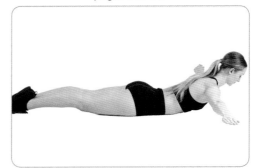

Back Burner
pages 56–57

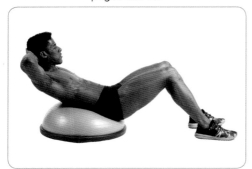

Balance Ball Crunch
262–263

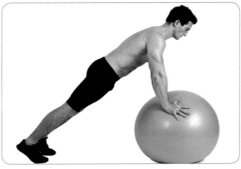

Balance Push-Up
pages 274–275

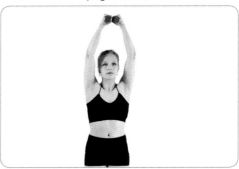

Ballet Biceps
pages 158–159

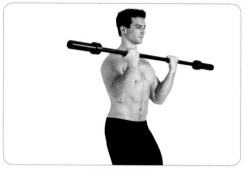

Barbell Curl
pages 172–173

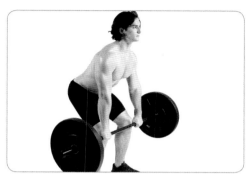

Barbell Deadlift
pages 148–149

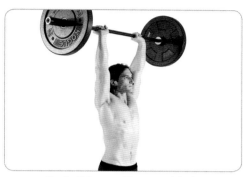

Barbell Power Clean and Jerk
pages 216–217

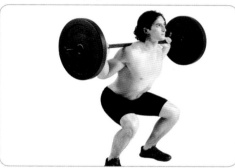

Barbell Squat
pages 208–209

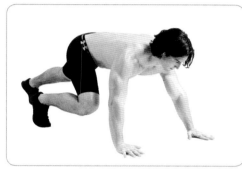

Bear Crawl
pages 60–61

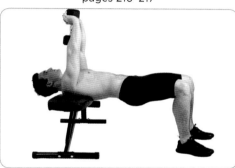

Bent-Arm Dumbbell Pullover
pages 178–179

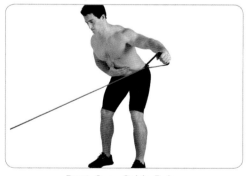

Bent-Over Cable Raise
pages 236–237

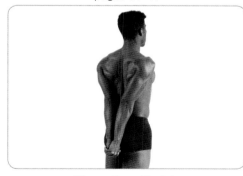

Biceps-Pecs Stretch
page 27

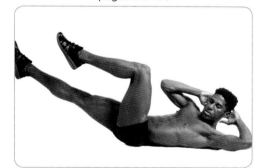

Bicycle Crunch
pages 82–83

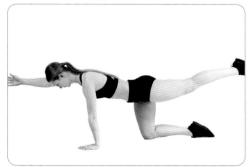

Bird Dog
pages 38–39

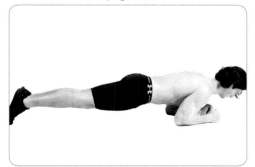

Body Saw
pages 88–89

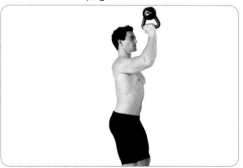

Bottom-Up Kettlebell Clean
pages 168–169

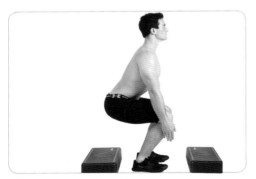

Box Jumps
pages 298–299

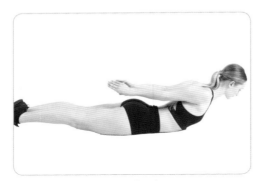

Breast Stroke
pages 54–55

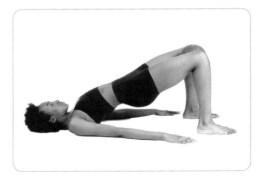

Bridge
pages 96–97

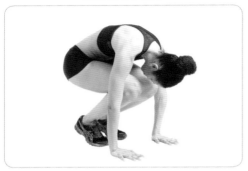

Burpee
pages 130–131

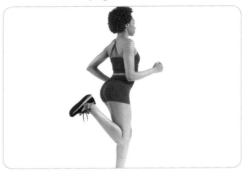

Butt Kick
pages 110–111

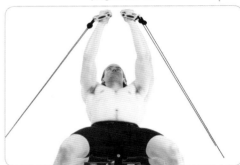

Cable Crossover Fly
pages 254–255

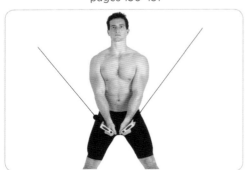

Cable Decline Fly
pages 252–253

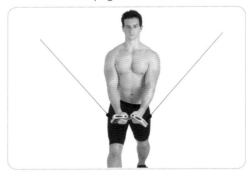

Cable Fly
pages 250–251

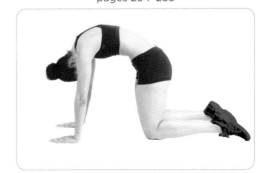

Cat-to-Cow Stretch
pages 34–35

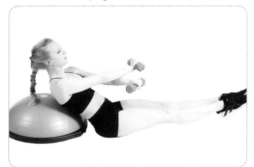

C-Curve Arm Cross
pages 186–187

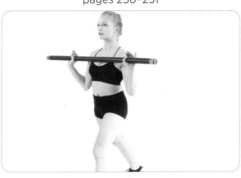

Clean-and-Press
pages 210–211

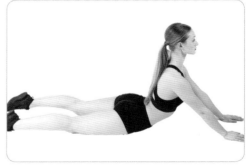

Cobra Stretch
pages 36–37

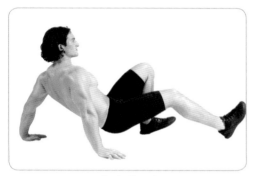

Crab Crawl
pages 62–63

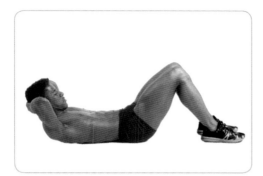

Crunch
pages 76–77

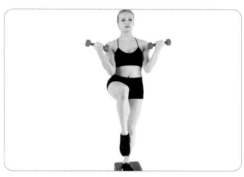

Curling Step-and-Raise
pages 212–213

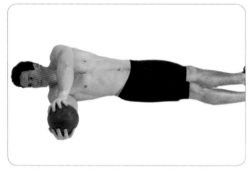

Diagonal Crunch with Medicine Ball
pages 264–265

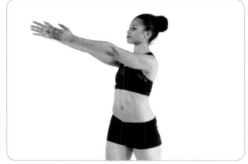

Diagonal Reach
pages 74–75

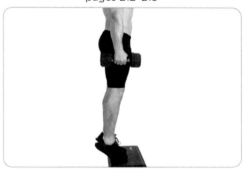

Dumbbell Calf Raise
pages 194–195

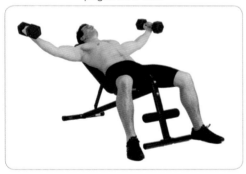

Dumbbell Fly
pages 180–181

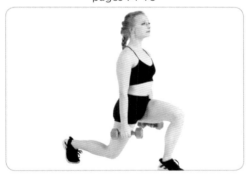

Dumbbell Lunge
pages 198–199

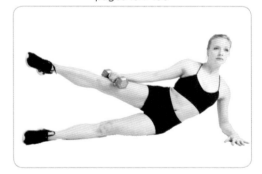

Dumbbell Lying Hip Abduction
pages 196–197

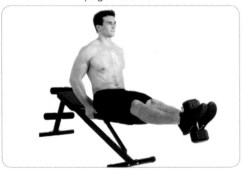

Dumbbell Shin Raise
pages 192–193

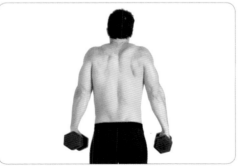

Dumbbell Shrug
pages 134–135

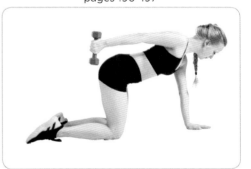

Dumbbell Triceps Kickback
pages 164–165

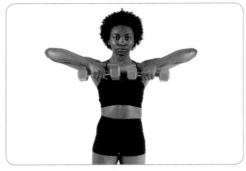

Dumbbell Upright Row
pages 138–139

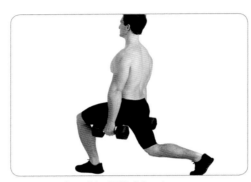

Dumbbell Walking Lunge
pages 200–201

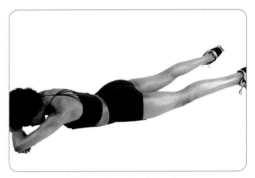

Extension Heel Beats
pages 98–99

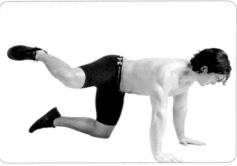

Fire Hydrant In-Out
pages 94–95

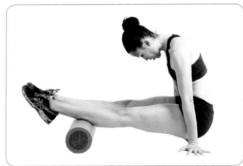

Foam Roller Abdominal Rollback
pages 280–281

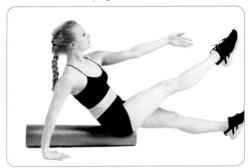

Foam Roller Diagonal Crunch
pages 282–283

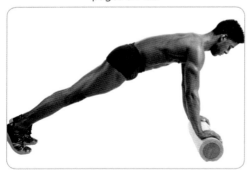

Foam Roller Push-Up
pages 306–307

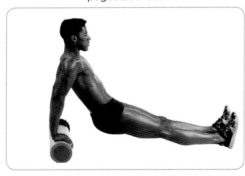

Foam Roller Triceps Dip
pages 248–249

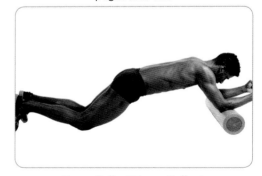

Foam Roller Triceps Rollout
pages 278–279

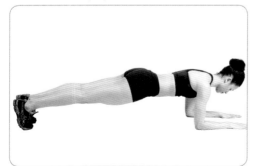

Forearm Plank
pages 112–113

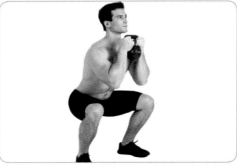

Goblet Squat
pages 206–207

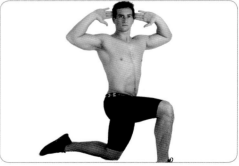

Half-Kneeling Rotation
pages 40–41

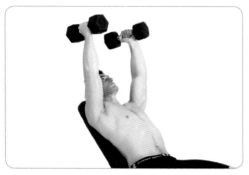

Hammer-Grip Press
pages 176–177

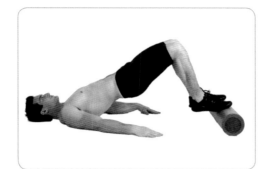

Hamstrings Pull-In
pages 296–297

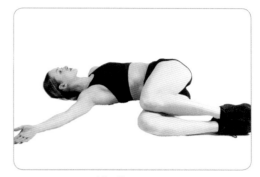

Hip Crossover
pages 50–51

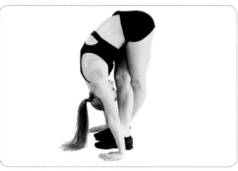

Iliotibial Band Stretch
pages 32–33

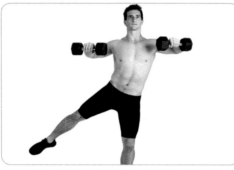

Knee Raise with Lateral Extension
pages 214–215

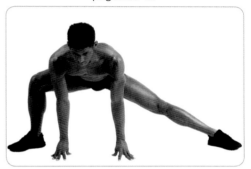

Lateral Lunge Stretch
pages 28–29

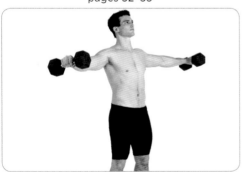

Lateral Shoulder Raise
pages 156–157

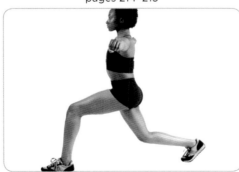

Lateral-Extension Reverse Lunge
pages 102–103

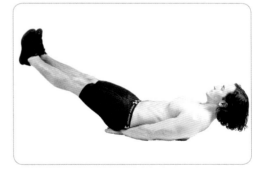

Leg Levelers
pages 86–87

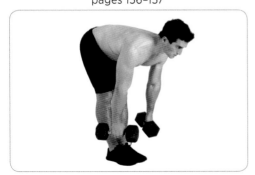

Lower-Back Extension
pages 150–151

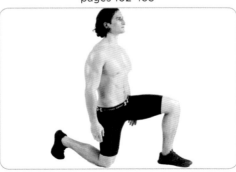

Lunge
pages 100–101

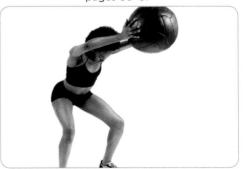

Medicine Ball Slam
pages 312–313

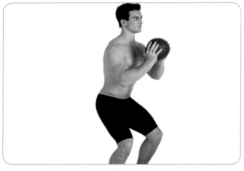

Medicine Ball Squat to Press
pages 314–315

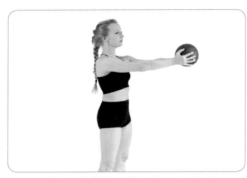

Medicine Ball Standing Russian Twist
pages 266–267

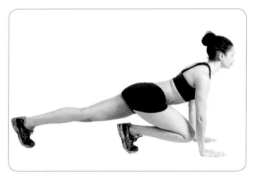

Mountain Climber
pages 126–127

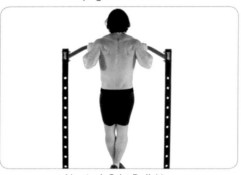

Neutral-Grip Pull-Up
pages 222–223

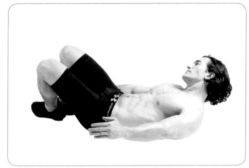

Penguin Crunch
pages 80–81

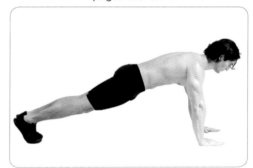

Plank
pages 114–115

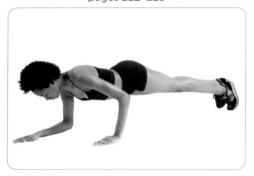

Plank-Up
pages 116–117

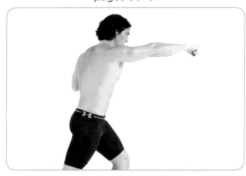

Power Punch
pages 64–65

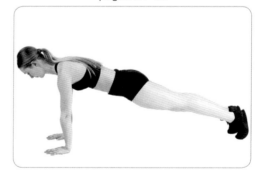

Push-Up
pages 68–69

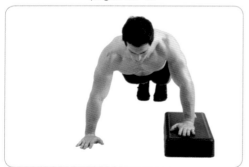

Push-Up Hand Walk-Over
pages 304–305

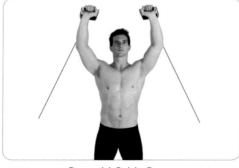

Pyramid Cable Press
pages 234–235

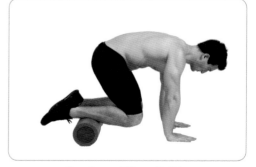

Quadruped Knee Pull-In
pages 284–285

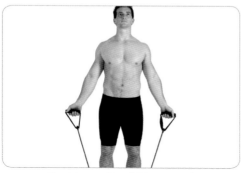

Resistance Band Biceps Curl
242–243

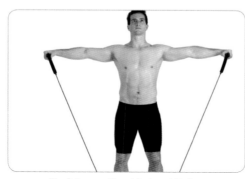

Resistance Band Lateral Raise
pages 240–241

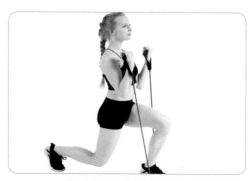

Resistance Band Lunge
pages 288–289

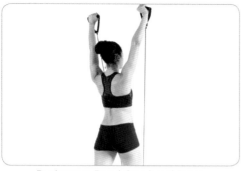

Resistance Band Overhead Press
pages 238–239

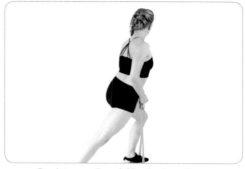

Resistance Band Single-Arm Row
pages 244–245

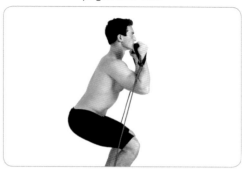

Resistance Band Squat
pages 286–287

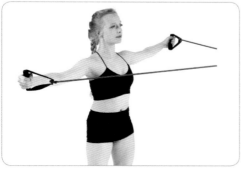

Resistance Band Standing Fly
pages 258–259

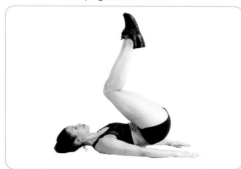

Reverse Crunch
pages 78–79

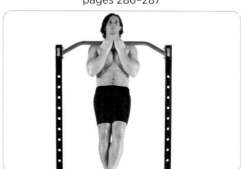

Reverse-Grip Pull-Up
pages 226–227

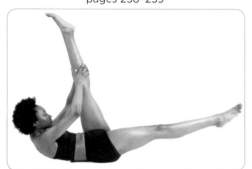

Scissors
pages 84–85

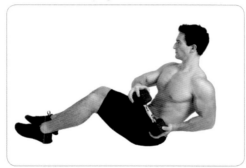

Seated Dumbbell Russian Twist
pages 184–185

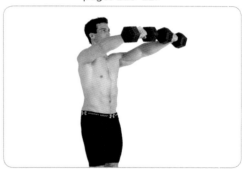

Shoulder Flexing
pages 154–155

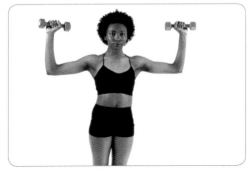

Alligator Crawl
pages 58–59

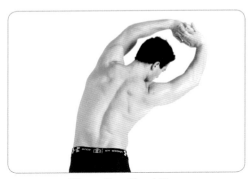

Alternating Chest Press
pages 256–257

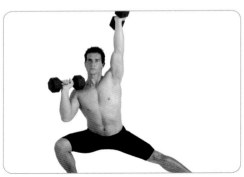

Alternating Floor Row
pages 142–143

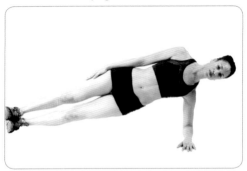

Side Plank
pages 120–121

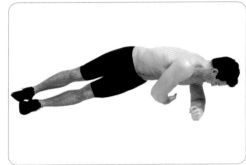

Alternating Hammer Curl
pages 160–161

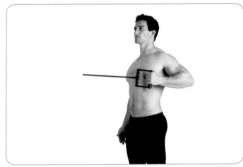

Alternating Kettlebell Press
pages 166–167

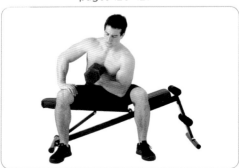

Alternating Kettlebell Row
pages 146–147

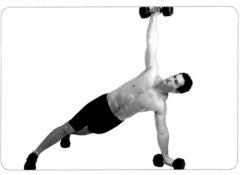

Alternating Renegade Row
pages 190–191

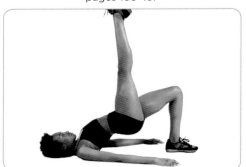

Arm-Reach Plank
pages 118–119

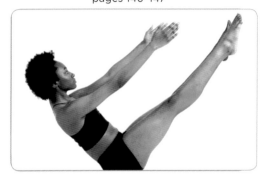

Back Burner
pages 56–57

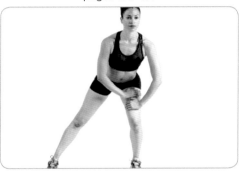

Balance Ball Crunch
262–263

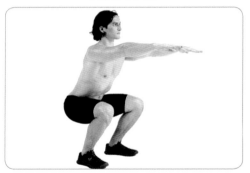

Balance Push-Up
pages 274–275

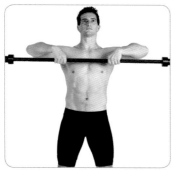

Ballet Biceps
pages 158–159

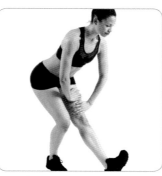

Barbell Curl
pages 172–173

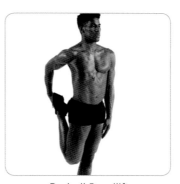

Barbell Deadlift
pages 148–149

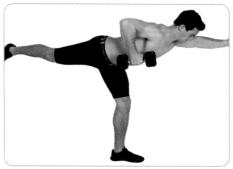

Barbell Power Clean and Jerk
pages 216–217

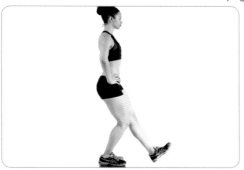

Barbell Squat
pages 208–209

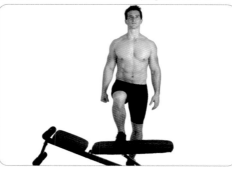

Bear Crawl
pages 60–61

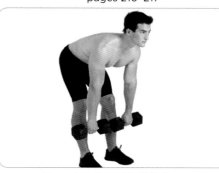

Bent-Arm Dumbbell Pullover
pages 178–179

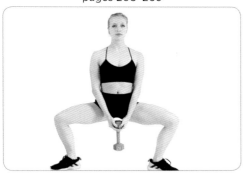

Bent-Over Cable Raise
pages 236–237

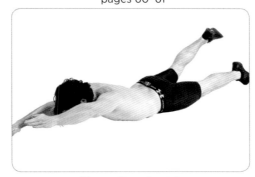

Biceps-Pecs Stretch
page 27

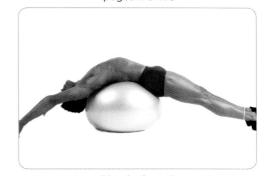

Bicycle Crunch
pages 82–83

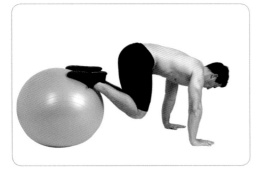

Bird Dog
pages 38–39

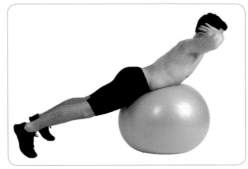

Body Saw
pages 88–89

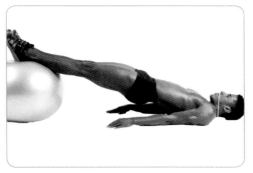

Bottom-Up Kettlebell Clean
pages 168–169

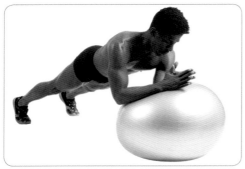

Swiss Ball Circles
pages 268–269

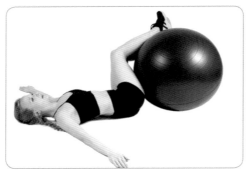

Swiss Ball Crossover
pages 220–221

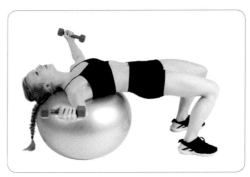

Swiss Ball Fly
pages 182–183

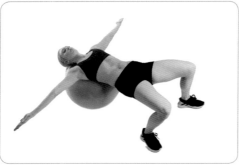

Swiss Ball Lateral Roll
pages 310–311

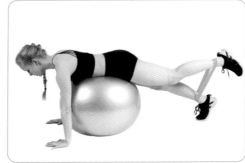

Swiss Ball Loop Extension
pages 290–291

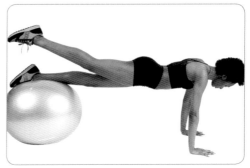

Swiss Ball Plank with Leg Lift
pages 308–309

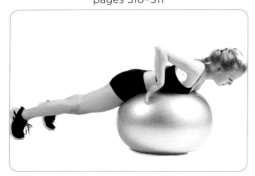

Swiss Ball Prone Row with External Rotation
pages 228–229

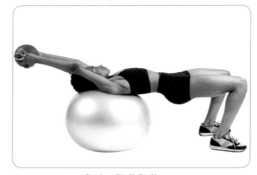

Swiss Ball Pullover
pages 144–145

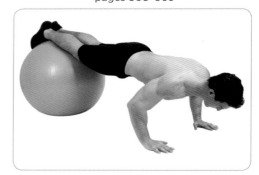

Swiss Ball Push-Up
pages 260–261

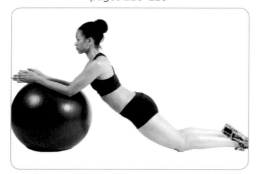

Swiss Ball Rollout
pages 272–273

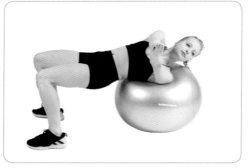

Swiss Ball Russian Twist
pages 276–277

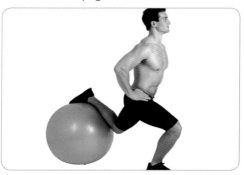

Swiss Ball Split Squat
pages 294–295

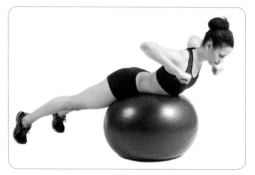

Swiss Ball W
pages 246–247

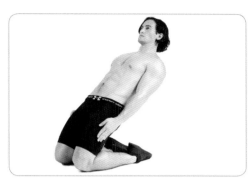

Thigh Rock-Back
pages 90–91

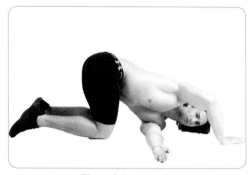

Thread the Needle
pages 48–49

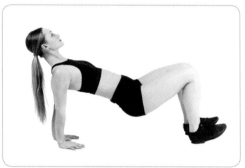

Triceps Dip
pages 66–67

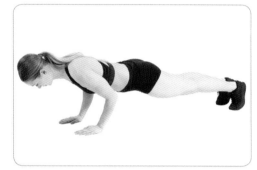

Triceps Push-Up
pages 72–73

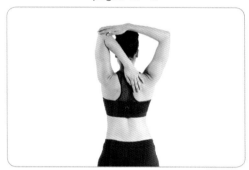

Triceps Stretch
page 26

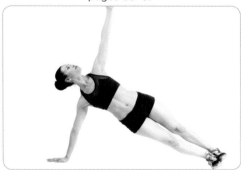

T-Stabilization
pages 124–125

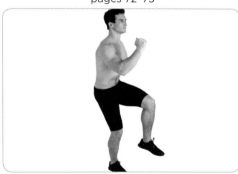

Up-Down
pages 128–129

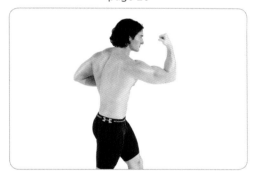

Uppercut
page 65

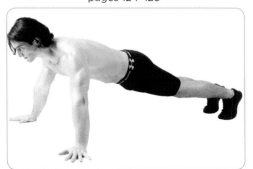

Wide Push-Up
pages 70–71

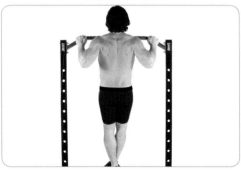

Wide-Grip Pull-Up
pages 224–225

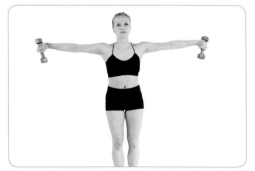

Zipper
pages 174–175

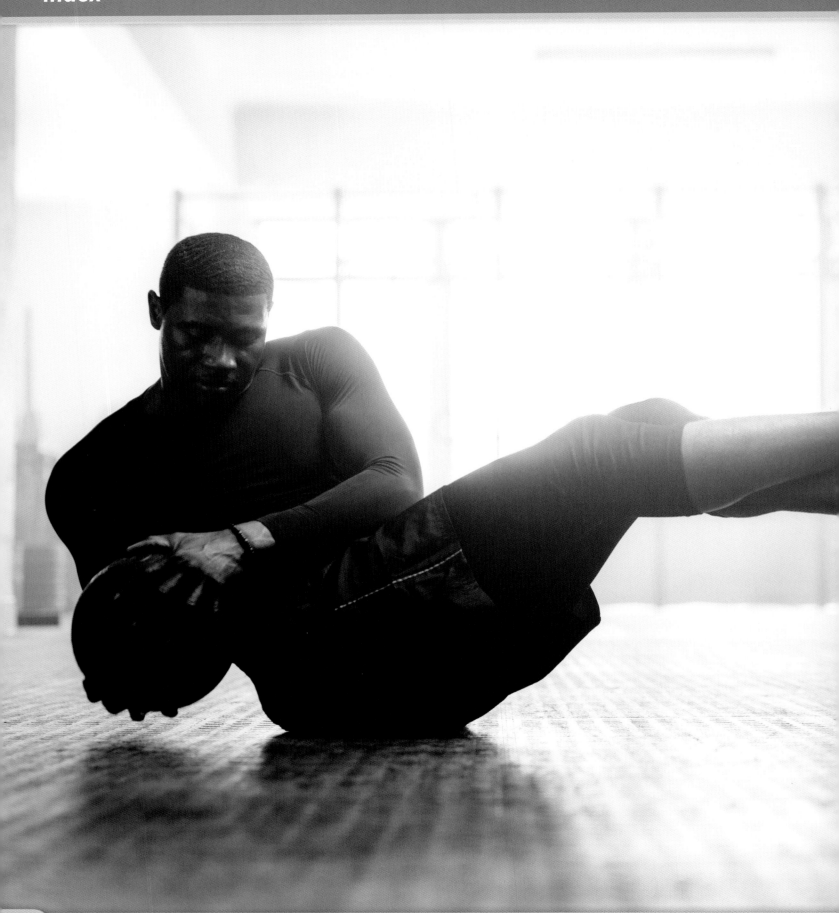

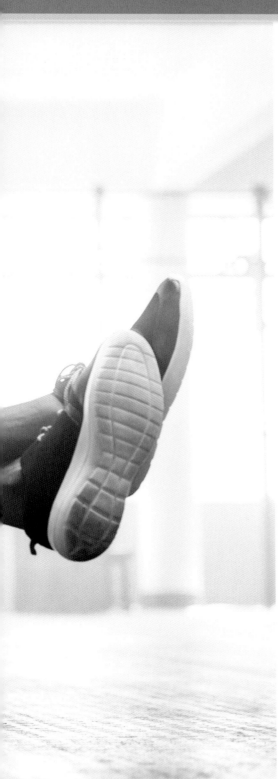

Index

A

abdominals, 37, 39, 83, 85, 89, 91, 93, 95, 97, 117
  upper, 45, 80, 273
Alligator Crawl, 58
Alternating Chest Press, 256
Alternating Floor Row, 142, 188
Alternating Renegade Row, 190

B

Balance Ball Crunch, 262
Ballet Biceps, 158
Barbell, 149, 171–73, 209, 217
  Curl, 172
  Deadlift, 148
  Power Clean and Jerk, 216
  Squat, 208
  Standing Row, 170
Bear Crawl, 60, 62
bench
  flat, 178–79, 192–93
  incline, 176–77, 180–81, 254–55
  Step-Up, 302
body bar, 210–11
Body Saw, 88
box
  Jumps, 298
  Push-Up Hand Walk-Over, 304
  Step-Down, 300
Breast Stroke, 54
Bridge, 96–97, 108
Burpee, 130
Butt Kick, 110

C

cable
  Alternating Chest Press, 256
  Bent-Over Raise, 236
  Crossover Fly, 254
  Decline Fly, 252
  Fly, 250
  Pyramid Press, 234
  Seated Chest Press, 255
C-Curve Arm Cross, 186
chest
  lower, 179, 253–55
  middle, 181
  muscles, 177
  upper, 54, 160, 172, 177, 216, 230, 251
Chin-Up, 226
Clean-and-Press, 210
core, 69, 73, 87, 95, 113, 143, 145, 185, 247, 251
  muscles, 84, 92, 184, 210, 266
  stability, 48
  stabilizers, 185
  strength, 278–79, 310
Crab Crawl, 62
Crunch, 76, 78, 80, 82, 264, 282
  Balance Ball, 262
  Bicycle, 82
  Diagonal with Medicine Ball, 264
  Foam Roller Diagonal, 282
  Penguin, 80
  Reverse, 78
Curling Step-and-Raise, 212

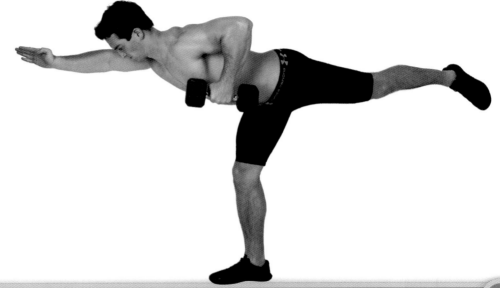

Index

D

Diagonal Reach, 74
dumbbell, 134, 136, 138, 164–65, 179, 184–85, 192–93, 197, 205
  Alternating Hammer Curl, 160
  Alternating Floor Row, 142
  Ballet Biceps, 158
  Bent-Arm Pullover, 178
  Calf Raise, 194
  C-Curve Arm Cross, 186
  Curling Step-and-Raise, 212
  Fly, 180
  Hammer-Grip Press, 176
  Knee Raise with Lateral Extension, 214
  Lateral Shoulder Raise, 156
  Lower-Back Extension, 150
  Lunge, 198
  Lying Hip Abduction, 196
  Seated Russian Twist, 184
  Shin Raise, 192
  Shoulder Flexing, 154
  Shoulder Press, 152
  Shrug, 134
  Side Lunge and Press, 202
  Single-Arm Concentration Curl, 162
  Single-Arm T-Row, 188
  Standing Single-Leg Row, 140
  Stiff-Legged Deadlift, 136
  Sumo Squat, 204
  Swiss Ball Fly, 182
  Swiss Ball Pullover, 144
  Swiss Ball W, 246
  Triceps Kickback, 164
  Upright Row, 138
  Walking Lunge, 200

E

exercises
  back, 48–58, 134–50
  Body-Weight, 46–131
  Chest, 68–72, 174–82, 251–61
  Core, 74–92, 184–90, 263–85
  Equipment, 218–314
  Flexibility, 24–45
    See also Stretch
  Leg and Glutes, 94–110, 192–208, 292
  Total-Body, 112–30, 210–16, 305–15
  Weighted, 132–217
Extension Heel Beats, 98

F

Fire-Hydrant In-Out, 94
foam roller, 218, 248–49, 278–85, 296–97, 306–7
  Abdominal Rollback, 280
  Diagonal Crunch, 282
  Hamstrings Pull-In, 296
  Push-Up, 306
  Quadruped Knee Pull-in, 284
  Triceps Dip, 248
  Triceps Rollout, 278

H

Half-Kneeling Rotation, 40
Hammer-Grip Press, 176, 180
Hamstrings Pull-In, 296
Hip Crossover, 50
hips, 28, 30, 32, 53

K

kettlebell, 146, 169, 207
  Alternating Press, 166
  Alternating Renegade Row, 190
  Alternating Row, 146
  Bottom-Up Clean, 168
  Goblet Squat, 206
Knee Raise with Lateral Extension, 214

L

Lateral Shoulder Raise, 156
Leg Levelers, 86
Lower-Back Extension, 150
Lunge, 100, 104, 202
  Dumbbell, 198
  Dumbbell Walking, 200
  Lateral-Extension Reverse, 102
  Resistance Band, 288
  Side, 104, 202
  Side and Press, 202
  Skater's, 104

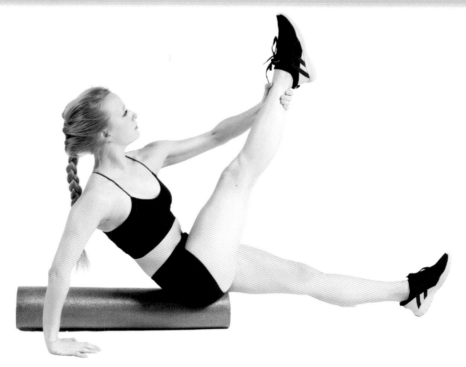

M

medicine ball, 97, 145, 264–67, 312–15
    Diagonal Crunch, 264
    Squat to Press, 314
    Standing Russian Twist, 266
    Slam, 312
Mountain Climber, 126

O

obliques, 41, 43, 51, 81, 267

P

pectorals, 59, 61, 67, 183, 257, 259, 261, 275
Plank, 112, 114–15, 118, 188, 190
    Arm-Reach, 118
    Forearm, 112, 116, 118–19
    Plank-Up, 116
    Side, 120, 122
    Side with Reach-Under, 122
    Swiss Ball with Leg Lift, 308
plyo box, 298–301
Power Punch, 64
Pull-Up, 222, 224, 226
    Neutral-Grip, 222
    Reverse Grip, 226
    Wide-Grip, 224
pull-up bar, 222–27
Push-Up, 68, 70, 72, 130, 270, 284, 304
    Balance, 274
    basic, 70, 72
    Burpee, 130
    classic, 260
    Foam Roller, 306
    Hand Walk-Over, 304
    modified, 70
    position, 274, 304
    strength, 155
    Swiss Ball, 260
    Swiss Ball Atomic, 270
    Triceps, 72
    Wide, 70

Q

Quadruped Knee Pull-In, 284

R

resistance band, 218, 232–33, 238–39, 241–43, 245, 256–59, 286–91
    Alternating Chest Press, 256
    Biceps Curl, 242
    Lateral Raise, 240
    Lunge, 288
    Overhead Press, 238
    Single-Arm Pull, 232
    Single-Arm Row, 244
    Squat, 286
    Standing Fly, 258
    Swiss Ball Loop Extension, 290
Routines
    Arm, 320
    Artillery, 354
    Back, 324, 326
    Balance, 356
    Baseball, 338
    Chest, 322, 326
    Cycling, 340
    Dance, 342
    Foam Roller, 358
    Football, 344
    Full-Body, 336
    Functional Chest/Back, 326
    Glutes, 322, 334
    Hero, 360
    Marathon Running, 346
    Military, 362, 364, 366
    Obliques, 330
    Postural, 368
    Rectus Abdominis, 328
    Resistance, 370
    Shoulder, 318
    Sprinting, 348
    Stretch, 372
    Swimming, 350
    Swiss Ball, 374
    Tennis, 352
    Thighs, 332

S

Scissors, 84
Shoulder Flexing, 154
Shoulder Press, 152, 158
Single-Arm Concentration Curl, 162
Single-Arm T-Row, 188
Single-Leg Gluteal Lift, 108
Single-Leg V-Up, 92
spine, 35, 41, 53, 55
Squat, 106, 130, 148, 204, 294, 314
    Barbell, 208
    Goblet, 206
    Medicine Ball to Press, 314
    Resistance Band, 286
    Sumo, 204
    Swiss Ball Split, 294
    Thrust, 130
Step-Down, 300
Step-Up, 302
stretch, 26–28, 30–32, 34, 36, 44, 52, 99

Index

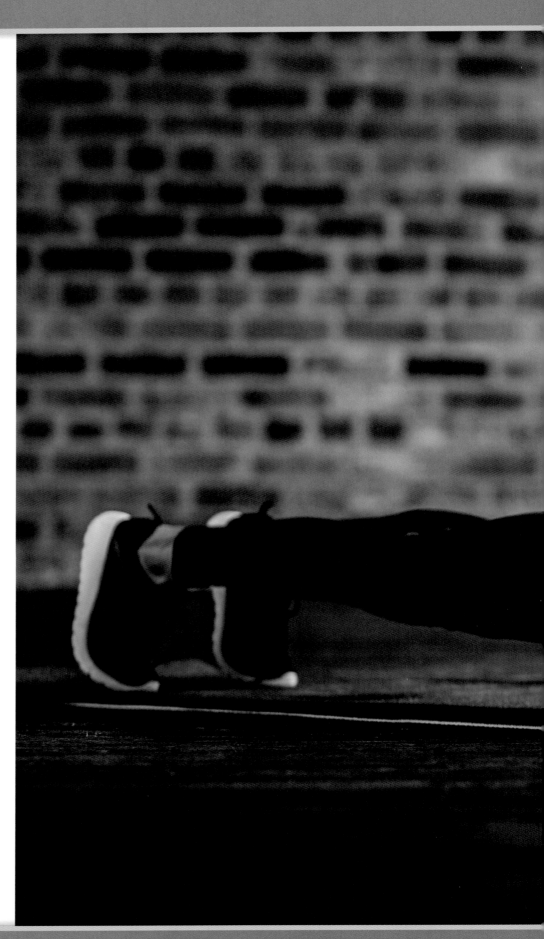

Biceps-Pecs, 27

Bird-Dog, 38

Cat-to-Cow, 34

Cobra, 36

Half-Kneeling Rotation, 40

Iliotibial Band, 32

Lateral Lunge, 28

Lunge, 100

Side Bending, 42

Standing Hamstrings, 31

Standing Quadriceps, 30

Swiss Ball Abdominal, 44

Triceps, 26

Swimmer, 52

Swiss ball, 144–45, 182–83, 220–21, 228–31, 246–47, 260–61, 268–77, 290, 292–95, 308–11

Atomic Push-Up, 270

Back Extension, 230

Balance Push-Up, 274

Bridge, 292

Circles, 268

Crossover, 220

Fly, 182

Lateral Roll, 310

Loop Extension, 290

Plank, 308

Plank with Leg Lift, 308

Prone Row with External Rotation, 228

Pullover, 144

Push-Up, 260

Rollout, 272

Russian Twist, 276

Split Squat, 294

W, 246

T

Thigh Rock-Back, 90

Thread the Needle, 48

Triceps Dip, 66

T-Stabilization, 124

U

Up-Down, 128

Uppercut, 65

Z

Zipper, 174

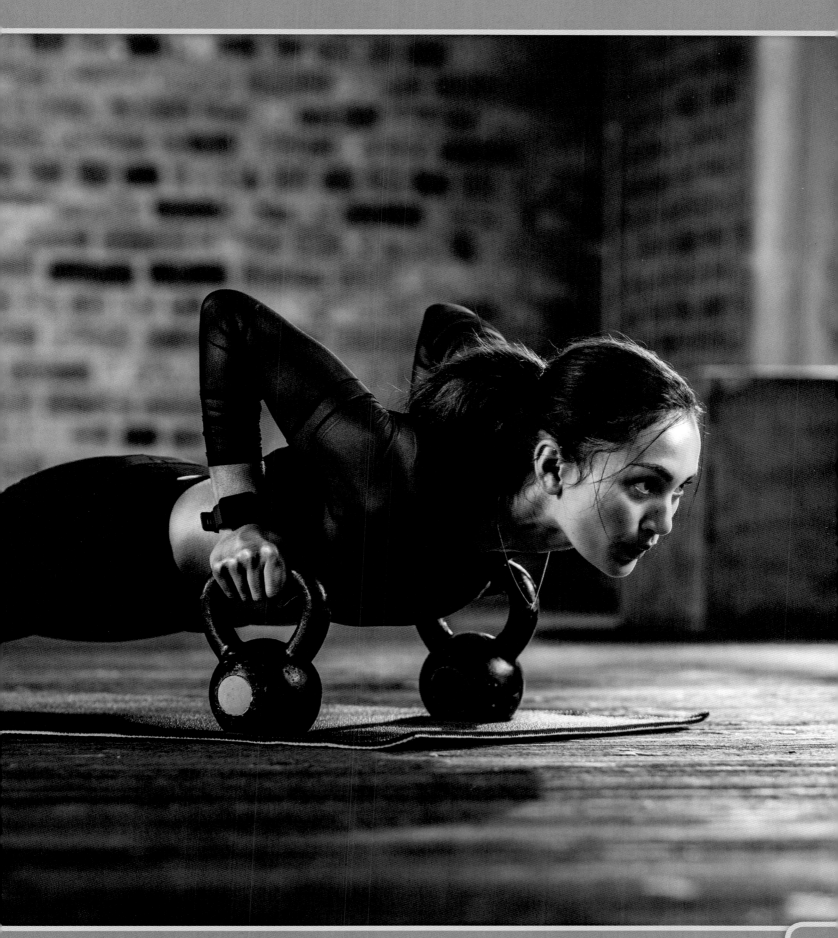

Credits & Acknowledgments

Photography

Naila Ruechel

Models

Alex Geissbuhler
Alyssa Cebulski
Conor Fallon
Dayzjah Thomas
Jessica Gambelluri
Lloyd Knight
Natasha Diamond-Walker

Additional Photography

Page 4 Microgen/Shutterstock.com
Page 7 Akhenaton Images/Shutterstock.com
Page 9 ESB Professional/Shutterstock.com
Page 11 Mitch Gunn/Shutterstock.com
Page 13 MilanMarkovic78/Shutterstock.com
Page 14 marilyn barbone/Shutterstock.com
Page 15 Flamingo Images/Shutterstock.com
Page 17 Karin Jaehne/Shutterstock.com
Page 18 Yuricazac/Shutterstock.com
Page 19 Syda Productions/Shutterstock.com
Page 24–25 fizkes/Shutterstock.com
Pages 46–47 Rocksweeper/Shutterstock.com
Pages 132–133 oneinchpunch/Shutterstock.com
Pages 218–219 nd3000/Shutterstock.com
Pages 316–317 Andrey_Popov/Shutterstock.com
Pages 376–377 aumnat/Shutterstock.com
Pages 394–395 Jacob Lund/Shutterstock.com
Pages 398–399 Jacob Lund/Shutterstock.com

Illustrations

All anatomical illustrations by Adam Moore, Hector Diaz/3DLabz Animation Limited
Full-body anatomy and insets by Linda Bucklin/Shutterstock.com

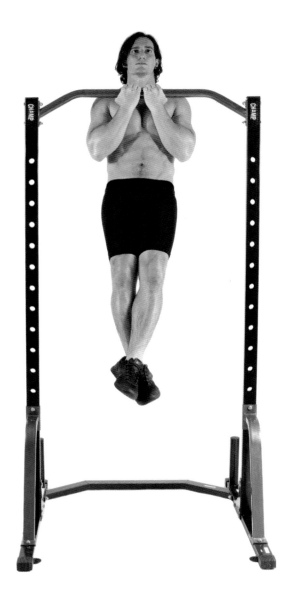